Global Health
Issues, Challenges, and Global Action

Lecture Notes

Elizabeth A. Armstrong-Mensah

Georgia State University/Morehouse School of Medicine
Atlanta, Georgia, US

WILEY Blackwell

Library of Congress Cataloging-in-Publication Data

Names: Armstrong-Mensah, Elizabeth A., author.
Title: Lecture notes. Global health : issues, challenges, and global action/ Elizabeth A. Armstrong-Mensah.
Other titles: Global health : issues, challenges, and global action
Description: Chichester, West Sussex ; Hoboken, NJ : John Wiley & Sons Inc., 2017. | Includes bibliographical references and index.
Identifiers: LCCN 2016047330 | ISBN 9781119110217 (pbk.) | ISBN 9781119110231 (Adobe PDF) | ISBN 9781119110224 (ePub)
Subjects: | MESH: Global Health | Cost of Illness | Environmental Health
Classification: LCC RA441 | NLM WA 530.1 | DDC 362.1–dc23
LC record available at https://lccn.loc.gov/2016047330

A catalogue record for this book is available from the British Library.

Global Health
Lecture Notes

This book is dedicated to William Armstrong-Mensah, David Armstrong-Mensah, Joseph Yankson, Rose Yankson, and Anthony Yankson.

Contents

Contents

Preface

Global health is an emerging interdisciplinary field of study, research, and practice whose scope, objectives, resources, and training requirements remain unclear to many. While it is now more apparent that we live in an increasingly globalized interconnected world, where countries and organizations form partnerships to address the host of health issues that confront the world, the lines of demarcation between what pertains and relates to the domains of international and global health unfortunately remain unclear to some. What is unsettling is how some consider global health as no different from that of international health; the health-related field the world focused on prior to global health. International health and global health share a few things in common, but they are very different in many respects. An understanding of these differences sets one on the path to knowing what global health is and what it is not, as well as its goals and required skill sets.

With this misconception and death of information comes the need for dialogue and literature to shed more light on this burgeoning field. Hence the authoring of this book. A global health textbook should contain a wide enough range of relevant topics with sufficient depth to provide a solid foundation and knowledge of the field. It should also adequately focus on the challenges posed by the global health issues they discuss and the global actions and strategies in place to address them. Global Health – Issues, Challenges, and Global Action does just that. It provides an appropriate mix and range of global health topics in one volume, with sufficient depth to provide clarity and a good grounding in the field. This book presents and clarifies the concept of global health, defines its scope, and shows how different it is from international health. It additionally introduces readers to key global health concepts and pertinent global health issues that confront both developed and developing countries. Using a multidisciplinary approach, the book further reveals the critical links between health, disease, and socioeconomic development, as well as the global efforts under way to address the global health issues and challenges it discusses.

Global Health – Issues, Challenges, and Global Action is intended as an introductory text in global health and is based on first-hand global health issues I personally observed and experienced after over 20 years in the developing world, and over 15 years in the developed. It is also the result of undergraduate and graduate courses I taught at Emory University, Morehouse School of Medicine, and Georgia State University. It is hoped that the book will increase the global health knowledge base and skills of undergraduate and graduate students who may or may not have taken a course in global health, and for faculty and practitioners of global health as they pursue careers in global health practice, education, and research.

The book comprises 16 interrelated chapters. Chapter one, which is essentials of global health outlines the features of global health, shows how it is different from international health, and why it is a relevant field of study in current times. Chapters two and three discuss the effects of globalization on global health and noncommunicable diseases. Chapter four focuses on the global burden of disease, chapter five on culture, behavior, and global health, and chapter six on water, sanitation and global health. Chapter seven presents information on global hunger, nutrition, and food security, and chapter eight features human rights and how they relate to global health. Chapters nine and ten deal with natural disasters and complex humanitarian emergencies, and gender, sexual and reproductive health. In chapters eleven and twelve, health systems and health systems financing are discussed followed by ethics in global health research in chapter thirteen. The last three chapters focus on the just ended United Nations Millennium Development Goals and their impact on global health, global health partnerships and governance, and evaluating global health projects.

Elizabeth A. Armstrong-Mensah

Acknowledgments

I am indebted to my husband and son for their encouragement, patience, and support throughout this journey.

Essentials of global health

Learning Objectives

By the end of this chapter, you will be able to:

✔ Define global health;

✔ List and explain at least two key global health concepts;

✔ Discuss at least two defining features of global health;

✔ Explain the difference between international health and global health;

✔ Explain the significance of global health in today's world.

Summary of key points

Global health is an emerging interdisciplinary field of study, research, and practice whose scope, objectives, and training requirements remain unclear to many around the world. Preceded by three other health-related fields, it is at present, the main health focus of the world. This notwithstanding, there are ongoing debates about what global health is and whether it is different from its predecessor, international health. Although a few similarities exist between global health and international health, they are different on several domains. This chapter traces the evolution of global health. It discusses the concept of global health and explains some key terms associated with it. It further highlights the difference between global health and international health, and draws attention to the significance of global health in the twenty-first century and beyond.

Evolution and concept of global health

Prior to the evolution of global health, the world experienced and focused on three health-related fields: tropical medicine (also known as colonial medicine), public health, and international health. These fields emerged at various points in time in response to environmental, political, and economic factors (see Figure 1.1).

Tropical medicine

The first health-related field the world experienced and focused on was tropical medicine.

Tropical medicine is a branch of medicine that focuses on identifying, diagnosing, preventing, and treating diseases most prominent in tropical regions of the world. Specifically, it focuses on infectious and

---

Global Health: Issues, Challenges, and Global Action Lecture Notes, First Edition. Elizabeth A. Armstrong-Mensah.

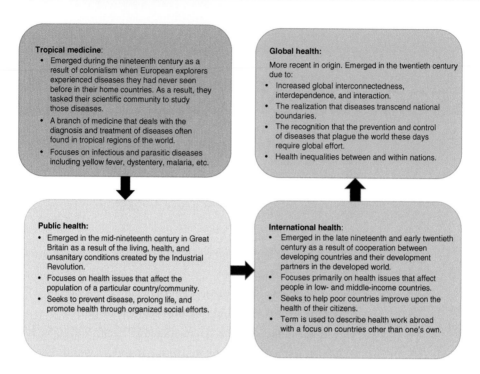

Tropical medicine:
- Emerged during the nineteenth century as a result of colonialism when European explorers experienced diseases they had never seen before in their home countries. As a result, they tasked their scientific community to study those diseases.
- A branch of medicine that deals with the diagnosis and treatment of diseases often found in tropical regions of the world.
- Focuses on infectious and parasitic diseases including yellow fever, dystentery, malaria, etc.

Global health:
More recent in origin. Emerged in the twentieth century due to:
- Increased global interconnectedness, interdependence, and interaction.
- The realization that diseases transcend national boundaries.
- The recognition that the prevention and control of diseases that plague the world these days require global effort.
- Health inequalities between and within nations.

Public health:
- Emerged in the mid-nineteenth century in Great Britain as a result of the living, health, and unsanitary conditions created by the Industrial Revolution.
- Focuses on health issues that affect the population of a particular country/community.
- Seeks to prevent disease, prolong life, and promote health through organized social efforts.

International health:
- Emerged in the late nineteenth and early twentieth century as a result of cooperation between developing countries and their development partners in the developed world.
- Focuses primarily on health issues that affect people in low- and middle-income countries.
- Seeks to help poor countries improve upon the health of their citizens.
- Term is used to describe health work abroad with a focus on countries other than one's own.

Figure 1.1 Health-related fields prior to global health.

parasitic infestations including yellow fever, dysentery, and malaria, and utilizes an individual clinical approach towards population disease prevention and management. Entomology, parasitology, clinical medicine, epidemiology, and community health are the major disciplines associated with early tropical medicine (Giles & Lucas, 1998).

In the mid-fifteenth century, during the Age of Discovery, Portuguese and Spanish explorers made successful voyages to the Americas and to the coasts of Africa, East Asia, India, and the Middle East. Their success spurred other European nations to embark on similar voyages. Thus, by the sixteenth century, European nations had begun to scramble for, partition, and colonize many regions around the world including Africa among themselves (see Figure 1.2). Many of the countries they colonized were located in the tropics. The hot climate and environmental conditions of the tropics negatively affected the health of the European colonists. They experienced many infectious diseases including malaria, yellow fever, dengue fever, and diarrheal diseases not prevalent in their home countries.

European colonists coined the term "tropical medicine" to describe the host of unfamiliar diseases they experienced in the tropics (MacFarlane *et al.*, 2008;

Warwick, 1998). They challenged scientists in their home countries to research and tackle those diseases. This effort culminated in the establishment of the first two schools of tropical medicine in 1898: the Liverpool School of Tropical Medicine and later, the London School of Hygiene and Tropical Medicine. The establishment of these two institutions was groundbreaking and pivotal in that, it led to a greater acceptance of the germ theory, which postulated that diseases in the tropics were caused by germs and not by climate, or poison in the air as some scientists at the time believed.

The development of the germ theory increased European momentum towards colonialism. European colonists came to realize that they could continue to colonize countries in the tropics if they could find a way to prevent and treat the germs that caused diseases in that area. Thus, the goal of the newly established schools of tropical medicine was to train colonial medical officers to treat tropical diseases inorder to make the colonies more habitable for economic exploitation and expansion (Baronov, 2008).

Following the establishment of the first two schools of tropical medicine, other schools of tropical medicine were established around the world. Today, there are several schools, institutions, and departments

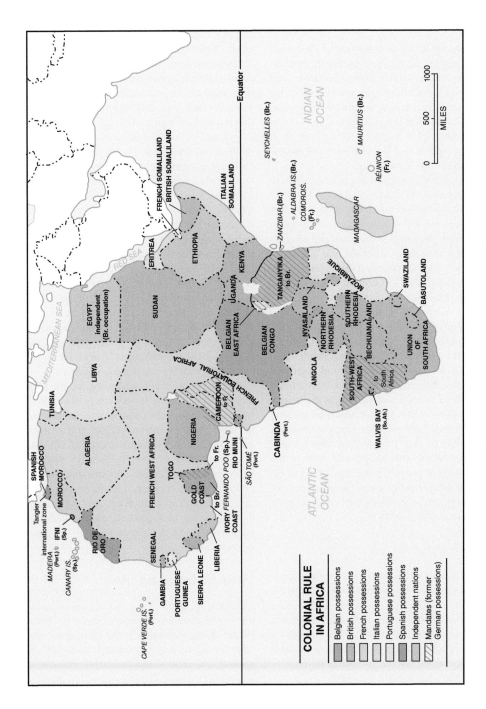

Figure 1.2 Map showing European colonization of Africa.
Source: de Blij H. J., and Muller, P. O. (n.d.).

devoted to the study of tropical medicine. Some of these include the Institute of Tropical Medicine and International Health in Berlin, the Institute of Tropical Medicine in Antwerp, the Institute of Tropical Medicine in Nagasaki, and the Department of Tropical Medicine at Tulane University in the United States of America. In the mid-twentieth century, many doctors and scientists from the tropical and subtropical regions of Africa, Asia, and Latin America went to Europe for training in tropical medicine. Upon returning to their home countries, they incorporated portions of tropical medicine into their educational curricula and founded research institutions devoted to tropical medicine.

Tropical medicine developed as a necessary part of the colonial system (Tropical Medicine, 2001). In order to sustain the territorial expansion of their empires in the tropics, it was necessary for European colonists to have the ability to diagnose and successfully treat the dozens of diseases and infections unique to the tropics that plagued them. Coining the term "tropical medicine" symbolized colonist recognition of the differences in disease and risk factors between the indigenous populations of the tropics and populations from Europe. The postulation and acceptance of the germ theory following the establishment of the first schools of tropical medicine in England and Liverpool, triggered and validated European perceptions that they were superior intellectually, technologically, and socially to the people in the tropics, especially those in Africa, whom they saw as suffering from various tropical diseases (Farley, 1991). It was this outlook that caused Europeans to believe that they could address the health problems of people in the developing world without their involvement, hence the emergence of international health in the late nineteenth and early twentieth century (Crozier, 2007).

Public health

The second health-related field the world experienced and focused on following tropical medicine is public health: a science that focuses on preventing disease, promoting health, and prolonging life among populations as a whole. Public health first emerged in Britain in response to the health and unsanitary conditions presented by the Industrial Revolution. It later spread to other parts of the world.

With the emergence of the Industrial Revolution in the late eighteenth century, many people mass migrated from rural areas to urban centers in search of well paying industrialized jobs in factories. By the early nineteenth century, the impetus created by the Industrial Revolution led to the overcrowding of cities, lodging houses, shelters, and homes, and in the process, created unforeseen sanitary and public health problems including the outbreak of cholera, tuberculosis, and diphtheria. Until John Snow, a British doctor, traced the cholera epidemic in London to a contaminated water pump on Broad Street in 1885, and until Edwin Chadwick learned that removing the pump handle would bring about a drastic reduction in the incidence and prevalence of cholera, no one knew exactly why people in the cities of London were getting sick. The discoveries of Snow and Chadwick, coupled with Chadwick's 1842 landmark *Report on the Inquiry into Sanitary Conditions of the Laboring Population of Great Britain,* contributed to revealing the public health challenges facing England and strengthened the debate on the need for government involvement in the preservation of the health of its people. Thus, in the mid-nineteenth century, the British government took steps to reform health and to improve upon the health of its citizens. This effort culminated in the passing of the first Public Health Act in 1848, and the coining of the term "public health" to distinguish government effort to preserve and protect the health of its citizens or the public from private actions.

The invention of the steam engine, the spinning jenny, and the power loom were at the heart of the Industrial Revolution. These inventions mechanized the factory system and created a shift from the manual production of goods in cottage industries, to the mass production of goods in factories powered by steam engines. Although the Industrial Revolution improved upon systems of transportation, production, communication, banking, and the standard of living for many in England, it also resulted in harsh employment and living conditions for the poor and working classes.

International health

International health is the third health-related field the world experienced and focused on following public health. Emerging in the late nineteenth and early twentieth century, international health seeks to prevent and control communicable diseases, water and sanitation-related diseases, improve upon nutrition, and reduce maternal and child mortality in the developing world through the promotion, support, and strengthening of international health programs including immunization and family planning. The term "international health" is often used to describe health work abroad with governments and nongovernmental organizations (NGOs) in the developing world. It is also used to portray bilateral associations between two or more countries in which countries in the developed world provide much needed health assistance to countries in the developing world.

Unlike tropical medicine that was borne out of European imperial repression, international health can be said to have been borne out of European benevolence towards the developing world. The question often asked about international health is whether it is truly a foreign policy effort by the international community to improve the health of people in the developing world, or whether it is a health field driven by clandestine European capitalist interests (Fidler, 2008). Whatever its intent, international health provided and continues to provide the necessary assistance needed by many developing countries to meet the health and development needs of their citizens.

Global health

The health-related field the world is currently focusing on is global health. Global health emerged in the latter part of the twentieth century as a result of increased global interconnectedness, interaction, interdependence, and the recognition by the global community of the global reach of diseases and disease risk factors. Prior to the twentieth century, nations were primarily concerned about health issues that affected them. What happened elsewhere was unfortunate. These days, this worldview is not only obsolete, but no longer feasible as it has become apparent that the health status of people in one part of the world is directly linked to the health of people in another part of the world.

The concept of global health

While global health is very much discussed these days, it is important to note that the association of the term "global" with "health", is not entirely new. The term was first used in conjunction with health in 1955, by the newly created United Nations (UN) World Health Organization (WHO) in its attempt to eradicate malaria from the world through the Global Malaria Eradication Program. WHO Public Affairs Committee pamphlet of 1958, also used the term "The World Health Organization: Its Global Battle against Disease," and in 1971, a report for the US House of Representatives was titled *The Politics of Global Health*. After these and a few other associations, the term "global" was not used again in relation to health until around the mid-twentieth century when it evolved as a defined health-related field.

Like many disciplines, there is no agreed definition of what global health is. Macfarlane *et al.* (2008) define global health as the "Worldwide improvement of health, reduction of disparities, and protection against global threats that disregard national borders," whereas the United States Institute of Medicine defines global health as "Health problems, issues, and concerns that transcend national boundaries, may be influenced by circumstances or experiences in other countries, and are best addressed by cooperative actions and solutions."

To WHO, global health is "The health of populations in a global context which transcends the perspectives and concerns of individual nations," and to Rowson and his colleagues, it is:

A field of practice, research, and education focused on health and the social, economic, political, and cultural forces that shape it across the world. The discipline has an historical association with the distinct needs of developing countries but it is also concerned with health-related issues that transcend national boundaries and the differential impacts of globalization. It is a cross-disciplinary field, blending perspectives from the natural and social sciences to understand the social relationship, biological processes, and technologies that contribute to the improvement of health worldwide. (Rowson *et al.*, 2007)

Despite their variations, a common thread that runs through the above definitions of global health is the fact that it is a field of health that transcends national boundaries, and which requires global collaboration to address the health issues that plague the world. For the purpose of this book, global health may be defined as a field of study, research, and practice of health issues that transcend national boundaries through the transfer of global risk factors for which global collaboration and action is needed. Its aim is to improve and reduce health inequities within and between countries.

Key global health concepts

There are several global health concepts that are germane to understanding the field. A few of the most widely used terms are described in this section.

Developing countries

Also referred to as the South or the Global South, developing countries have certain characteristics in common. They are generally agrarian societies with low levels of industrialization. Their average per capita income, literacy rates, and life expectancy are low, while their population growth rates and mortality rates are high. Poverty, undernutrition, unstable governments, poor infrastructure, and low levels of urbanization are additional characteristics of developing countries. While low- and middle-income countries are all referred to as developing countries, there are vast differences in their economies. According to the July 1, 2014, World Bank classification of world economies, low-income countries have a gross national income (GNI) per capita of $1045 or less, whereas middle-income countries have a GNI per capita of more than $1045, but less than $12746. Afghanistan, Benin, Cambodia, Ethiopia, and Liberia are examples of low-income countries, and China, Ghana, Mauritius, Turkey, and Yemen are examples of middle-income countries.

Developed countries

Unlike developing countries, developed countries are generally highly industrialized societies with high-performing market economies. Their per capita income and literacy levels are high and population growth rate is low. Mortality rates are low, life expectancy is generally high, and majority of people live in urban areas. Developed countries have stable democratic governments and good infrastructure. They are also referred to as the North, Global North, or high-income countries. According to the July 1, 2013, World Bank classification of the world's economies, developed countries have a GNI per capita of $12746 or more. Austria, Denmark, France, the United Kingdom, and the United States are examples of developed countries. Just like low- and middle-income countries, there are differences in GNI per capita among developed countries (World Bank, 2015).

Disease control

Disease control is the deliberate reduction of disease incidence, prevalence, morbidity, and mortality to a locally acceptable level. With disease control, continued interventions are needed to maintain reductions. Onchocerciasis or river blindness is an example of a disease that is being controlled locally in certain parts of the world. Between 1974 and 2002, river blindness was brought under control in affected communities in West Africa through the work of the Onchocerciasis Control Program. Disease control was achieved through the spraying of black fly larvae with insecticide and through the large-scale distribution of ivermectin in endemic areas (World Health Organization, 2016a).

Disease elimination

Disease elimination is the deliberate reduction to zero of the incidence of a specified disease in a defined geographical area. Like disease control, disease elimination requires continued intervention measures to maintain reductions gained (Dowdle, 1999). In 2010, Vietnam and Myanmar in East Asia, took steps to eliminate maternal and neonatal tetanus, and in 2013, WHO confirmed the elimination of onchocerciasis from Colombia, in South America (Carter Center, 2016; Centers for Disease Control and Prevention, 2016).

Disease eradication

Disease eradication is the deliberate permanent reduction to zero of the worldwide incidence of infection caused by a specific agent. With disease eradication, continued intervention measures are not needed. To date, smallpox is the only disease that has been eradicated globally. Some global disease eradication initiatives currently underway focus on guinea worm and polio. These initiatives were declared global goals in 1986 and 1988, respectively. According to the Carter Center, there were only four cases of guinea worm globally as of May 2016: three in Chad and a case in Ethiopia, and according to global polio surveillance data, 34 cases of polio were reported in 2015: 28 from Pakistan and six from Afghanistan.

Global burden of disease

Global burden of disease is the measure of the amount of disease, disability, and mortality in the world as measured in disability adjusted life years (DALYs).

Global burden of disease varies by country, region, age, sex, and income level. Communicable and non-communicable diseases and injury account for a huge part of the global burden of disease. Cancer and heart disease were among the leading causes of morbidity and mortality worldwide in 2012 (World Health Organization, 2015b).

Global health inequity

Global health inequity is the difference in health status between people in different parts of the world and among people living within the same country. This inequity is often due to social and economic inequalities, such as education, income, race, and sex. Social and economic conditions determine the extent to which people will access health facilities in the event of illness and the extent to which they will receive quality healthcare in time of need.

Global health issues

Global health issues are the health problems that affect or concern many countries such as Ebola disease, malaria, sexually transmitted diseases, obesity, and HIV/AIDS. They are also global collaborative actions to tackle and address health problems and challenges, such as the Global Malaria Eradication Program and the Global Polio Eradication Initiative.

Global health partnerships

Global health partnerships are collaborative relationships between governments, donors, NGOs, and a variety of private-sector organizations dedicated to the pursuit of a shared health goal. The Global Alliance for Vaccines and Immunization (GAVI) and the Global Fund to Fight AIDS, Tuberculosis and Malaria (GFTAM) are examples of global health partnerships formed to tackle childhood vaccine preventable diseases, and HIV/AIDS, tuberculosis, and malaria.

Global health risk factors

Global health risk factors are conditions or behaviors that increase the possibility of disease, disability, or injury worldwide. They are also conditions that can exacerbate or worsen existing health conditions. Globally, high blood pressure, smoking tobacco, and obesity are risk factors for heart disease. The lack of access to safe water supply, improved sanitation, and hygiene are risk factors for schistosomiasis, guinea-worm disease (dracunculiasis), and bilharzia (Prüss-Üstün *et al.*, 2004).

Globalization

Globalization is the process of increased global interconnectedness and interdependency as a result of political, social, and cultural integration. Through its processes, globalization may positively or negatively impact the health of populations.

Millennium Development Goals (MDGs)

The Millennium Development Goals are a set of eight goals with targets and indicators identified by the UN Millennium Project in 2000 and adopted by UN Member States to eliminate poverty and to significantly improve health and environmental outcomes for disadvantaged populations around the globe by the year 2015.

World Health Organization geographic regions

Member States of the UN WHO are grouped into six epidemiological regions (African, Americas, Eastern Mediterranean, Europe, South East Asia, and West Pacific), based on the Global Burden of Disease (GBD) regional classification system (see Figure 1.3). Each WHO region has a regional office that works actively with the countries it oversees to develop and implement strategies for the control and prevention of diseases as part of WHO's global response to disease prevention and control.

The WHO African regional office is located in The Congo, and is responsible for 47 African countries including Algeria, Botswana, Cameroun, Ethiopia, Ghana, and Zimbabwe. That of the Eastern Mediterranean region is located in Egypt, and works with 21 countries including Afghanistan, Iran, Iraq, Jordan, Kuwait, Libya, Saudi Arabia, and Yemen. The European and Americas WHO regional offices are located in Denmark and Washington DC, and are in charge of 53 and 35 countries, respectively. Countries in the WHO European Region include Albania, Belgium, Cyprus, Israel, Netherlands, and the United Kingdom, and those in the Americas Region include Argentina, Canada, Cuba, Honduras, Peru, United States of America, and Venezuela. In the Southeast, the WHO regional office is headquartered in India and works with 11 countries including Bangladesh, Indonesia, Sri Lanka, and Timor-Leste. The Philippines is where the WHO Western Pacific regional office is located. It serves 27 countries including Australia, Japan, New Zealand, Singapore, and Vietnam.

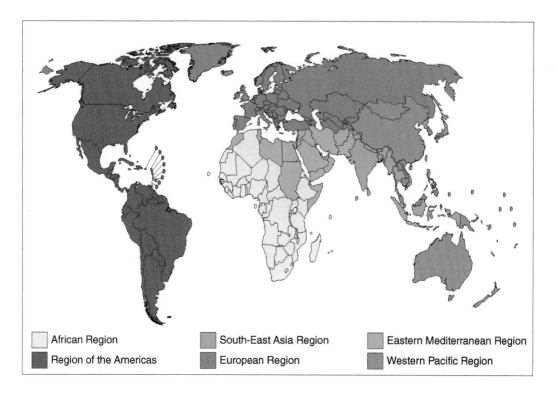

Figure 1.3 WHO regions.
Source: World Health Organization Regional Offices (2016b), with permission.

Defining features of global health

Just as developed and developing countries have features that define them, global health also has a set of features that defines and differentiates it from other disciplines. The defining features of global health lie in its mission, geographical reach, level of cooperation, health content, health conditions, health response, and range of disciplines.

Mission

The mission of global health is to achieve health equity for all within and across countries through the reduction of disparities and the removal of political, economic, social, and environmental determinants that negatively impact health and determine health outcomes.

Health inequities exist when by reason of the wealth of their economies, people living in developed countries have higher life expectancies at birth and reduced maternal mortality rates than people living in developing countries. Health inequities are also present when within the same country, the infant mortality rate of mothers with no education is higher than for those with at least secondary education. Health inequities are not naturally determined. They are socioeconomically determined and can therefore be addressed.

Geographic reach

Geographically, global health focuses on health issues and concerns that transcend national boundaries and which affect many countries around the world directly or indirectly. While the Ebola epidemic that started in 2014 was largely limited to the West African countries of Guinea, Liberia, and Sierra Leone, the global community got involved as it became apparent that if not controlled, the epidemic could spread to other parts of the world and cause a global pandemic of epic proportions.

Level of cooperation

The nature and scope of diseases affecting people around the world these days are such that no one country has the resources and ability to address them single-handedly. The emergence of HIV/AIDS, avian influenza, Ebola disease, and severe acute respiratory syndrome underscore this fact. To tackle and address these health issues, countries and organizations around the world have had to form partnerships and pool funds, expertise, and human resources.

Health content and health conditions

Addressing both communicable and noncommunicable diseases is at the core of global health. In the early part of the twentieth century, the burden of disease in developing countries was primarily due to communicable diseases such as malaria, cholera, and tuberculosis, whereas those in developed countries were due to noncommunicable diseases including cardiovascular diseases, cancers, respiratory diseases, and diabetes. The status quo however changed by the latter part of the twentieth century; people in the developed and developing world now experience both communicable and noncommunicable diseases, thanks to globalization and global interconnectedness (World Health Organization, 2015a).

Health response

Prior to the emergence of global health, bilateral organizations and development practitioners in the developed world responded to health issues in the developing world with a top-down approach. They believed that they alone had the knowledge and skills to tackle and address the health issues in the developing world. Therefore, they required developing countries to standby while they tackled the health issue they had come to address. With the emergence of global health, the nature of health response has shifted from an entirely top-down approach towards one that is horizontal; more inclusive of local people, their communities, institutions, and organizations. The response to the 2014 Ebola disease outbreak, is an example of such a shift.

Range of disciplines

Global health utilizes a multidisciplinary approach. From a medical perspective, it describes the pathology, diagnosis, and treatment of major global diseases, and from an epidemiological perspective, it focuses on patterns, causes, and effects of health and disease in defined populations. From an economic perspective, global health emphasizes the cost and financing of health programs and interventions, and from a sociological perspective, it

shows how cultural beliefs and practices influence perceptions and health outcomes of populations. From a political economy perspective, global health highlights who owns what, controls whom, and who makes decisions that impact the health of a population.

Global versus international health

There are ongoing debates on the differences between global health and international health. According to a school of thought, the two fields are one and the same; the only difference is that of semantics. According to another school of thought, the two fields are not the same. This section presents the view that both fields are for the most part different in terminology and across several domains, and should therefore not be used interchangeably (see Table 1.1).

The mission of global health is to eliminate health disparities and achieve health equity among and within nations whereas the mission of international health, on the other hand, is primarily to help individual nations deal with their health issues. As a consequence, global health programs and interventions on HIV/AIDS prevention, seek to make antiretroviral therapy available to all populations in societies at risk, both rich and poor while international health programs focus on how a developed country can help a developing country deal with health problems that are unique to it, or to a few countries.

In terms of geographical reach, global health focuses on health issues that directly or indirectly transcend national boundaries, whereas international health focuses on health issues in countries other than one's own, especially in low- and middle-income countries. Global health focuses on the commonalities of health issues and concerns across countries of the world; international health focuses on their differences.

Global health and international health vary when it comes to the issue of health conditions. Global health focuses on the transfer of health risks precipitated by globalization while international health focuses on the health needs of poor nations. By contrast, international health focuses on the control of communicable diseases, maternal and child health, poor nutrition, and water- and sanitation-related diseases, whereas global health focuses on these health issues in addition to other noncommunicable diseases that affect the whole world including HIV/AIDS, cardiovascular diseases

Table 1.1 Differences between global health and international health.

Domains	Global health	International health
Mission	Achieve health equity among nations and for all people	Seeks to help poor people of developing nations
Geographical reach	Focuses on health issues that transcend national boundaries	Focuses on health issues of countries other than one's own – especially developing ones
	Focuses on commonalities between countries rather than their differences	Focuses on differences between countries rather than their commonalities
Level of cooperation	Depends on multilateral cooperation for the development and implementation of solutions to global health issues	Depends on bilateral cooperation for the development and implementation of solutions to health issues
Health conditions	Focuses on the global transfer of health risks	Focuses on risk factors within a country
Health content	Focuses on diseases/ health issues that affect the world; both communicable and noncommunicable	Focuses on the control of communicable diseases (tropical diseases, water and sanitation and maternal, and child health)
Range of disciplines	Highly multidisciplinary	Embraces a few disciplines

(like heart attacks and stroke), cancers, chronic respiratory diseases (such as chronic obstructive pulmonary disease and asthma), and diabetes.

Global health, unlike international health, realizes that the health issues confronting the world are such that no one nation can address them alone. As a result, global health practitioners work to develop partnerships to pool together resources and technical expertise to tackle and address prevalent and or emerging health issues that threaten the world's population.

In responding to health issues in developing countries, international health practitioners assume a vertical top-down approach. They come in as the experts with the funds, knowledge, and technical know-how, to help a country address its health problem or epidemic. With global health, the approach is different. The response and strategy to health is horizontal, collaborative, and inclusive.

Significance of global health in today's world

Given the extent to which the world is currently interconnected, all countries are vulnerable to disease threats, therefore ignoring global health issues is not an option. Diseases do not respect national boundaries. Through modern trade and transportation, diseases that originate in one part of the world can

spread with alarming speed across the world. Each year, over 500 million people travel across international borders by aircraft alone, expediting the import and export of diseases like essential commodities. The emergence and spread of the avian flu pandemic and HIV/AIDS attest to this fact.

Health and disease are closely associated with human, economic, and social development. The fact is, no matter the country one originates from, the wellbeing of people in the world depends to a large extent on how health issues are managed around the world. As a result, high on WHO's agenda is the issue of global health security; the desire to secure a world that is free from the threats posed by infectious diseases, so as to reduce human suffering, the loss of human life, and the negative impact of ill health on economic development. To facilitate the achievement of global health security, WHO in 2005, established the International Health Regulations, an international legal instrument that is binding on 196 countries across the globe, including all the Member States of WHO. The regulations help the international community prevent and respond to acute public health risks that have the potential to cross borders and threaten people worldwide.

For foreign direct investments (FDI), international trade, and the global economy to thrive, the collective health of populations is vital. Although the primary pull factors for FDI in the developing world have been identified to include cheap raw material costs, deregulated environments, and economic and political stability, the most significant factors are really the health of the nation and the nonexistence of disease risk factors.

Due to globalization, people are migrating to cities from rural areas in huge numbers, therefore making cities potential breeding grounds for global epidemics. In 2007 alone, over 50% of the world's population was living in towns and cities. Current trends show that the numbers may continue upwards. As urban populations grow with no concomitant provision of increased facilities and amenities such as solid waste disposal, and safe water and sanitation to meet the needs of people, the public health consequences could be great and costly.

Social and economic conditions affect people's lives, determines their risk for illness, and the actions they can take to prevent illness. Global health seeks to achieve health equity among nations and for all people by removing disparities and promoting a population-based approach to health.

Discussion points

1 What is global health?
2 How does global health differ from international health?
3 What are the defining features of global health? Briefly explain each feature.
4 In your opinion, is global health of relevance in this present time? Why?
5 Describe the health-related fields that preceded global health.
6 To what extent is global health a multidisciplinary field of study?
7 The mission of global health is to achieve health equity among nations and for all people. Is this feasible? Explain your response.
8 How did public health emerge?
9 Tropical medicine developed as a necessary part of the colonial system. Discuss.
10 List and explain four key global health concepts.

REFERENCES

Baronov, D. (2008) *The African Transformation of Western Medicine and the Dynamics of Global Cultural Exchange*, Temple University Press, Philadelphia, PA.

Carter Center (2016) *Guinea Worm Case Totals*, http://www.cartercenter.org/health/guinea_worm/case-totals.html (accessed October 14, 2016).

Centers for Disease Control and Prevention (2016) *Updates on CDC's Polio Eradication Efforts*, http://www.cdc.gov/polio/updates/(accessed October 14, 2016).

Crozier, Anna (2007) *Practising Colonial Medicine: The Colonial Medical Service in British East Africa*, I. B. Tauris, London.

de Blij, H. J., and Muller, P. O. (n.d.) *Realms, Regions and Concepts*, http://www.cabinda.net/Berlin_Conference.htm (accessed October 19, 2016).

Dowdle, W. R. (1999) The principles of disease elimination and eradication. *Morbidity and Mortality Weekly Report (MMWR)* **48**(SU01), 23–27.

Farley, J. (1991) *Bilharzia: A History of Imperial Tropical Medicine*, Cambridge University Press, New York, NY.

Fidler, D. P. (2008) After the revolution: global health politics in a time of economic crisis and threatening future trends. *Global Health Governance* **2**(2), 1–21.

Gilles, H. M., and Lucas, A. O. (1998) Tropical medicine: 100 years of progress. *British Medical Bulletin* **54**(2), 269–280.

Macfarlane, S. B., Jacobs, M., and. Kaaya, E. E. (2008) The name of global health: Trends in academic institutions. *Journal of Public Health Policy* **29**, 383.

Prüss-Üstün, A., Kay, D., Fewtrell, L., and Bartram, J. (2004) Unsafe water, sanitation and hygiene. *Comparative Quantification of Health Risks* **2**, 1321–1352, http://www.who.int/publications/cra/chapters/volume2/1321-1352.pdf?ua=1 (accessed October 14, 2016).

Rowson, M., Hughes, R., Smith, A., *et al.* (2007) *Global health and medical education – definitions, rationale and practice*. Unpublished work.

Tropical Medicine (2001) *The Oxford Illustrated Companion to Medicine* (3rd edn.). Oxford University Press, Oxford.

Warwick, A. (1998) Where is the Postcolonial History of Medicine? *Bulletin of the History of Medicine* **72**, 522–530.

World Bank (2015) *Updated Income Classification*, http://data.worldbank.org/news/2015-country-classifications (accessed October 14, 2016).

World Health Organization (2015a) *Non-Communicable Diseases*. Fact sheet no. 355, http://www.who.int/mediacentre/factsheets/fs355/en/(accessed October 14, 2016).

World Health Organization (2015b) *Cancer*. Fact sheet no. 297, http://www.who.int/mediacentre/factsheets/fs297/en/(accessed October 14, 2016).

World Health Organization (2016a) *Onchocerciasis*. Fact sheet no. 374, http://www.who.int/mediacentre/factsheets/fs374/en/(accessed October 14, 2016).

World Health Organization (2016b) *WHO Regional Offices*. Retrieved June 20, 2016, from http://www.who.int/about/regions/en/(accessed October 14, 2016).

FURTHER READING

Arnold, D. (1996) *Warm Climates and Western Medicine: The Emergence of Tropical Medicine*, Rodopi, Atlanta, GA.

Mendis, K., Rietveld, A., Warsame, M., *et al.* (2009) From malaria control to eradication: The WHO perspective. *Tropical Medicine and International Health* **14**(7), 802–809.

Weatherby, J. N., Evans, E. B., Gooden, R., *et al.* (2003) *The Other World: Issues and Politics of the Developing World* (5th edn.), Longman, New York, NY.

2

Globalization, infectious diseases, and global health

Learning objectives

By the end of this chapter, you will be able to:

✔ List and explain at least two factors that contribute to the emergence and re-emergence of infectious diseases;

✔ Discuss the effects of globalization on health;

✔ Identify and explain at least two health challenges due to globalization;

✔ List and explain at least two strategies for dealing with health issues caused by globalization.

Summary of key points

In an increasingly interconnected world where national borders are being eroded and where fast transportation has made it easy for people to travel from one country to another, diseases, both emerging and re-emerging, have also been able to spread easily to several parts of the world at alarming rates. Globalization can be held accountable for disease transmission around the world, but it must be noted that, prior to its occurrence, people transmitted diseases to different parts of the world, but at a slower pace. While globalization has improved the wealth of nations, it has also brought in its wake, practices that negatively impact health outcomes. This chapter opens with a brief overview of the epidemiological transition. Next, it presents a timeline of disease transmission through human history and then goes on to discuss emerging and re-emerging infectious diseases, as well as the effects of global trade on health. Health challenges associated with globalization, and global strategies in place to address them are also discussed.

Epidemiological transition

Postulated by the epidemiologist Abdel R. Omran in 1971, the epidemiological transition theory outlines phases in human development, which describe a shift in demographic and disease profiles of populations over time, from predominantly famine and infectious diseases, to chronic degenerative noncommunicable diseases. According to Omran's theory, countries experience an epidemiological transition as they progress from 'developing' to 'developed'. Related to this progression is the development of modern healthcare systems and medications like antibiotics, which, in addition to reducing infant mortality rates and increasing average life expectancy, can cause chronic degenerative diseases in humans.

Omran's epidemiological transition theory has three phases. First is the Age of Pestilence and Famine represented by hunting and gathering, where mortality rates were high due to infectious diseases and where

---

Global Health: Issues, Challenges, and Global Action Lecture Notes, First Edition. Elizabeth A. Armstrong-Mensah.
© 2017 John Wiley & Sons Ltd. Published 2017 by John Wiley & Sons Ltd.

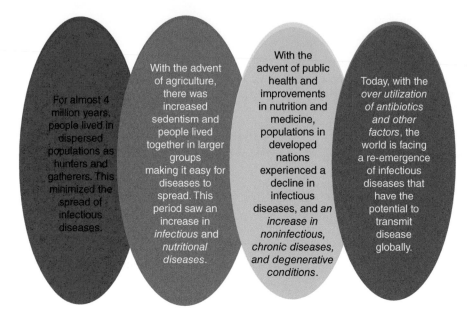

Figure 2.1 The epidemiological transition.

the average life expectancy at birth was between 20 and 40 years. Second is the Age of Receding Pandemics, represented by the emergence of agriculture and sedentism, where mortality rates gradually dropped due to reductions in the frequency of epidemics and where the average life expectancy at birth was between 30 and 50 years. Third is the Age of Degenerative and Man-Made Diseases, represented by chronic diseases experienced by humans in present times and where mortality rates continue to decline (Omran, 1971). Omran's theory has been criticized. Some of his critics question the accuracy and reliability of his theory to the health situation of populations in low- and middle-income countries, which although are at the first or second phase of transition, suffer from both infectious and noninfectious chronic degenerative diseases (McCracken and Phillips, 2012). The three phases of Omran's epidemiological transition theory are further discussed in the rest of this section, preceded by a brief synopsis of the baseline – the Paleolithic era (see Figure 2.1).

The baseline: Paleolithic era

In the Paleolithic era, people hunted animals, fished, and gathered wild berries and plants for food. They lived a nomadic life, moving from place to place in search of food and settling for brief periods in places where they found sustenance. The settlements of hunters and gatherers were small, sparsely populated (about 20–30 clans), and far apart from each other. This made it difficult for pathogens and infectious diseases to spread easily. Hunters and gatherers suffered from diseases related to their environment, such as Chagas disease, mosquito spread encephalitis, rabies, sleeping sickness (trypanosomiasis), and yellow fever, as well as from the wounds they sustained from the animals they hunted.

The first epidemiological transition: Age of Pestilence and Famine

Following the Paleolithic era, was the Age of Pestilence and Famine. In about 10 000 BC, hunters and gathers in Mesopotamia (present-day Iraq) discovered that they could produce food by planting the seeds of some of the food they gathered. This discovery, along with the development of specialized farming skills, advanced farming tools, and the domestication of animals, such as goats, sheep, and later cattle and pigs, led to what has been dubbed the Neolithic Age or Agricultural Revolution. With the ability to produce food for themselves, hunters and gathers moved away from a nomadic lifestyle to a sedentary agrarian existence in villages and communities in great numbers. The additional discovery of irrigation and food storage methods led to surplus food production and increased the population size of communities. Food production in the Age of Pestilence and Famine focused on select cereals including rice, wheat, and barley. In general, people who lived in the Paleolithic era were healthier than those who lived in the Age of Pestilence and Famine. This was because the diet of the people in the former age was more balanced and varied than that consumed by people in the latter. In the Age of Pestilence and Famine people suffered from nutritional diseases.

Infectious diseases including measles, mumps, pneumonia, smallpox, tuberculosis (TB), and typhoid, and zoonotic diseases from domesticated animals and vectors, were the prevailing diseases and the cause of mortality in this age. Living together in large numbers and in close proximity facilitated the spread of diseases within communities and to new regions. This phase was called the Age of Pestilence and Famine because, epidemics, famines, and wars caused mortalities and infectious diseases were prevalent, claiming the lives of many, especially children.

The second epidemiological transition: Age of Receding Pandemics

The second epidemiological transition was the Age of Receding Pandemics, which began with the Industrial Revolution. During this age, diseases from the first phase of the epidemiological transition continued to coexist with newly appearing noninfectious chronic degenerative diseases. In time, the status quo changed. With increased economic growth, access to clean water and improved sanitary sewage, together with advances in nutrition, public health, medicine, science, and technology, infectious disease and mortality rates began to drop and stabilize. As a result of preventing and controlling infectious diseases through immunization programs, improved hygiene, and the utilization of antimicrobials, populations began to live longer and to experience chronic degenerative diseases, such as diabetes, heart disease, and stroke. This phase of the epidemiological transition was referred to as such because it saw drastic reductions in infectious disease prevalence and mortality, and an increase in chronic degenerative diseases.

Chronic degenerative diseases are particularly prevalent in societies undergoing a shift from "developing" to "developed." In these countries, it is common for some segments of society to be experiencing the second phase of the epidemiological transition while others experience the first.

The third transition: Age of Chronic Diseases

The Age of Chronic Diseases is the third epidemiological transition that the world is currently experiencing. It is characterized by the continued presence of noncommunicable chronic degenerative and man-made diseases, the emergence and re-emergence of infectious diseases, and antibiotic-resistant diseases. This stage of the epidemiological transition is also characterized by fast transportation systems that facilitate the rapid and extensive transmission of pathogens and diseases across the world within a short space of time (Manju, 2015).

The concept of globalization

For many years, countries were economically, socially, and politically self-sufficient. Economically, they produced the food and raw materials they needed and did not need to depend on outside sources. Socially, some countries were closed off from the rest of the world and observed their own customs. Politically, although countries had arrangements or treaties among themselves, they were not as far reaching and as myriad as they are today.

Things have changed; countries are no longer in a state of autarky. Economies of the world have become so integrated and interdependent that countries now greatly depend on each other for a variety of goods, ideas, information, services, and technology among other things. This interdependence and interconnectedness is what is referred to as globalization.

Like many other fields of study, there is no generally agreed definition of what globalization is. According to Brown *et al.* (2006), globalization is "The process of increasing economic, political, and social interdependence, and integration as capital, goods, persons, concepts, ideas, and values cross state boundaries." To Labonte *et al.* (2004), "Globalization, defined at its simplest, describes the constellation of processes by which nations, business and people are becoming more connected and interdependent across the globe through increased economic integration and communication exchange, cultural diffusions (especially of Western culture) and travel." For Giddens (1991), "Globalization can thus be defined as the intensification of worldwide social relations which link distant localities in such a way that local happenings are shaped by events occurring many miles away and vice versa." Wide-ranging as these definitions of globalization appear to be, they underscore the economic, political, and social connectivity of countries globally.

Evolution and features of globalization

From existing literature, it is clear that there is no consensus on when the phenomenon of globalization emerged. According to Andre Gunder Frank, an economic historian and sociologist, there was a "single global world economy and a worldwide division of labor and multilateral trade from 1500 onward." Jerry Bentley disagrees with Gunder Frank. To Bentley, globalization began prior to 1500 – in 1492 when Christopher Columbus stumbled upon the Americas, and in 1498, when Vasco da Gama sailed around the Southern tip of Africa. Economic historians including James Tracey are skeptical of Bentley's claims. Tracey questions the connection between countries in the sixteenth and seventeenth centuries after the voyages of Columbus and da Gama and holds that there was no economic integration during those times and therefore, dismisses those periods as the beginning of globalization (Bentley, 1996). From the perspective of the World Bank, there have been three waves of globalization. The first wave occurred in 1870, precipitated by reduced trade barriers and improved transportation technology, which lasted until the start of World War I in 1914. This wave resulted in the vast migration of people around the world. The second wave occurred from 1950 to 1980 and was characterized by multilateral trade agreements among only developed countries. The third and current wave of globalization, also known as modern globalization, commenced in 1980 due to the adoption of trade liberalization by some developing countries with the aim of drawing foreign capital.

Modern globalization is characterized by transborder information flow via the internet, e-mail, mobile phones, and satellite TV; international trade through trade agreements like the General Agreement on Tariffs and Trade (GATT), World Trade Organization (WTO), the North American Free Trade Agreement (NAFTA), Asia-Pacific Economic Cooperation (APEC), Economic Community of West African States (ECOWAS) and the European Union (EU); global banking; and the international flow of capital. Additional features of modern globalization are international travel and tourism, international technology transfer, population movement (e.g., migration and displacements), and cultural assimilation (e.g., diet, clothes, and lifestyle).

Disease and human history

As mentioned in the introductory section of this chapter, globalization is considered by some as accountable for the emergence, re-emergence, and transmission of diseases. While this notion has credence, it is pertinent to note that diseases spread across the globe through various means long before globalization occurred. In the first century AD, merchants and travelers were able to travel from Britain and Spain in the west, to China and Japan in the east. Trade routes, such as the Silk and Spice Routes facilitated the movement of raw materials, foodstuffs, and luxury goods over long distances via animals or by sea, from areas with excess to areas where they were needed. The trade routes made it possible for diseases to be transferred from one place to another. In the second century, smallpox spread along the caravan routes between Rome and Asia. In the fourteenth century, the bubonic plague (Black Death) spread from China to Western Asia and Europe through trade, claiming the lives of an estimated 25 million people in Europe and 12 million people in China.

Around the third century, troops of Alexander the Great brought leprosy from India to Greece. By the thirteenth century, leprosy had reached epidemic proportions in medieval Europe through the crusaders and travelers. In the fifteenth century, the first recorded case of syphilis occurred in Naples and in the sixteenth century, Europeans exploring the Americas carried infectious diseases with them. These diseases killed a third of the Native American population who had no immunity against measles and chickenpox.

In the seventeenth century (1699), yellow fever hit the American colonies of Charleston and Philadelphia in the United States. Mortality rates were staggering and almost brought life to a standstill. In the eighteenth century, smallpox was used as a weapon of war by the British against the United States. When the American army besieged Quebec City in 1776, the British sent recently variolated (inoculated / infected) prostitutes into Canadian encampments. Consequently, approximately 5000 American soldiers contracted smallpox. This event caused the American army to retreat, leaving Quebec in the hands of Britain.

In the nineteenth century (1816), the first cholera pandemic occurred in Bengal and then spread across India. It also spread to China, Indonesia, and the Caspian Sea in Europe before receding. Hundreds of thousands of Indians and 10 000 British troops died as a result of the pandemic (Crosby, 1989). In the twentieth century (between 1918 and 1920), the Spanish flu pandemic occurred. There were over 20 million mortalities in Africa, China, India, and Russia. Close troop quarters, massive troop movements, and jubilation after World War I, hastened the spread of the pandemic. In the twentieth century (1981), the first known human immunodeficiency virus (HIV) cases were detected by the Centers for Disease Control and Prevention (CDC). This marked the official beginning of the HIV and the acquired immune deficiency syndrome (AIDS) epidemic.

Emerging and re-emerging infectious diseases

Irrespective of medical and technological advances in present times, infectious diseases, both new and re-emerging, continue to pose significant threats to human health. Infectious diseases are caused by a specific infectious agent or its toxic product that results from transmission of that agent or its products from an infected person, animal, or reservoir to a susceptible host, either directly or indirectly. Cholera, dengue fever, Ebola disease, HIV/AIDS, leprosy, malaria, measles, neonatal tetanus, poliomyelitis, typhoid, and yaws are examples of infectious diseases.

Emerging infectious diseases

Emerging infectious diseases are diseases that have not occurred in humans before, but have been recently recognized as distinct diseases due to an infectious agent. They are also newly identified and previously unknown infectious agents that cause public health problems either locally or internationally. Avian flu (H5N1), HIV/AIDS, and severe acute respiratory syndrome (SARS) are diseases that emerged for the first time in certain parts of the world.

Avian flu is a viral infection that occurs in birds. The virus is able to mutate and infect humans. The first known case of avian flu occurred in Hong Kong in 1997. It killed millions of poultry throughout Africa, Asia, and Europe. By 2011, avian flu had killed 306 people in 12 countries. HIV/AIDS is believed to have originated from nonhuman primates (chimpanzee and sooty magabeys) in Africa. It is believed that strains of the primate version of the immunodeficiency virus (simian immune deficiency virus) crossed the species barrier into humans through the consumption of bush meat and other practices, resulting in HIV/AIDS. The first recognized cases of HIV/AIDS occurred in the United States in 1981. In 2015, an estimated 36.7 million people were living with HIV/AIDS and about 1.1 million people died from AIDS-related illnesses globally (Joint United Nations Programme on HIV and AIDS, 2016). From the onset of the HIV/AIDS epidemic, cumulatively, about 78 million people have been infected with HIV and an estimated 25 million have died from AIDS-related illnesses.

Re-emerging infectious diseases

Re-emerging infectious diseases are those diseases that have been around for decades or centuries, but have come back in a different form or at a different location (Morens *et al.,* 2004). They are also infectious diseases that had once fallen to such low levels that they were no longer considered public health threats, but are now showing upward incidence or prevalence globally. Ebola disease, malaria, and TB are examples of re-emerging infectious diseases.

Ebola disease has been around since the 1970s. The first known case occurred in 1976 in the Democratic Republic of Congo and Sudan, claiming 280 and 151 lives, respectively. It re-emerged in Gabon and Cote d'Ivoire in 1994, in South Africa in 1996, in Uganda in 2000, and in the Democratic Republic of Congo again in 1977, 1995, 2007, 2008, 2012, and 2014. From March 2014 to mid 2016, Ebola re-emerged in the West African countries of Guinea, Liberia, Sierra Leone, Mali, and Nigeria, and in the European countries of Italy, Spain, and the United Kingdom. A few cases were also reported in the United States. Cumulatively, Ebola mortalities as of June 2015, was 27,550. Figure 2.2 provides an overview of the countries affected by Ebola since 1976, and mortality rates for the 2014 to 2016 outbreak.

Malaria has been around for over 4000 years. The disease is caused by the bite of the female anopheles mosquito. In the 1950s, WHO attempted to eradicate malaria from the world, but was unsuccessful due to a number of factors including the noninvolvement of

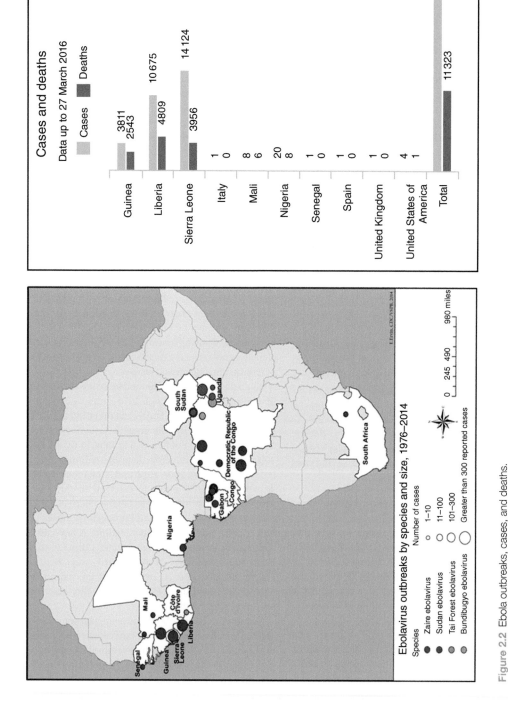

Figure 2.2 Ebola outbreaks, cases, and deaths.

Sources: Centers for Disease Control and Prevention, http://www.cdc.gov/vhf/ebola/outbreaks/history/distribution-map.html (accessed 21 October 2016); World Health Organization, http://apps.who.int/ebola/ebola-situation-reports (accessed October 21, 2016), with permission.

the community at large, the fact that the malaria program had to be implemented with rigid fidelity to a very detailed standard manual of operations, and the fact that research on the disease was considered unnecessary (Henderson, 1999). In the early 1960s, malaria was almost eradicated from India, but re-emerged as a major public health issue. In India, malaria kills over 200 000 people on an annual basis (Dhingra *et al.*, 2010). Globally, approximately 198 million cases of malaria were reported in 2013. In that same year, there were an estimated 584 000 malaria-related deaths. In 2014, 97 countries were malaria endemic. According to WHO estimates released in September 2015, there were 214 million cases of malaria in 2015 and 438 000 deaths. Worldwide, 80% of malaria deaths occur in 15 countries, mainly in sub-Saharan Africa (World Health Organization, 2015).

Following HIV/AIDS, TB is the second disease that causes death by a single infectious agent. Prior to the emergence of the HIV epidemic, TB infection rates had fallen to between 1 and 5% per year in developing countries. The emergence of the HIV epidemic reversed this trend. Thus, by 2013, about 9 million people around the world were infected with TB and an estimated 1.5 million had died from TB. In 2013, the highest increases in new TB cases occurred in South-East Asia and the Western Pacific regions, accounting for 56% of new cases. Multidrug-resistant TB (MDR-TB) has also contributed to the re-emergence of TB, as standard anti-TB drugs have become ineffective owing to either inappropriate treatment, incorrect use of anti-TB drugs, or the utilization of poor-quality TB medicines.

Contributing factors to the emergence and re-emergence of infectious diseases

The emergence and re-emergence of infectious diseases are caused by a number of factors including the nature of disease agents, the environment, human activity, commerce, technology, and international travel. The ability of microbial agents to mutate, adapt, and resist drugs meant to control and treat them, and the ability of vectors to resist pesticides, cause infectious diseases such as gonorrhea, malaria, H5N1, and TB to persist, emerge, or re-emerge globally.

Environmentally, deforestation and land use compel animals to live in close proximity to humans thereby, creating opportunities for disease agents to breach species barriers. The emergence of Lyme disease in the United States and Europe was probably caused by reforestation, as it increased the deer population and the deer tick, the vector of Lyme disease. The movement of people into these deer-infested areas placed populations at risk for Lyme disease (Barbour and Fish, 1993). Global warming alters the natural habitats of animals and vectors, and allows diseases to re-emerge and spread to different geographic areas. For example, hot temperatures in Ravenna, Italy, in 2007, caused tiger mosquitos to migrate to that city and spread the chikungunya virus to the northeastern parts of the country for the first time. This culminated in 197 deaths. Subsequent to the 2007 outbreak, chikungunya also occurred in France and Croatia (World Health Organization, 2016). Agricultural projects, though necessary for economic growth and social wellbeing, sometimes set the stage for the re-emergence of infectious diseases. The re-emergence of over 100 000 cases of Korean hemorrhagic fever in China on an annual basis, is the result of human contact with the Hantavirus in the urine, saliva, or feces of infected field mice (*Apodemus agrarius*) during rice harvesting.

Human activity, including migration and settlement in hitherto uninhabited areas, exposes populations to new pathogens, insects, and animals already present in the environment. It also causes new diseases carried by migrant populations to be introduced into the new environment and to vulnerable populations living in the chosen area of settlement. Urbanization and its concomitant problems of overcrowding, substandard housing, unsafe water, and poor sanitation, puts populations at risk for numerous infectious diseases. International trade and travel also contribute to the emergence and re-emergence of infectious diseases. Through commercial activities in the sixteenth and seventeenth century's, ships transporting slaves from West Africa to the New World, brought yellow fever and its vector, the *Aedes aegypti* mosquito, to the new territories (Morse, 1995).

The liberalization of the airline industry has made air travel affordable and has thus, dramatically amplified the volume of global travel. It has been estimated that about one million people travel internationally every day and a comparable number travel between developed and developing countries each week (Sutherst, 2004). Lengthy nonstop flights accelerate the spread of emerging and re-emerging infectious diseases, as passengers sit in close proximity to one another for prolonged periods. The outbreak of SARS which occurred in 2003, is an example of the rapid spread of a previously unknown disease through air travel by an infected person.

World trade and global health

International trade facilitates the spread of infectious diseases and crossborder health risks. In the fourteenth century, Black Death (bubonic plague) was spread along shipping routes from the arid plains of Central Asia, along the Silk Road to Crimea, and throughout the Mediterranean and Europe by oriental rat fleas living on black rats who were regular passengers on merchant ships. The Black Death killed an estimated 30 to 60% of the total population of Europe.

Global trade in illicit drugs such as cannabis, cocaine, heroin, and opioids, negatively impact human lives and productivity. In 2012, about 183 000 drug-related deaths were reported globally, accounting for a mortality rate of 40 deaths per million among a population aged 15–64 years (World Health Organization, 2014). Opioids are the primary contributors to the global statistics on drug-related deaths. Alcohol consumption is another area where the globalization of trade has created health risks. The harmful use of alcohol causes socioeconomic burdens on societies, facilitates violence, and causes liver cirrhosis, some cancers, and injuries (Beaglehole and Yach, 2003).

The implementation of the World Trade Organization's (WTO) agreement on Trade Related Aspects of Intellectual Property Rights (TRIPS) extends patent protection on new drugs, which are usually expensive, for a minimum of 20 years. As a result, TRIPS limits and undermines access to new medicines, especially by poor populations living in the developing world. Global trade in livestock and poultry may have contributed to the outbreak of mad cow disease in the Northern hemisphere and avian influenza in Asia.

Effects of globalization on health

Globalization positively and negatively affects health outcomes in developed and developing countries. On a positive note, globalization has increased access to medicines, medical information, technology, and the training of healthcare professionals. Through medical tourism, globalization enables patients in developed countries to travel across borders to less developed countries to receive a wide range of medical services at a fraction of the cost in their home countries.

Through telemedicine – medical consultation via video conferencing or the transmission of still images to medical personnel – patients are able to obtain medical care from healthcare professionals in various parts of the world. Telemedicine also connects healthcare professionals in remote rural areas with healthcare professionals around the world for distance learning (Kvedar et al., 2006; Mishra, 2003; Vassallo et al., 2001), and facilitates cross-site, intercountry, and across-country collaboration and networking (Geissbuhler et al., 2003; Kifle et al., 2006).

Globalization has helped to improve patient heath through online support groups. Results of a survey on online social networking features showed that features such as friending and sharing of personal stories on blogs were helpful in meeting the emotional needs and support of people who were ill (Chung, 2014). Studies conducted by researchers at the University of Netherlands and Luephana University on mortality rates, using the Maastricht Globalization Index (MGI) as a gauge to measure associations between globalization and health in a nation, showed that countries with high levels of globalization had lower infant, under five, and adult mortality rates than those with low levels of globalization. Scientists attributed this outcome to the attainment of higher education, growing GDP, improved neonatal care, and access to sanitation by globalized nations.

Improved communication technologies have made real-time disease surveillance possible, thus making it easier for countries to alert relevant authorities and entities of the outbreak of diseases and, more broadly, to share information on health issues.

On a negative note, globalization enhances crossborder transmission of diseases, facilitates the marketing of harmful illicit products such as cocaine and heroin, and promotes the adoption of unhealthy lifestyles including smoking, alcohol abuse, and the consumption of unhealthy foods. Globalization also encourages privatization of healthcare, which has the tendency to increase healthcare costs, and facilitates the migration of trained medical professionals in developing countries to developed countries, in search of better livelihoods and opportunities.

Health challenges due to globalization

A major health-related problem associated with globalization is the increased public health responsibilities on nations. Prior to the easy movement of people around the world, the governments of various countries focused on preventing, controlling, and treating diseases that were indigenous to their populations. Through international travel, some deadly infectious diseases, have been able to spread rapidly around the globe. As a result, these governments now have to deal with their indigenous health issues plus those foreign to them. In addition to increased health responsibilities, governments also have to be proactive. They have to anticipate global health threats and put in place appropriate mechanisms including real-time surveillance systems to protect the health of their citizens. These efforts not only cost money, but also require resources and technical expertise that are not readily available in many developing countries.

International trade has made it possible for a number of goods to cross borders every day. This has increased the risk for tainted food products, illegal black market goods, and diseases to be transported and transmitted. Due to trade in illegal drugs, there were over 50 million users of heroin, cocaine, and synthetic drugs worldwide in 2000. These drugs can cause withdrawal symptoms, functional abnormalities of the brain, heart problems, and long-term brain damage among others.

Global action and strategies

Emerging and re-emerging infectious diseases

The World Health Organization launched the Global Outbreak Alert and Response Network (GOARN) in 2000 to protect the world from threats of infectious diseases. Consisting of a network of technical institutions, research institutes, universities, international health organizations, and technical networks willing to contribute and participate in internationally coordinated responses to infectious disease outbreaks, GOARN seeks to assist countries with disease-control efforts by ensuring rapid and appropriate technical support to affected populations, investigating and characterizing events, assessing risks of rapidly emerging epidemic disease threats, and supporting national outbreak preparedness by ensuring that responses contribute to sustained containment of epidemic threats.

Since 2000, WHO and GOARN have responded to over 50 events worldwide with over 400 experts providing field support to about 40 countries. GOARN

has helped to build consensus on guiding principles for international outbreak alert and response. It has established operational protocols to standardize field logistics, security and communications, and has also streamlined administrative processes to ensure rapid mobilization of field teams.

Travel and health

Global travel exposes people to a wide range of health risks and diseases. In an attempt to protect the world from global infectious disease threats, WHO launched the International Health Regulations (IHR) in 1969 and later updated it in 2005. The old IHR applied to only three diseases: cholera, yellow fever, and the bubonic plague. With increased trade and travel in the 46 years since the last major revision, the updated rules focus on preventing and protecting against the international spread of diseases, while minimizing interference with world travel and trade.

The IHR are a legally binding international agreement that govern the role of WHO and its 195 Member States in identifying, sharing information about, and responding to public health events that may have international consequences. The regulations provide guidance and encourages developed and developing countries to work together to develop appropriate surveillance and response capacities to prevent and address health concerns.

Global food safety

The Global Food Safety Initiative (GFSI) was launched in 2000 in response to a number of food safety crises, when consumer confidence was at an all-time low. The GFSI is a private business-driven initiative established and managed by the Consumer Goods Forum, an international trade association, to improve food safety management systems and the delivery of safe food to consumers worldwide. The GFSI's activities include the definition of food safety requirements along the entire food supply chain, from feed distribution and packaging, to capacity development programs for small and/or less developed businesses, so as to facilitate access to local markets, and the training of food safety auditors to equip them with the knowledge, attitudes, and skills that competent auditors should possess. The GFSI provides a platform for collaboration between some of the world's leading food safety experts, from retailers, manufacturers, and food service companies, to service providers associated with the food supply chain, international organizations, academia, and the government. Since its establishment, GFSI experts have been collaborating in numerous technical working groups to tackle food safety issues defined by GFSI stakeholders.

The Codex Alimentarius Commission established by the Food and Agricultural Organization (FAO) and WHO in 1963, develops harmonized international food standards, guidelines, and codes of practice to protect the health of consumers and to ensure fair practices in the food trade.

The Commission also promotes coordination of all food standards work undertaken by international, governmental, and nongovernmental organizations. Codex Alimentarius officially covers all foods – processed, semi-processed or raw – and particularly, foods that are marketed directly to consumers. It contains general standards for food labeling, food hygiene, food additives, pesticide residues, and procedures for assessing the safety of foods derived from modern biotechnology. It also contains guidelines for governmental import and export inspection and certification systems for food.

Discussion points

1 List and discuss the three phases of the epidemiological transition.
2 Which health conditions are more prevalent in the second phase of the epidemiological transition. Why is this the case?
3 What is the link between globalization and health?
4 What are emerging infectious diseases? How are they different from re-emerging infectious diseases?
5 How do environmental factors and human activities contribute to the emergence and re-emergence of infectious diseases?
6 How does international trade impact global health?
7 Discuss how globalization affects health positively and negatively.
8 Why is food safety a global health issue?
9 What are some of the challenges posed by globalization on health?
10 What strategies or actions are in place to address the impact of globalization on health?

REFERENCES

Barbour, A. G., and Fish, D. (1993) The biological and social phenomenon of Lyme disease. *Science* **260**, 160–166.

Beaglehole, R., and Yach, D. (2003) Globalization and the prevention and control of non-communicable disease: the neglected chronic diseases of adults. *The Lancet* **362**(9387), 903–908.

Bentley, J. (1996) Cross-cultural interaction and periodization in world history. *American Historical Review* **101**, 749–770.

Brown, T. M., Marcos, C., and Fee, E. (2006) The World Health Organization and the transition from "international" to "global" public health. *American Journal of Public Health* **96**(1), 62–72.

Chung, J. E. (2014) Social networking in online support groups for health: how online social networking benefits patients. *Journal of Health Communication* **19**(6), 639–659.

Crosby, A. W. (1989) *America's Forgotten Panidemic: The Influenza of 1918*, CambridgeUniversity Press, Cambridge.

Dhingra, N., Jha, P., Sharma, V. P., *et al.* (2010) Adult and child malaria mortality in India: A nationally representative mortality survey. *The Lancet* **376**, 1768–1774.

Geissbuhler, A., Ly, O., Lovis, C., and L'Haire, J. (2003) Telemedicine in western Africa: Lessons learned from a pilot project in Mali: perspectives and recommendations. *AMIA Annual Symposium Proceedings* **2003**, 249–253.

Giddens, Anthony. (1991) *The Consequences of Modernity*, Stanford University Press, Palo Alto, CA.

Henderson, D.A. (1999) Eradication:Lessons from the past. *Morbidity and Mortality Weekly Report (MMWR)* **48**(1), 16–22.

Joint United Nations Programme on HIV and AIDS. (2016) *Global AIDS Update 2016*, http://www.unaids.org/en/resources/documents/2016/Global-AIDS-update-2016 (accessed October 14, 2016).

Kifle, M., Mbarika. V., and Datta P. (2006) Telemedicine in sub-Saharan Africa: The case of teleophthalmology and eye care in Ethiopia. *American Society for Information Science and Technology* **57**(10), 1383–1393.

Kvedar, J., Heinselmann, P. J., and Jacques, G. (2006) Cancer diagnosis and telemedicine:A case study from Cambodia. *Annals of Oncology* **17**(8), S37–42.

Labonte, R., Schrecker, T., Sanders, D., and Meeus, W. (2004) *Globalization, Health and Development: The Right Prescription*, University of Cape Town Press, Cape Town.

Manju, P. (2015) *Epidemiological Transition*, http://www.slideshare.net/ManjuPilania/jepidemiological-transition-43609219?from_action=save (accessed October 14, 2016).

Mc Cracken, K., and Phillips D. R. (2012) *Global Health: An Introduction to Current and Future Trends*, Routledge, London.

Mishra, A. (2003) Telemedicine in otolaryngology : An Indian perspective. *Indian Otolaryngology and Head and Neck Surgery*, **55**(3), 211–212.

Morens, D. M., Folkers, G. K, and Fauci, A. S. (2004) The challenge of emerging and reemerging infectious diseases. *Nature* **430**, 242–249.

Morse, S. S. (1995) Actors in the emergence of infectious diseases. *Emerging Infectious Diseases* **1**(1), 1–15.

Omran A. R. (1971) The epidemiologic transition: theory of the epidemiology of population change. *Milbank Quarterly* **49**, 509–538.

Sutherst, R. W. (2004) Global change and human vulnerability to vector-borne diseases. *Clinical Microbiology Reviews* **17**(1), 136–173.

Vassallo, D. J., Hoque, F., Farquharson Roberts, M., *et al.* (2001) An evaluation of the first years' experience with a low-cost telemedicine link in Bangladesh. *Telemedicine and Telecare* **7**(3), 125–138.

World Health Organization (2014) *World Drug Report*, https://www.unodc.org/documents/wdr2014/World_Drug_Report_2014_web.pdf (accessed October 15, 2016).

World Health Organization (2015) *Malaria*. Fact sheet, http://www.who.int/malaria/media/world-malaria-report-2015/en/(accessed October 15, 2016).

World Health Organization (2016) *Chikungunya*. Fact sheet no. **327**, http://www.who.int/mediacentre/factsheets/fs327/en/(accessed October 15, 2016).

FURTHER READING

Ibeki, M. (2011) *Black Death*, http://www.bbc.co.uk/history/british/middle_ages/black_01.shtml (accessed October 14, 2016).

3

Noncommunicable diseases

Learning objectives

By the end of this chapter, you will be able to:

✔ List and describe at last two types of noncommunicable diseases;

✔ List and discuss the causes of at least two noncommunicable diseases;

✔ Describe risk factors associated with at least two noncommunicable diseases;

✔ List and explain at least two challenges associated with noncommunicable diseases;

✔ Describe global action and strategies to address noncommunicable diseases.

Summary of key points

Unlike communicable diseases, noncommunicable diseases (NCDs) are not contagious and therefore, cannot be transmitted from an infected person to another person. They are often inherited, or may arise from genetic abnormalities, lifestyle, behavioral, or environmental factors. Globally, NCDs are becoming major contributors to the burden of disease and the leading cause of mortalities, yet unfortunately, they tend to be neglected. In the past, NCDs were considered as diseases of rich developed countries. With globalization, this notion is no longer valid, as populations in developing countries now suffer from the double burden of communicable and NCDs. Noncommunicable diseases have adverse human, social, and economic consequences, and can be costly to manage. This chapter focuses on NCDs particularly what they are, types, risk factors, their health and economic burden, challenges, and global strategies and action in place to address them.

The concept of noncommunicable diseases

Noncommunicable diseases are a group of health conditions or diseases that are caused by acute infection, which often result in chronic consequences that progress slowly over time and usually require long-term management, or lifetime treatment and care. Sometimes referred to as "chronic diseases," NCDs are distinguished from infectious diseases primarily because of their noninfectious nature and not because of how long they last. While NCDs are not infectious diseases, they may be caused by an infectious agent, as is the case with HIV/AIDS.

Global Health: Issues, Challenges, and Global Action Lecture Notes, First Edition. Elizabeth A. Armstrong-Mensah.
© 2017 John Wiley & Sons Ltd. Published 2017 by John Wiley & Sons Ltd.

In September 2011, NCDs were formally recognized by the United Nations (UN) and placed high on the global development agenda as major diseases that threaten economies and societies. Prior to 2011, the world's focus was mainly on infectious diseases.

Types of noncommunicable diseases

The World Health Organization (WHO) has identified four main types of NCDs: cardiovascular disease, cancers, noninfectious diseases of the respiratory system, and diabetes. These types of NCDs account for 82% of total global NCD deaths. Other health conditions considered as clusters of NCDs are injuries and mental health disorders. Behavioral factors such as alcohol abuse, excessive tobacco use, physical inactivity, and unhealthy diet are some of the risk factors associated with the occurrence of NCDs.

Cardiovascular diseases

Cardiovascular or heart diseases are an assortment of diseases, disorders, and conditions that affect the human heart and blood vessels. The human heart is a muscle tissue about the size of a fist that pumps blood through the cardiovascular system (a network of arteries and veins) throughout the body. Running along the surface of the heart are coronary arteries, which provide the heart with a constant flow of oxygen that it needs to pump blood effectively.

There are several types of cardiovascular diseases: abnormal heart rhythms or arrhythmias, cardiac arrest, cardiomyopathy, coronary artery disease, congestive heart failure, myocardial infarction, heart valve disease, pericarditis, pulmonary embolism, and stable angina pectoris. Some cardiovascular diseases are discussed below.

Abnormal heart rhythms or arrhythmias

Arrhythmias is the irregular beating of the heart, where the heart beats less or faster than the normal 50 to 100 beats per minute. This heart condition is caused by coronary artery disease, electrolyte imbalance in the blood, changes in the heart muscle, and

injury from a heart attack among others. Types of arrhythmias are premature atrial contractions, which are additional beats that originate in the atria, premature ventricular contractions (PVCs), which are skipped heartbeats brought on by stress, too much caffeine, exercise, or electrolyte imbalance, and ventricular tachycardia (V-tach), which is a rapid heart rhythm from the lower chambers (or ventricles) of the heart that prevents the heart from adequately pumping blood throughout the body. Palpitations, pounding in the chest, dizziness, and fainting are some of the symptoms associated with arrhythmias.

Cardiac arrest

Cardiac arrest is loss of life as a result of the sudden stoppage of the heart. It often occurs in adults aged 35–45 years and is more prevalent in men than in women. Children rarely experience cardiac arrest. Signs and symptoms that precede sudden cardiac arrest are immediate and drastic. In most cases, cardiac arrest occurs without warning. Where there are symptoms, they include sudden collapse, no pulse, no breathing, loss of consciousness and at times, fatigue, fainting, blackouts, dizziness, chest pain, and shortness of breath.

Coronary artery disease

Coronary artery disease is the result of plaque buildup in the coronary arteries over a period of time. The buildup narrows the arteries and prevents oxygen-rich blood from getting to the heart. When plaque blocks a blood vessel in the brain, an ischemic stroke can occur, and when the blood vessel bursts in the brain, it could lead to hemorrhagic stroke. Angina, burning, numbness, fullness, squeezing or painful feeling in the left shoulder, arms, neck, back, or jaw, are the most common symptoms of coronary artery disease. Other symptoms are nausea, palpitations, shortness of breath, and rapid heartbeat.

Myocardial infarction

Myocardial infarction or heart attack is the permanent damage or death of the heart muscle caused by a blood clot in the arteries that completely blocks off blood supply to the heart. Symptoms of a heart attack may last for 30 minutes or longer and include discomfort, pain in the chest, arm, or below the breastbone, sweating, nausea, vomiting, dizziness, shortness of breath, or rapid or irregular heartbeat. On some occasions, there are no symptoms.

Economic burden of cardiovascular disease

The global economic burden of cardiovascular diseases, both direct and indirect, is compelling. In 2012, the global estimated cost for heart failure was $108 billion with about $65 billion in direct costs and approximately $43 million in indirect costs. In the United States, the total cost of cardiovascular treatment, medication, and lost productivity due to disability in 2010, was approximately $444 billion. Cardiovascular diseases were estimated to cost the Russian Federation a total of about RUR 836.1 billion (€24 517.8 million) in 2006 and RUR 1076 billion (€24 400.4 million) in 2009. Approximately 15% in 2006 and 21% in 2009 of cardiovascular disease costs in Russia were direct costs and about 86% and 79%, respectively were indirect costs.

Cancer

Also called malignancy, cancer is a group of diseases that involve the abnormal or out-of-control growth of cells that crowd out normal cells and invade or spread to other parts of the body. The human body is made up of trillions of cells. These cells grow and divide to form new cells as and when the body needs them. Cancer is said to have developed when the normal cell process breaks down and when abnormal, grown, or damaged cells survive when they should die, and when new cells form that are not needed by the body. The extra cells that grow can divide without ceasing and may form growths called tumors or masses of tissue. Many cancers form solid tumors, some of which are benign (noncancerous) and some of which are malignant (cancerous – these can spread into, or invade nearby tissues). Cancerous tumors are malignant tumors.

Cancer can originate from almost anywhere in the human body. Some cancerous cells can break off from the original tumor and travel through the blood or the lymph system to distant places in the body and form new tumors. For example, cancer cells in the lung can travel to the bones and grow there. When lung cancer spreads to the bones, doctors still refer to it as lung cancer because it started in the lung, the primary site. When cancer cells spread, it is known as metastasis (see Figure 3.1) (National Cancer Institute, 2015).

Causes of cancer

Cancer is a genetic disease that can be inherited from parents or can arise from errors that occur as cells divide. It may also occur as a result of damage to DNA caused by environmental exposure to

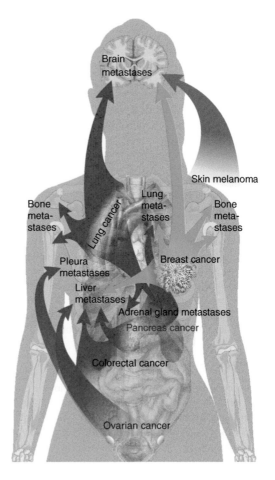

Figure 3.1 Cancer metastasis.
Source: Image courtesy of Mikael Häggström/ Wikimedia Commons.

chemical substances in tobacco smoke or by radiation from ultraviolet rays from the sun (National Cancer Institute, 2015). Each person's cancer has a unique combination of genetic changes, which tend to affect three main types of genes – proto-oncogenes, tumor-suppressor genes, and DNA repair genes. These genetic changes are sometimes referred to as "drivers" of cancer.

Proto-oncogenes facilitate normal cell growth and division. When they are altered, or become more active than they should, they may become cancer-causing genes (or oncogenes), and thus, allow cells to grow and survive when they should not. Like proto-oncogenes, tumor suppressor genes are involved in controlling cell growth and division. Cells with certain alterations in tumor suppressor genes may divide uncontrollably and cause cancer. DNA repair genes are involved with fixing damaged DNA. Cells with mutations in these genes tend to develop additional mutations in other genes, which together may cause the cells to become cancerous (National Cancer Institute, 2015). In certain parts of the world, tumors may develop into cancer because of the lack of screening and early detection services, as well as the lack of knowledge of early signs and symptoms by healthcare providers.

Types of cancer

Studies show that there are over 100 types of cancers, including bone marrow, breast, cervical, colon, lung, ovarian, and prostate cancer. Cancers are usually named after the organs or tissues where they form. As mentioned earlier, lung cancer is described as such because it starts in cells of the lung, and brain cancer because it originates in cells of the brain. Cancers may also be described by the type of cell that forms them, for example epithelial carcinoma.

Breast cancer

Breast cancer is a malignant tumor that develops in the cells of the breast. Most of these tumors start in the inner lining of the milk ducts or the lobules, which supplies milk (Nordqvist, 2016). Breast cancer is prevalent in women and men, but more so in the former. A man's lifetime risk of developing breast cancer is about one in 1000.

It is unclear what causes breast cancer. In women, it may be caused by aging (over 80% of breast cancers in females occur among women aged 50 years and above), genetics (women who carry the BRCA1 and BRCA2 genes have a higher probability of developing breast cancer), a history of previous breast cancer and benign tumors, dense breast tissue, cosmetic implants, estrogen and radiation exposure, or alcohol consumption.

An early symptom of breast cancer is usually an area of thickened tissue or a lump in the breast. Additional symptoms of breast cancer are swelling and pain in the armpit or breast that are unrelated to a woman's menstrual period, redness of the breast skin, a rash around (or on) the nipples, discharge from the nipple, which may sometimes contain blood, and changes in the appearance (sunken or inverted) of the nipple and size or shape of the breast.

In men, breast cancer also originates from the breast and is more widespread among men aged 65 years or more, and in some cases among men younger than 20 years. In men, breast cancer may be caused by

estrogen (which binds to the cancer cells stimulating cell growth and multiplication), Klinefelter's syndrome (a condition where baby boys are born with much higher levels of estrogen than normal), genetics, or mutated genes (the BRAC2 mutation) (Kraft, 2015).

Common symptoms of male breast cancer include the appearance of a lump in the breast, often painless, and less common symptoms include nipple retraction, ulceration, and discharge from the nipple. Where the cancer has spread, symptoms may include breast pain, bone pain, and swelling of the lymph nodes (glands) near the breast, usually in or around the armpit (Kraft, 2015).

Breast cancer accounts for 16% of all female cancers and 23% of invasive cancers in women. Globally, an estimated 18% of all cancer deaths among women and men are from breast cancer. The rate of breast cancer is higher in developed countries than in developing countries. This is because of the fact that women with breast cancer in developed countries live longer than those in developing countries and because of differences in lifestyle and eating habits. In the United States, 232 340 female and 2240 male breast cancers are reported annually, with about 39 620 fatalities.

Cervical cancer

Cervical cancer occurs when abnormal cells develop and spread in the cervix: the lower part of the uterus. Chronic genital human papillomavirus (HPV) can bring about changes in the cells of the cervix, which may lead to cervical cancer. Globally, over 90% of cervical cancers are caused by an HPV infection. Cigarette smoking, having multiple sexual partners and many children, the utilization of birth control pills for a long time, and a weak immune system, increase exposure to HPV. Nicotine increases the growth rate of HPV. As cervical cancer progresses, there may be unusual vaginal discharge, vaginal bleeding between periods, bleeding after menopause, and bleeding or pain during sex. Cervical cancer is most prevalent in women in their mid-50s. However, girls who engage in sexual activity before age 16 or within a year of menstruation are at high risk of developing cervical cancer.

Cervical cancer is the fourth most prevalent cancer in women, especially in developing countries. In 2012, about 84% of cervical cancer cases occurred in this part of the world with Malawi accounting for the highest rate followed by Mozambique and the Comoros. North America and Oceania recorded the lowest number of cases. Globally, 528 000 new cases of cervical cancer were diagnosed in 2012 (Farley *et al.*, 2012; see also http://www.wcrf.org/int/cancer-facts-figures/data-specific-cancers/cervical-cancer-statistics, accessed October 15, 2016). In 2008, cervical cancer accounted for 21% of the total newly diagnosed cancers in females in Africa and was the leading cause of cancer death (21 600) in women in Eastern Africa.

Leukemia

Cancer that begins in the blood-forming tissue of the bone marrow and spreads to other parts of the body is called leukemia. Unlike most cancers, this type of cancer does not form solid tumors. Instead, huge numbers of abnormal white blood cells (leukemia cells and leukemic blast cells) build up in the blood and bone marrow and crowd out normal blood cells, which make it more difficult for oxygen to reach body tissues, control bleeding, or fight infections. There are four main types of leukemia: acute, chronic, lymphoblastic, or myeloid. The classification into acute and chronic leukemia is based on how quickly the disease degenerates, and the further classification into lymphoblastic, or myeloid is based on the type of blood cell the cancer starts in.

Leukemia usually occurs in young children and in people older than 60 years. It also occurs in people who smoke, have undergone previous chemotherapy or radiation therapy, people infected with the human T-cell leukemia virus, and people with myelodysplasctic (a blood disorder) and Down syndrome. Symptoms of leukemia include fever, infection, excessive bruising, fatigue, physical exercise intolerance, abdominal pain, weight loss, abnormal bleeding, enlargement of the lymph nodes, spleen and / or liver, and weakness.

Lung cancer

Lung cancer is a type of cancer that originates in the cells lining the bronchi and parts of the lung, such as the bronchioles or alveoli. It occurs when cells of the lung become abnormal and begin to grow out of control. There are over 20 types of cancerous tumors that originate in the lung. The two main types are small-cell lung cancer and nonsmall cell lung cancer. Small-cell lung cancer, also called oat cell cancer, grows rapidly, is generally found in only one lung, and has the tendency to spread quickly to other organs in the body. Nonsmall cell lung cancer is the most common type of lung cancer and accounts for about 75% of all lung cancer cases. This type of lung cancer is further divided into squamous cell carcinoma, adenocarcinoma, and large-cell carcinoma among others.

Squamous cell carcinoma, also known as epidermoid carcinoma, often begins in the bronchi and does not spread as quickly as other types of lung cancer. Adenocarcinoma usually begins on the outer edges of the lungs and under the lining of the bronchi. It often occurs in people who have never smoked. Large cell carcinomas are a group of cancers with large, abnormal-looking cells, which can occur anywhere in the lungs (Sharecare, 2016).

Lung cancer develops over many years and is strongly associated with smoking cigarettes, cigars, and pipes, second-hand smoke, and exposure to asbestos and radon gas. Symptoms often appear after a tumor has grown or even spread. Although symptoms vary from person to person, common signs include coughing up blood, back pain, repeated pneumonia or bronchitis, chest pain, hoarseness, and exhaustion. In 2012, 1.8 million new cases of lung cancer were diagnosed globally, with Hungary, Serbia, and the Democratic Republic of Korea accounting for the highest rates respectively. Also in 2012, 210 828 people in the United States were diagnosed with lung cancer: 111 395 men and 99 433 women and in that same year, an estimated 58% of lung cancer cases occurred in developing countries.

Approximately 1.6 million new cases of lung cancer occurred worldwide in 2008, accounting for about 13% of total cancer diagnoses. Men in North America, Europe, Eastern Asia, Argentina, and Uruguay had the highest lung-cancer incidence rates, while men in sub-Saharan Africa had the lowest rates. Among women, lung cancer rates in that year were highest in North America, Northern Europe, Australia, New Zealand, and China.

Prostate cancer

Prostate cancer develops in the prostate: a walnut-sized gland in the male reproductive system that wraps around the male urethra. It is the most common and leading cause of death in men. Prostate cancer often occurs among men over 65 years and is rare among men under the age of 40. Family history, genetics, diet, and obesity can cause prostate cancer. In some men, symptoms do not occur until years after the cancer has developed. Where there are symptoms, they manifest in the form of urinary frequency, difficulty starting or stopping urination, interrupted or weak or slow urinary stream, blood in urine or in semen, discomfort with urination or ejaculation, or intense pain in the lower back, hips, or thighs. In 2012, over 1.1 million cases of prostate cancer were recorded globally. This accounted for about 8% of all new cancer cases. Martinique had the highest rate, followed by Norway and France. An estimated 68% of prostate cancer cases in 2012 occurred in developed countries (see http://www.wcrf.org/int/cancer-facts-figures/data-specific-cancers/prostate-cancer-statistics, accessed October 15, 2016).

Economic burden of cancer

The economic costs associated with cancer are direct, or related to productivity and administration, and can be substantial for patients, their families, and society. Direct cancer costs include outpatient and doctor fees, hospitalization and prescription medication payments, insurance premiums, and the cost of care and rehabilitation. Productivity and nonmedical costs manifest in the form of patient days missed from work due to disability (temporary or permanent), loss of wages by family members providing care, increased healthcare costs due to the premature death of qualified staff, and expenses such as transportation, child or elder care, housekeeping assistance, and wigs (Mackay *et al.*, 2006). Administrative and other financial costs comprise government and nongovernment costs such as cancer screening and prevention services, community palliative care, special education, counseling and support programs, educational materials, and funeral costs. In 2008, the global cost of cancer-related premature death and disability was $895 billion (CancerConnect, n.d.). In 2010, medical care expenditures for cancer survivors in the United States was about 137.4 billion (National Cancer Institute, National Institutes of Health, and Department of Health and Human Services, 2010).

Respiratory diseases

Breathing is a basic function of the body, yet people who suffer from respiratory diseases are not able to perform this function easily. The term "respiratory diseases" refers to a series of conditions that affect the respiratory system, such as the lungs, bronchial tubes, upper respiratory tract, trachea, or the pleural cavity. Respiratory diseases include asthma, common colds, cystic fibrosis, emphysema, inflammatory lung diseases, laryngitis, obstructive lung diseases, pneumonia, restrictive lung diseases, respiratory tract infections, pleural cavity diseases, pulmonary vascular diseases, and tuberculosis (TB). Allergies, low immunity, changes in climatic conditions, excessive air pollution, exposure to smoke, asbestos, harsh chemicals, dust, pollen and fibers, genetic factors (where one or both of the parents have chronic respiratory diseases),

inadequate lung development before birth or during childhood, and the presence of bacterial, viral or fungal infections, can cause respiratory diseases. Common symptoms associated with different types of respiratory diseases include difficulty breathing, coughing, swelling, and throat ache.

According to the Forum of International Respiratory Societies report entitled *World: Realities of Today – Opportunities for Tomorrow*, five respiratory conditions – asthma, chronic obstructive pulmonary disease, acute respiratory infections, TB, and lung cancer – primarily contribute to the global burden of respiratory disease. Millions of people suffer from chronic respiratory conditions globally. Of this number, four million (especially those in developing countries), die prematurely each year (World Health Organization, 2013b). Infants and young children are especially vulnerable to respiratory diseases. In 2013, almost three million children, largely those under the age of five, died from pneumonia and lower respiratory tract infections (see Figure 3.2).

In 2012, TB infected an estimated 8.6 million people and claimed the lives of 1.3 million people mainly in sub-Saharan Africa. While the global burden of childhood TB is unknown, it is known that an estimated 10 to 15% of cases in endemic areas occur in infants and children. Multi-drug-resistant TB has become a global health issue. In 2012, about 450 000 new cases occurred, culminating in 170 000 deaths (Bryce *et al.*, 2005). Globally, respiratory diseases account for about 25% of all deaths worldwide owing primarily to the lack of access to immunization, medications, or the inability of the healthcare system to provide care.

Economic burden of respiratory diseases

In the European Union (EU), chronic obstructive pulmonary disease (COPD) and asthma contribute significantly to the economic burden of respiratory diseases when it comes to healthcare services. Together, these diseases cost about EUR 20 billion each for healthcare and EUR 25 billion and 15 billion, respectively for lost productivity. Lung cancer, COPD, followed by pneumonia and asthma result in the greatest losses from disability and premature mortality. In 2012 and 2013, a study conducted with patients who were accessing TB services from ten clinics in four provinces in South Africa recorded an average total annual individual income of $111.83 or 12% of annual individual presymptom income. This was 53% of the average patient's healthcare costs

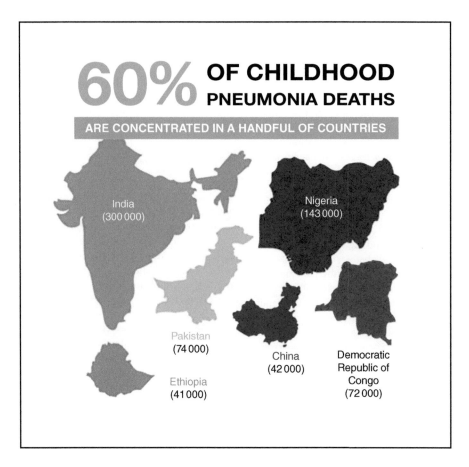

Figure 3.2 Global childhood pneumonia deaths.
Source: World Health Organization (2016b), with permission.

for TB diagnosis and treatment. The study also found that patients starting TB treatment were receiving 22% of the average patient's presymptom income.

Diabetes

Often referred to as diabetes, diabetes mellitus is a group of metabolic diseases in which the level of blood sugar (glucose) in the human body is abnormal. In the human body, the pancreas, produces a hormone called insulin. This hormone helps the body to use sugars (glucose) produced from carbohydrates consumed. When the body has more sugar than it needs, insulin helps to store the excess in the liver and releases it as and when the body needs it. Insulin thus helps to balance body sugar levels and to keep it at a normal range. In situations where the human body does not produce enough insulin, or is unable to use the insulin it produces, it may lead to hyperglycemia

(high blood sugar), a condition that can result in lifelong health problems if blood sugar levels stay elevated for a long period of time.

The two main types of diabetes are type 1 diabetes and type 2 diabetes. A third type, gestational diabetes, only occurs during pregnancy. Type 1 diabetes, an autoimmune disease, typically occurs in children and adolescents, hence its previous name: juvenile diabetes. However, it may occur among people of any age. Type 1 diabetes is caused by a lack of insulin owing to attacks on insulin-producing beta cells by the body's immune system (white blood cells/T cells). While the destruction of the beta cells may take place over several years, symptoms of type 1 diabetes often develop within a short period of time. Latent autoimmune diabetes (LADA) is a slowly developing kind of type 1 diabetes in adults, which usually occurs after the age of 30. People with LADA may produce their own insulin, but may at some point need insulin shots or an insulin pump to control their blood glucose levels. Type 1 diabetes may lead to health complications such as high blood pressure, cardiovascular disease, stroke, skin and mouth infections, gastroparesis (delayed gastric emptying), a type of neuropathy, sexual dysfunction, and depression.

Type 2 diabetes is the most common type of diabetes, accounting for 90 to 95% of all diabetes cases. With this kind of diabetes, the body does not respond properly to insulin – it becomes resistant to insulin. Type 2 diabetes is primarily caused by being obese or overweight, having excessive abdominal fat (which has the tendency to change the way the body responds to insulin), eating calorie-dense and refined foods, physical inactivity, sleep disturbances that can affect the body's balance of insulin and blood sugar, and genetics.

Patients with type 1 diabetes are ten times more at risk of heart disease than healthy patients. If left untreated, diabetes can cause serious health complications including heart disease, blindness, kidney failure, and lower extremity amputations. In the United States, diabetes is the seventh leading cause of death. Symptoms of high blood sugar include frequent urination, increased thirst, and increased hunger.

There are about 347 million people with diabetes worldwide. In 2014, 9% of adults aged 18 years and older had diabetes. Over 80% of diabetes deaths occur in developing countries.

In certain countries, type 2 diabetes accounts for almost 50% of newly diagnosed cases in children and adolescents. According to studies, type 2 diabetes, once rare in children, is now on the increase worldwide.

Economic burden of diabetes

Studies show that the national economic burden of prediabetes and diabetes in the United States was $218 billion in 2007. This estimate covers medical costs ($153 billion) and reduced productivity ($65 billion). The average annual cost per diagnosed diabetes case was $9975 and $443 for prediabetes medical costs (Dall *et al.*, 2010). In 2000, WHO African region incurred a total economic loss of $25.51 billion (PPP) associated with 7.02 million cases of diabetes. The estimated total annual cost of diabetes in Latin America and the Caribbean is $65.216 billion (direct cost $10.721 billion and indirect cost $54.495 billion).

Mental illness

Mental illness is a psychological or behavioral phenomenon that leads to disorder or disability that is not part of normal development. Mental illness can occur when the brain (or part of the brain) is not working well or is working in the wrong way. When the brain is not working properly, one or more of its functions will be disrupted (see Figure 3.3). When these functions significantly disrupt a person's life, we say that person has a mental disorder or a mental illness.

Mental illness is caused by a variety of factors, including biological, psychological, environmental and poor nutrition. Biologically, a person's genes may predispose them to mental illness. Experts believe that many mental illnesses are associated with abnormalities in genes and with an imbalance of special chemicals in the brain called neurotransmitters. Neurotransmitters help nerve cells in the brain to communicate with each other. When these chemicals are out of balance, or are not working properly, messages may not make it through to the brain correctly, and thus cause certain symptoms of mental illness. It must however be noted that, the fact that a person inherits a susceptibility to a mental illness does not necessarily mean that they will become mentally challenged. Brain defects, injury, poor fetal brain development, microcephaly, and trauma can result in the development of certain mental conditions.

Psychologically, severe psychological trauma suffered as a child, emotional, physical, or sexual abuse,

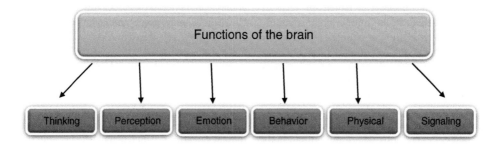

Figure 3.3 Functions of the brain.

the loss of a parent or loved one, and neglect may contribute to mental illness. On the environmental front, mental illness may be triggered by divorce, dysfunctional family life, feelings of inadequacy, low self-esteem, anxiety, anger, loneliness, changing of jobs or schools, social or cultural expectations, substance abuse, and physical abuse. Poor nutrition and the exposure to toxins, such as lead, may also contribute to the development of mental illness.

Types of mental illness

There are various types of mental illness. These may be classified into common and uncommon. Common mental illnesses are anxiety, mood disorder, psychotic disorders, eating disorders, impulsive control, and addiction disorder. Uncommon mental illnesses include Landau syndrome, boanthropy, and autophagia.

Anxiety

To be anxious before taking an exam, interviewing for a job, or getting on a plane is a normal human emotion. However, to have an anxiety disorder is not a normal emotion. This is because, it can result in conditions that cause distress and interfere with a person's ability to lead a normal life. One is said to have anxiety disorder when their response to a situation is inappropriate, or when the anxiety interferes with their normal functioning. People with anxiety disorders often react to certain objects or situations with fear and dread. Physically, they are nervous and have rapid palpitations, muscle tension, nausea, dizziness, sweating, and insomnia. Anxiety disorders may be caused by a combination of factors including changes in the brain and stressors in the environment.

Mood disorder

Also referred to as affective disorder, mood disorder is characterized by persistent fluctuations of feelings of extreme happiness to extreme sadness. Depression and bipolar disorder are the most common examples of mood disorders. People are said to have depression if they have a state of low mood and aversion to activity that affects their thoughts, behavior, feelings, and sense of wellbeing. Depressed people may feel sad, anxious, empty, hopeless, helpless, worthless, guilty, irritable, ashamed, or restless. They may also lose interest in activities that once gave them pleasure, lose their appetite or overeat, have difficulty concentrating, remembering details

or making decisions, and may contemplate, attempt, or commit suicide. Insomnia, excessive sleeping, fatigue, aches, pains, digestive problems, or reduced energy are some of the symptoms people with depressed moods may exhibit. To be bipolar is to have a chemical imbalance in the brain that causes one to experience extreme mood swings, from hyper highs to depressive low points.

Psychotic disorders

People are diagnosed with psychotic disorders when they have distorted awareness and thinking that causes them to hallucinate (experience images or sounds that are unreal, or hear voices) or be delusional (a false belief that the person with the disorder accepts as true, despite contrary evidence). Schizophrenia is a psychotic disorder and so are eating disorders. Eating disorders involve extreme emotions, attitudes, and behaviors related to weight and food that negatively impact one's physical and mental wellbeing. They include anorexia nervosa, bulimia nervosa, and binge eating disorder.

Impulsive control and addiction disorders

People suffering from impulsive control and addiction disorders are unable to resist urges, or impulses to do things that could potentially be harmful to themselves or others. Some people with this condition ignore responsibilities and relationships due to their addiction to substances like alcohol and illicit drugs. Others become pyromaniacs (start fires), kleptomaniacs (steal for reasons other than personal use or financial gain), and compulsive gamblers.

Mental disorders account for five of the top ten global burden of diseases. Worldwide, about 450 million people have a mental health problem and over 75% of this number live in developing countries (World Health Organization, 2001). About 85% of patients with serious mental disorders in the developing world, do not receive treatment. One in four British adults experiences at least one diagnosable mental health problem in a given year. Around 16 individuals for every 100 000 people worldwide commit suicide as a result of some underlying mental disorder. In the United States, 11 individuals for every 100 000 people commit suicide as a result of an underlying mental disorder. In a given year, about 20.9 million American adults aged 18 and older experience a mood disorder. White men who are 85 years and above have the highest suicide rates.

Economic burden of mental health

In 2002, mental illness accounted for over $190 billion in lost personal earnings primarily arising from lost workplace productivity in the United States. The total mental illness costs incurred by individuals, employers, and governments in England is about GBP 105.2 billion a year (Centre for Mental Health, 2010). In the EU the cost of mental illness was an estimated EUR 240 billion (excluding dementia) in 2004 (Andlin-Sobocki et al., 2015; Kaplan & Laing, 2004). The impact of the cost on the EU economy was an estimated 3–4% reduction of total gross domestic product (GDP) (Gabriel & Liimatainen, 2000).

Noncommunicable disease risk factors

Alcohol abuse

Alcohol abuse involves drinking on a continuous basis irrespective of the repeated social, physical, legal, and mental problems the practice causes. Alcohol abuse may occur due to one's genetic makeup, the environment in which one was raised, emotional health, or because of instability and stressful change such as a breakup, retirement, or other loss. Alcohol abuse may also be the result of the level of economic development, culture, availability of alcohol, and the noneffectiveness of alcohol related policies. Alcohol abuse has social and economic consequences.

Socially, intoxication, dependence, or alcohol abuse often leads to social ostracization, stigma, poor performance of social roles (including parenting, relationships, and friendships), dysfunction in family life, and facilitates risky and violent behavior, suicide, and homicide. Economically, alcohol abuse may cause absenteeism from work, lack of productivity, unemployment, the loss of earnings, financial problems, and barriers to accessing healthcare.

Alcohol consumption

Alcohol consumption is the drinking of beverages containing ethyl alcohol. All over the world, people consume alcohol for a variety of reasons: for religious purposes, for its physiological and psychological effects, to socialize, celebrate, or to relax. While drinking alcohol is not necessarily a problem, excessive drinking is, as it can result in a range of negative consequences.

The most common alcoholic beverages consumed globally are beer, sprits, and wine, with spirits being the most consumed (about 50%). Other alcoholic beverages made from fermented sorghum, maize, millet, rice, or cider are also consumed. The alcohol content in beer ranges from as low as 2% to as high as 8%. In most lager or ale-type beers, the alcohol content can be between 4 to 5%. Wines such as burgundy, Chianti, and chardonnay, usually contain between 8 and 12% alcohol, though some varieties have a higher alcohol content, ranging from 12 to 14%. Spirits, such as vodka, rum, and whiskey, usually contain the most alcohol-between 40 and 50%.

Alcohol consumption varies from county to country, with high-income countries recording the highest alcohol per capita consumption (APC) and the highest prevalence of heavy episodic drinking (the consumption of 60 or more grams of pure alcohol on at least one single occasion at least monthly) (World Health Organization, 2014). About 16% of drinkers worldwide aged 15 years and above engage in heavy episodic drinking. In 2010, pure alcohol consumption among people aged 15 years and above was highest in Belarus (17.5 liters per capita), followed by Moldova (16.8), Lithuania (15.4), and Russia (15.1). Per capita consumption was lowest in Kuwait, Lybia, Namibia, and Pakistan: 0.1 l. On average, people aged 15 and above consume about 6.2 liters of pure alcohol per year. Men in the six WHO regions consume more alcohol than women. Globally, less than 50% of the world's population (38%) drinks alcohol.

Health risks

Alcohol has a strong effect on people. The magnitude of its effect varies from person to person depending on their drinking threshold, frequency of drinking and quantity drunk, age, gender, health status, and family history.

Alcohol immediately enters the bloodstream after the first sip, and its effects become manifest within 10 minutes of consumption. Alcohol increases the blood alcohol concentration (BAC) levels (the amount of alcohol present in the bloodstream) and can cause reduced inhibitions, slurred speech, motor impairment, confusion, concentration and respiratory problems, coma, and even death. Medically, alcohol abuse causes more than 200 diseases and injury conditions in individuals, as well as alcohol dependence, which may result in impaired physical coordination, consciousness and cognition, cirrhosis of the liver, cancers, alcohol poisoning, and neuropsychiatric conditions.

In the brain, alcohol interferes with the brain's communication pathways and causes disruptions in mood and behavior, and makes it harder for alcoholics to think clearly. In the heart, it damages the heart, and puts people at risk for cardiomyopathy (the stretching and drooping of heart muscle), arrhythmias (irregular heart beat), stroke, and high blood pressure. In the liver, heavy alcohol consumption negatively impacts the liver, causing steatosis, or fatty liver, alcoholic hepatitis, fibrosis, and cirrhosis. In the pancreas, alcohol produces toxic substances that can eventually lead to pancreatitis, a dangerous inflammation and swelling of the blood vessels in the pancreas that prevents proper digestion. Alcohol abuse predisposes people to certain cancers, namely cancers of the mouth, esophagus, throat, liver, and breast. It also has the tendency to weaken one's immune system, making the body vulnerable to disease.

Additionally, alcohol abuse brings about lifelong disability, intentional and unintentional injuries, traffic and workplace accidents, the scalding of children, mental health conditions, fetal alcohol syndrome (FAS), preterm birth complications in women, the incidence of infectious diseases such as TB and even death.

Global disease burden of alcohol abuse

Alcohol abuse is the world's third largest risk factor for global disease burden. It results in about 2.5 million deaths per year globally. About 320 000 youth between the ages of 15 and 29 die from alcohol-related causes annually. This corresponds to 9% of all deaths in that age group. An estimated 2.4% of all deaths in WHO African Region occurs as a result of injuries, cancer, cardiovascular diseases, and mental disorders associated with alcohol abuse.

In 2012, about 3.3 million (6%) of all global deaths were related to alcohol consumption. About 8% of these deaths were among males and 4% among females. Alcohol consumption among women is rising steadily due to economic development and changing gender roles (Grucza *et al.*, 2008). This has serious implications for women's health as they tend to experience more negative health outcomes (cancers, gastrointestinal diseases or cardiovascular diseases) than their male counterparts who consume the same amount of alcohol (Rehm *et al.*, 2006). Also in 2012, the total number of disability-adjusted life years (DALYs) lost to alcohol abuse was 139 million, accounting for 5% of the overall global burden of disease and injury. WHO European Region recorded the highest number of alcohol-related deaths and DALYs in that year.

Children, adolescents, and the elderly who consume a certain volume of alcohol are more likely to suffer alcohol-related harm than other age groups. Among children and adolescents, early alcohol initiation before the age of 14, has the tendency to impair health status, increase the risk for alcohol dependence at an older age, and cause unintentional injuries. Due to their age and physical status, alcohol consumption among the elderly often leads to alcohol-related falls. Alcohol-related burden of disease among the older population is increasing as global life expectancy has greatly improved.

Economic burden of alcohol abuse

Studies conducted on alcohol dependence in Europe revealed that the direct cost for the treatment of a single alcohol-dependent patient ranged from EUR 1591 to EUR 7702 per hospitalization, accounting for 0.04 to 0.31% of a country's GDP per annum. Indirect costs were greater than the direct costs, accounting for up to 0.64% of GDP per country annually (Laramée *et al.*, 2013). In 2002, the total direct annual cost (including deaths, illness, law enforcement, and loss of productivity) associated with alcohol abuse in Canada was about $14.6 billion. Alcohol abuse in that same year also accounted for $3.3 billion in direct healthcare costs.

Excessive alcohol consumption in the United States in 2006, cost states an average of $2.9 billion per annum. The cost to states ranged from about $420 million in North Dakota, to $32 billion in California. This accounts for an average cost of $1.91 per state for each alcoholic drink consumed. In 2010, the economic cost of excessive drinking in the United States was about $249 billion (Sacks *et al.*, 2015).

Tobacco use

Tobacco is used widely all over the world by people of all ages and by both sexes. Irrespective of its deleterious social, economic, and health effects, its use persists and is especially on the rise in developing countries where there are few or no restrictions on production, and where taxes on tobacco products are low.

Types of tobacco use

There are two types of tobacco use; smoking and non-smoking (see Figure 3.4). Smoking tobacco includes cigarettes, bidis, cigars, kreteks, pipes and sticks, and nonsmoking tobacco includes chewing tobacco, moist and dry snuff, and dissolvable smokeless tobacco products.

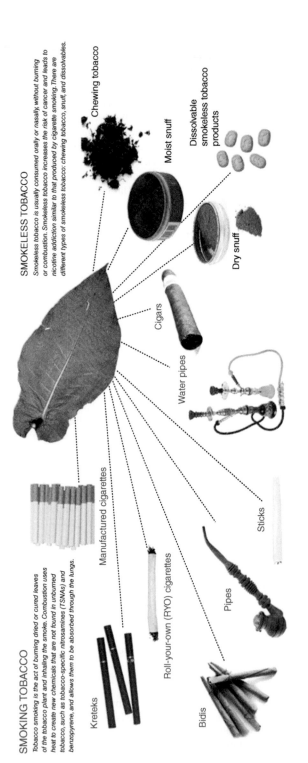

SMOKING TOBACCO

Tobacco smoking is the act of burning dried or cured leaves
of the tobacco plant and inhaling the smoke. Combustion uses
heat to create new chemicals that are not found in unburned
tobacco, such as tobacco-specific nitrosamines (TSNAs) and
benzopyrene, and allows them to be absorbed through the lungs.

Manufactured cigarettes

Kreteks

Roll-your-own (RYO) cigarettes

Bidis

Pipes

Sticks

SMOKELESS TOBACCO

Smokeless tobacco is usually consumed orally or nasally, without burning
or combustion. Smokeless tobacco increases the risk of cancer and leads to
nicotine addiction similar to that produced by cigarette smoking. There are
different types of smokeless tobacco: chewing tobacco, snuff, and dissolvables.

Chewing tobacco

Moist snuff

Dissolvable
smokeless tobacco
products

Dry snuff

Cigars

Water pipes

Figure 3.4 Types of tobacco.
Source: http://sites.saschina.org/mkarkkainen/2015/03/10/tobacco/ (accessed October 16, 2016).

Cigarettes are small cylindrically cut tobacco leaves manufactured or hand rolled in thin paper for smoking. They comprise approximately 600 ingredients and create over 700 chemicals when burned. About 69% of the chemicals in cigarettes are poisonous and are known to cause cancer. Bidis are small amounts of tobacco hand wrapped in dried temburni leaf and tied with a string. Regardless of their small size, the tar and carbon monoxide in bidis can be higher than that found in manufactured cigarettes. Cigars are made of air-cured and fermented tobacco. They come in various shapes, sizes, and forms; from cigarette sized cigarillos, to double coronas, cheroots, stumpen, chuttas and dhumtis. Kreteks are clove-flavored cigarettes, which have an anaesthetizing effect. Pipes are made of briar, slate, clay, or other substances. To use them, tobacco is placed in the bowl and inhaled through the stem, or sometimes through water. Sticks are made from sun-cured tobacco known as brus, and wrapped in cigarette paper.

Chewing tobacco, also known as plug, loose-leaf, and twist, is chewed. Moist snuff is taken orally and dry snuff is powdered tobacco that is inhaled through the nose or taken orally. Unlike chewing tobacco, dissolvable smokeless tobacco products dissolve in the mouth.

Standard cigarettes are the most commonly used type of smoked tobacco. Other smoked tobacco products, like bidis, kreteks, and shisha, are now gaining popularity.

Tobacco consumption

Cigarette smoking is the most prevalent type of tobacco consumption. It accounts for about 85% of all tobacco consumed worldwide. Prior to 1900, cigarette consumption was low. However, consumption rates increased substantially in the first half of the twentieth century, first among men and then later among women in developed countries. By 1950, a significant number of women and men were smoking in the United States and the United Kingdom. Between 1980 and 2012, global cigarette consumption stood at about 6.25 trillion (Doughton, 2014). In 1960, total cigarette consumption per capita was 4171, but dropped to 1232 cigarettes per capita in 2011.

Between 2008 and 2012, about 75% of all smokers lived in China, India, the EU, Indonesia, the United States, Russia, Japan, Brazil, Bangladesh, and Pakistan (Giovino et al., 2012; Zatoński and Mańczuk, 2010). At present, China is the world's major cigarette consumer with about 320 million smokers. Cigarette consumption in China continues to rise sharply (about 6 trillion cigarettes are smoked per year) and accounts for more than 2 trillion of worldwide total consumption. Smokers in China consume approximately 1.7 trillion cigarettes a year, or 3 million cigarettes a minute. In India, people mostly consume noncigarette products such as hand-rolled bidis and chewing tobacco (Jha et al., 2011). The demand for tobacco in India is likely to increase, but at a slower pace than in previous decades. Over 30% of Indonesia's population smokes, and more than 3% of children between the ages of 3 and 15 years in that country are active smokers. In Indonesia, a packet of cigarettes cost only $1.

Smoking in developed countries including Australia, Britain, Canada, and the United States is slowly waning due to increasing awareness of the negative health effects of smoking, smoking cessation programs, antismoking measures including antismoking campaigns, the banning of cigarette advertising, and increased taxation. While gains have been made in tobacco cessation in many developed countries, most developing countries continue to smoke, as cigarette cessation programs among other things are uncommon in these parts of the world.

Secondhand smoke

Secondhand smoke is the involuntary inhalation of smoke from burning tobacco products or from exhaled smoke by a smoker in the environment. Secondhand tobacco smoke causes over 600 000 premature deaths per year worldwide. About 31% of all secondhand smoke-related deaths occur among children and about 64% among women. Secondhand smoke causes frequent and severe asthma attacks, respiratory infections, ear infections, and sudden infant death syndrome (SIDS) among children. Smoking during pregnancy accounts for more than 1000 infant deaths annually.

Exposure to secondhand smoke causes fatalities in about 603 000 nonsmokers each year. Fourteen percent of nonsmokers in the EU are exposed to other people's smoke at home, and a third of working adults are exposed at the workplace. Exposure to secondhand smoke is estimated to cause about 7600 deaths per year in the EU. More 13–15 year olds in the WHO European Region are exposed to secondhand smoke at home than in any other part of the world. These youth are 1.5 to 2 times more likely to start smoking than children not exposed.

Nonsmokers who are exposed to secondhand smoke inhale the same cancer-causing substances and poisons as smokers. The inhalation of secondhand smoke has the tendency to damage cells in ways that set the cancer process in motion. Like smoking, continued exposure to secondhand smoke puts one at risk for lung cancer. In the United States, secondhand smoke causes more than 7300 lung cancer deaths among nonsmokers annually. In China, 100 000 people die from exposure to secondhand smoke annually.

Global disease burden of tobacco use

Tobacco smoking is the leading risk factor for NCDs and the second leading cause of death globally (Non-Communicable Disease Alliance, n.d.). Tobacco claims the lives of more than 14 500 people every day (Peto *et al.*, 1996), debilitates, and sickens many times that number of people. Indeed, the continuous use of tobacco prematurely shortens life by about 10 to 15 years and causes chain smokers to experience dyspnea and pain in their final years of life. WHO European Region has one of the highest proportions of tobacco-related deaths in the world; 16% of adults over the age of 30. This contrasts with the proportion of tobacco-related deaths in WHO African and Eastern Mediterranean regions: 3% and 7% respectively.

Annually, about 5 million people die from tobacco-related illnesses (Murray and Lopez, 1997). Globally, an estimated 5.4 million people died from tobacco-related illnesses in 2006. In 2008, tobacco use accounted for 22% of cancer deaths in general (1.7 million) and 71% of lung cancer deaths in particular (Eriksen *et al.*, 2012).

According to WHO, unless urgent measures are put in place to stave off the epidemic, the annual tobacco death toll could rise to over 8 million by 2030.

Health risks associated with tobacco use

Tobacco use is a risk factor for over 25 diseases including lung, oral, and other cancers, and chronic respiratory and cardiovascular diseases (particularly ischemic heart disease) among others (see Figure 3.5). In populations that have engaged in cigarette smoking for decades, about 90% of lung cancer, 15% to 20% of other cancers, 75% of chronic bronchitis and emphysema, and 25% of deaths from cardiovascular disease in people aged 35 to 69 years can be attributed to tobacco use (Peto *et al.*, 1994).

The pattern of tobacco-related diseases varies from country to country. In the United States, for

Tobacco use is a risk factor for six of the eight leading causes of death in the world

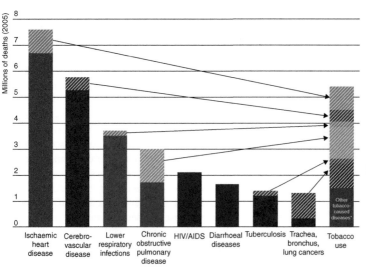

Hatched areas indicate proportions of deaths that are related to tobacco use and are coloured according to the column of the respective cause of death.

*Includes mouth and oropharyngeal cancers, oesophageal cancer, stomach cancer, liver cancer, other cancers, as well as cardiovascular diseases other than ischaemic heart disease and cerebrovascular disease.

Source: Mathers, C. D. and Loncar, D. (2006) Projections of global mortality and burden of disease from 2002 to 2030. *PLoS Medicine* **3**(11), e442. Additional information obtained from personal communication with C. D. Mathers.

Source of revised HIV/AIDS figure: AIDS epidemic update. Geneva, Joint United Nations Programme on HIV/AIDS (UNAIDS) and World Health Organisation (WHO), 2007.

Figure 3.5 Health risks associated with tobacco use.
Source: World Health Organization (2008), with permission.

example, tobacco-related vascular diseases and lung cancer are more prevalent (Jha and Chaloupka, 2000), whereas chronic respiratory diseases related to tobacco use are more prevalent in China. New research shows that women smokers have a 25% greater risk of coronary heart disease than their male counterparts. In India, smoking increases the risk of death from TB (Gajalakshmi and Peto, 1999).

Male smokers in China have a greater propensity to develop COPD than their male nonsmoker counterparts (Lin *et al.*, 2008). Figure 3.6 contains an array of health risks associated with smoking and second-hand smoke.

Economic burden of tobacco use

In addition to causing chronic diseases, tobacco use imposes financial costs on individuals, their families, and society as a whole. The economic costs associated with tobacco use are both direct and indirect. Direct costs are measurable and unambiguous costs related to smoking behavior, such as spending on treatment of smoking-related illnesses, the purchasing of medications, hospitalization, and outpatient visits. Indirect economic costs are the more difficult-to-measure costs including low productivity, lost wages, fires, and costs for cleaning and repainting homes and offices due to smoking. In 2011, the total economic cost of smoking in Vietnam was about 24679.9 billion dong (VND), or $1173.2 million – approximately 0.97% of the country's GDP. Direct inpatient and outpatient cost of care that same year was 9896.2 billion VND ($470.4 million) and 2567.2 billion VND ($122.0 million), respectively. Government spending resulting from tobacco use in Vietnam was 4534.3 billion VND ($215.5 million), accounting for 5.76% of Vietnam's healthcare budget for 2011. Indirect costs (productivity loss) due to morbidity and mortality were 2652.9 billion VND ($126.1 million) and 9563.5 billion VND ($454.6 million), respectively (Hoang *et al.*, 2016).

The total cost for transportation and caregiver costs for smoking tobacco-related illnesses in Vietnam amounted to $91.3 million. Cardiovascular diseases recorded the highest share of transportation costs. The total amount of income lost as a result of tobacco-related hospitalization and outpatient visits was $411.4 million (John *et al.*, 2004). Economically, tobacco use contributes to world hunger by diverting prime land away from food production, exacerbating poverty, and damaging the environment through deforestation.

Obesity

Obesity is an epidemic that is prevalent in all parts of the world. It is a condition of abnormal excessive fat accumulation in the adipose tissue of the human body, which negatively affects health. The terms "obesity" and "overweight" are sometimes used interchangeably, but they are two different things. Overweight simply means being over a weight that is set for one's height and bone structure. The terms overweight and obesity describe ranges of weight that are more than what is generally considered healthy for a person based on their height. They also draw attention to ranges of weight that have been shown to increase the likelihood of certain diseases and health problems.

Causes of obesity

Obesity is mainly caused by energy imbalance between calories consumed and calories expended. In adults, obesity is caused by a combination of biological, cultural, environmental, psychological, and social factors, as well as the overconsumption of energy-dense highly fatty foods, physical inactivity brought on by sedentism associated with the types of work people engage in, improved transportation, and urbanization. In children, obesity is caused by increased screen time (TV, videogames etc.), physical inactivity at school and home, less active travel (walking and cycling), the environment (bags of chips in the pantry), and genetics.

Calculating and interpreting obesity

Body mass index (BMI) is a measurement tool that is used to screen for high body fat. It compares a person's height to weight and indicates whether they are overweight, underweight, or at a normal healthy weight for their height. Body mass index is calculated the same way for adults and children, but interpreted differently. It is calculated by dividing a person's weight by the square of their height. It is expressed in either metric or US customary units (see Figure 3.7). In adults aged 20 years and older, one is said to be obese if their BMI is 30.0 or higher (see Table 3.1).

The BMI for children (2 to 19 years) is determined by using a BMI table that compares their weight and height on a growth chart (see Figure 3.8). Growth charts use a child's BMI, age, and sex to generate a BMI percentile. A BMI percentile shows how a child compares with other children of the same age in terms of weight and height. A score between the 85th and 95th percentile on a growth chart indicates that a

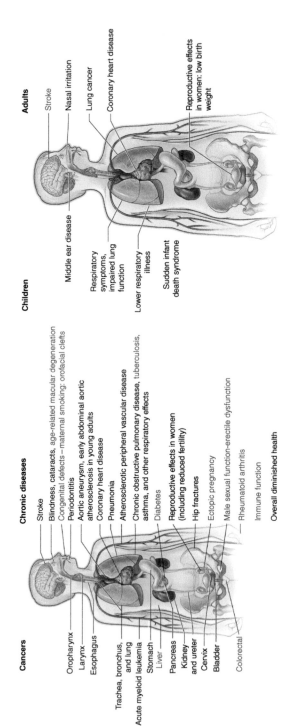

Cancers

Oropharynx
Larynx
Esophagus
Trachea, bronchus, and lung
Acute myeloid leukemia
Stomach
Liver
Pancreas
Kidney and ureter
Cervix
Bladder
Colorectal

Chronic diseases

Stroke
Blindness, cataracts, age-related macular degeneration
Congenital defects – maternal smoking: orofacial clefts
Periodontitis
Aortic aneurysm, early abdominal aortic atherosclerosis in young adults
Coronary heart disease
Pneumonia
Atherosclerotic peripheral vascular disease
Chronic obstructive pulmonary disease, tuberculosis, asthma, and other respiratory effects
Diabetes
Reproductive effects in women (including reduced fertility)
Hip fractures
Ectopic pregnancy
Male sexual function–erectile dysfunction
Rheumatoid arthritis
Immune function
Overall diminished health

Children

Middle ear disease
Respiratory symptoms, impaired lung function
Lower respiratory illness
Sudden infant death syndrome

Adults

Stroke
Nasal irritation
Lung cancer
Coronary heart disease
Reproductive effects in women: low birth weight

Figure 3.6 Health risks associated with smoking.
Source: Department of Health and Human Services (2014).

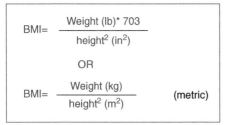

$$BMI = \frac{Weight\ (lb)^* \times 703}{height^2\ (in^2)}$$

OR

$$BMI = \frac{Weight\ (kg)}{height^2\ (m^2)} \quad \text{(metric)}$$

Figure 3.7 Calculating BMI.

Table 3.1 Interpreting BMI in adults 20 years and older.

BMI	Classification
< 18.5	Underweight
18.5–24.9	Normal or healthy weight
25.0–29.9	Overweight
30.0–34.9	Class I obesity
	(fat accumulation is higher than desirable)
35.0–39.9	Class II obesity
	(risk of weight-related health problems and even death)
≥ 40.0	Class III obesity
	(morbid obesity – extremely high risk of weight-related disease and premature death)

child is at risk of becoming overweight, and a score at the 95th percentile and above indicates that a child is obese. A healthcare provider would need to perform additional assessments to determine if excess fat in a child is a health problem.

Other methods of estimating body fat and body fat distribution include measurement of skin-fold thickness, calculating waist-to-hip circumference ratios, having an ultrasound or magnetic resonance imaging (MRI), or measuring waist circumference. A man whose waist circumference exceeds 40 inches and a nonpregnant woman whose waist circumference is over 35 inches are at a higher risk of developing obesity-related conditions.

Global burden of obesity

Until the past few decades, obesity was a condition primarily associated with the developed world. At present, obesity is a health condition that affects people in both developed and developing countries, with urban areas in the latter struggling with the so-called "dual burden" of obesity and underweight.

Obesity and overweight predispose people to ill health, disability, and even death. Globally, about 2.8 million people die annually from being overweight or obese. In 2010, overweight and obesity accounted for 3.4 million deaths, 3.9% of years of life lost to premature death, and 3.8% of disability-adjusted life years (DALYs) worldwide (Ng *et al.*, 2013). Majority of the world's population lives in regions where obesity and underweight claim the lives of more people than underweight. This is true of developed and most developing countries. In 2014, 50% of the world's obese population lived in only ten countries – the United States, China, India, Russia, Brazil, Mexico, Egypt, Germany, Pakistan, and Indonesia.

Between 1980 and 2014, the global prevalence of obesity more than doubled. In 2014 alone, over 1.9 billion adults aged 18 years and older were overweight and more than 600 million were obese. In 2013, 42 million children under the age of five were overweight or obese. Overweight and obesity rates in children in developing countries with emerging economies, is over 30% higher than that of children in developed countries (World Health Organization, 2016a). A study on obesity and overweight in adults and children conducted in 188 countries from 1980 to 2013, found that men in developed countries had higher obesity rates than women, with the converse being true in developing countries. The study also found that 62% of the world's obese people live in developing countries where the prevalence of overweight and obesity in childhood increased from 17% in 1980 to 24% in 2013 for boys, and from 16% to 23% for girls.

Health risks associated with obesity

People with BMIs over 30.0 are at risk of a menu of NCDs and conditions: cardiovascular diseases (mainly coronary artery disease, high blood pressure and stroke), which were the leading causes of death in 2012, type 2 diabetes, musculoskeletal disorders (especially osteoarthritis – a highly disabling degenerative disease of the joints), and some cancers (endometrial, breast, colon, kidney, gallbladder and liver). People who are obese are also at risk of high low-density lipoprotein (LDL) cholesterol, low high-density lipoprotein (HDL) cholesterol, or high levels of triglycerides, gallbladder disease, insulin resistance, sleep apnea, breathing problems, chronic inflammation, low quality of life, mental illness such as clinical depression, anxiety, and other mental

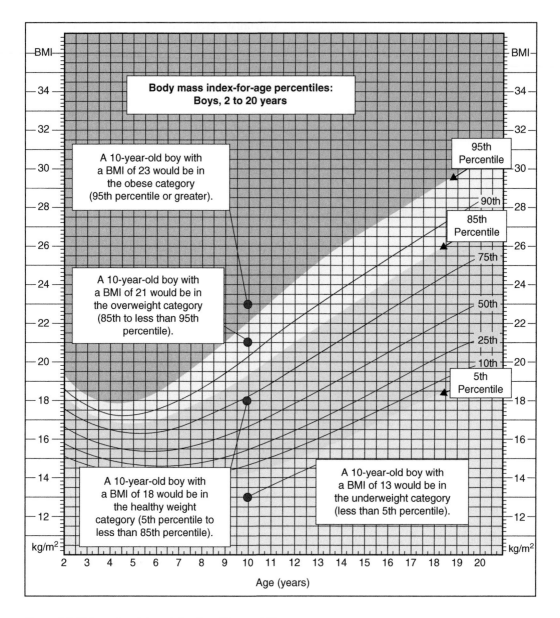

Figure 3.8 BMI numbers interpretation for a 10-year-old boy.
Source: Centers for Disease Control and Prevention, BMI-for-age growth chart, http://www.cdc.gov/healthyweight/assessing/bmi/childrens_bmi/about_childrens_bmi.html (accessed October 15, 2016).

disorders, body pain, and difficulty with physical functioning (Ng *et al.*, 2013).

Economic burden of obesity

According to the Public Health Agency of Canada (PHAC), the direct costs of obesity in Canada in 2008 came to about $2 billion, whereas losses from premature mortality were $2.63 billion (Anis *et al.*, 2010). Obesity- and overweight-related absenteeism and disability owing to productivity losses in Canada accounted for about $5 billion in 2006, and the annual total direct cost (healthcare and non-health care) per capita rose from $1472 for people of normal weight to $2788 for those who were obese. For Australians aged 30 years and above, the total direct cost was

$6.5 billion for overweight and $14.5 billion for obesity in 2005 (Colagiuri *et al.*, 2010).

Challenges of noncommunicable disease prevention and control

Alcohol abuse

The need for national policies and commitment to reduce the harmful use of alcohol, and the lack of global guidance and increased international collaboration to support and complement regional and national efforts on alcohol abuse reduction, are challenges in the fight against alcohol abuse.

Preventing and reducing the harmful use of alcohol is often not on the agenda of decision makers despite its serious effects on individual and public health. Additionally, in many developing countries, there is a discrepancy between the availability and affordability of alcoholic beverages, and country capability and capacity to meet the public health problems they cause. Furthermore, the implementation of interventions aimed at alcohol prevention tend to be transferred from developed to developing countries without appropriate tailoring to accommodate local contexts. This renders the interventions ineffective.

Tobacco use

Many smokers begin smoking at an early age, making juvenile tobacco use a challenge. This places enormous responsibility on countries and creates the need for a worldwide coordinated response to curb the problem.

Less than 11% of the world's population is protected from smoking tobacco use by comprehensive national smoke-free laws. Comprehensive healthcare services to support smoking cessation are available in only 19 countries, that is, 14% of the world's population. With over 1.3 billion tobacco users worldwide, countries would have to provide tobacco dependence treatment centers for more than 650 million people, which translates to a huge financial burden.

Tobacco is the most unregulated consumer product on the market today, exempt from important basic consumer protections, such as ingredient disclosure, product testing, accurate labeling, and restrictions on marketing to children. According to WHO, only

19 countries (15% of the world's population) meet the best practice for pictorial warnings, which include warnings in the local language that cover an average of at least half of the front and back of cigarette packs. No low-income country meets this best practice level. Only 19 countries have achieved banning tobacco advertising, promotion, and sponsorship, and only about 38% of countries have minimal or no restrictions at all. As few as 27 countries have tobacco tax rates greater than 75% of the retail price. Tobacco tax revenues are on average 154 times higher than spending on tobacco control. Many tobacco users, policymakers, and even governments in certain parts of the world are oblivious to the scope of economic and health conditions caused by tobacco use. This to some extent explains the low level of attention accorded tobacco control and prevention.

Obesity

Obesity and its associated diseases and conditions are largely preventable, nevertheless, poor diet, the presence of food deserts, low income, ignorance, inadequate infrastructure to support and promote physical activity, and the lack of supportive policies in the health, urban planning, environment, food processing, distribution, marketing, and education sectors are some of the current major global obesity challenges. On the individual level, people are not deliberate about increasing physical activity, consuming healthy foods (whole grains, fresh fruits and vegetables, healthy fats and protein) and beverages, and do not limit their consumption of refined grains, red meat, processed food and sugary beverages, cut down on the use of salt, limit television, visual gadget and other sitting time, or get adequate sleep.

Global strategies and action

At the global level, WHO, to prevent NCDs, launched the Global Action Plan for the Prevention and Control of NCDs for the period 2013 to 2020. This plan focuses primarily on the four WHO identified NCDs; cardiovascular diseases, cancer, chronic respiratory diseases, and diabetes, as well as the four shared behavioral risk factors – tobacco use, unhealthy diet, physical inactivity, and harmful alcohol use – which have the highest morbidity and mortality rates. WHO Global NCD Action Plan provides a road map and policy options for WHO Member States and other stakeholders. It calls for coordinated efforts towards the attainment of nine voluntary global targets, including a 25% relative reduction in premature mortality from cardiovascular diseases, cancer, diabetes or chronic respiratory diseases by 2025 at the local and global levels (World Health Organization, 2013a), a minimum relative reduction (10%) in the harmful use of alcohol depending on what is deemed appropriate within the national context, and a 30% relative reduction in tobacco use among persons aged 15 years and above.

WHO Global NCD Action Plan offers a menu of "best buy" or cost-effective, high-impact interventions for meeting the nine voluntary global targets including banning all forms of tobacco and alcohol advertising, replacing trans fats with polyunsaturated fats, promoting and protecting breastfeeding, and preventing cervical cancer through screening.

In 2015, WHO Member States began to set national targets and to measure progress towards the 2010 baselines reported in the 2014 Global Status Report on NCDs. In 2018, the UN General Assembly will convene a third high-level meeting on NCDs to take stock of national progress in attaining the voluntary global targets scheduled to be achieved by 2025.

In response to the tobacco epidemic, WHO established the Framework Convention on Tobacco Control (FCTC); the first global health treaty on Tobacco. The FCTC was adopted by the 56th World Health Assembly in May 2003 and became international law in February 2005. As of August 2009, 168 WHO Member States had signed up to become party to the convention.

The FCTC features internationally coordinated provisions to control tobacco use by raising the price of tobacco products, banning smoking in public places, restricting tobacco advertising and promotion, counteradvertising, and providing treatment and counseling for tobacco dependence (FCTC Convention Secretariat, 2009). To date, 44 of the 53 African WHO Member States have ratified the FCTC. This notwithstanding, just a few of these countries have implemented the tobacco control measures or policies according to the framework. In 2009, only seven countries (Botswana, Djibouti, Eritrea, Madagascar, Niger, South Africa and Sudan) had comprehensive advertising bans in place (Shafey *et al.*, 2009), four had introduced complete public smoking bans (Botswana, Guinea, Niger, and Uganda); and 12 had implemented moderate public smoking bans (Djibouti, Egypt, Eritrea, Libya, Madagascar, Mali, Mauritius, Morocco, Mozambique, Nigeria, South Africa, and Zimbabwe). Although these efforts are laudable,

they are unfortunately insufficient to address the tobacco use issues in Africa.

Discussion points

1 What NCDs are of prime concern to WHO. Describe them.
2 Discuss the global burden of two NCDs.
3 Describe the economic burden of two NCDs.
4 How is alcohol a risk factor for NCDs?
5 Why is tobacco use referred to as a global epidemic?
6 Is obesity a global health epidemic? Explain your response.
7 How is obesity calculated in children and adults and how are the numbers interpreted?
8 Which part of the world suffers the most from NCDs? Explain your response.
9 What are some of the challenges associated with NCDs?
10 What global actions and strategies are in place to address the issues related to NCDs?

REFERENCES

Andlin-Sobocki, P., Jonsson, B., Wittchen, H. U., and Olesen, J. (2015) Cost of disorders of the brain in Europe. *European Journal of Neurology* **12**(1), 1–27.

Anis, A. H., Zhang, W., Bansback, N., *et al.* (2010) Obesity and overweight in Canada: An updated cost-of-illness study. *Obesity Reviews* **11**(1), 31–40.

Bryce, J., Black, R. E., Walker, N., *et al.* (2005) Can the world afford to save the lives of 6 million children each year? *The Lancet* **365**, 2193–2200.

CancerConnect (n.d.) *Wordwide, Cancer has Biggest Economic Impact of Any Cause of Death*, http://news.cancerconnect.com/worldwide-cancer-has-biggest-economic-impact-of-any-cause-of-death/#_edn1 (accessed October 15, 2016).

Centre for Mental Health (2010) *Economic and Social Costs of Mental Health Problems in 2009/10*, https://www.centreformentalhealth.org.uk/economic-and-social-costs-2009 (accessed October 15, 2016).

Colagiuri, S., Lee,C. M., Colagiuri, R. *et al.* (2010) The cost of overweight and obesity in Australia. *Medical Journal of Australia* **192**(5), 260–264.

Dall, T. M., Zhang,Y., Chen, Y. J., *et al.* (2010) The economic burden of diabetes. *Health Affairs* **29**, 2297–2303.

Department of Health and Human Services (2014) *The Health Consequences of Smoking —50 Years of Progress: A Report of the Surgeon General*,

http://www.surgeongeneral.gov/library/reports/
50-years-of-progress/exec-summary.pdf (accessed
October 20, 2016).

Doughton, S. (2014) Global cigarette consumption,
number of smokers climbing. *The Seattle Times*
(January 7), http://www.seattletimes.com/seattle-
news/global-cigarette-consumption-number-of-
smokers-climbing/ (accessed October 15, 2016).

Economic Burden of Lung Disease (2016), http://www.
erswhitebook.org/chapters/the-economic-burden-
of-lung-disease/ (accessed October 15, 2016).

Eriksen, M., Mackay J, and Ross, H. (2012) *The
Tobacco Atlas* (4th edn.). American Cancer Society,
Atlanta, GA.

Farlay, J., Soerjomataram, I., Ervik, M., *et al.* (2012)
Cancer Incidence and Mortality Worldwide. IARC
CancerBase No. 11. International Agency for
Research on Cancer, Lyon.

FCTC Convention Secretariat (2009) *2009 Summary
Report on Global Progress in Implementation of the
WHO Framework Convention on Tobacco Control*,
http://www.who.int/fctc/FCTC-2009-1-en.pdf
(accessed October 15, 2016).

Ferkol, T. and Schraufnagel, D. (2014) The global
burden of respiratory disease. *Annals of the American
Thoracic Society* 11(3), 404–406.

Foster, N., Vassall,A., Cleary, S., *et al.* (2015) The
economic burden of TB diagnosis and treatment in
South Africa. *Social Science and Medicine* **130**,
42–50.

Gabriel, P., and Liimatainen, M. R. (2000) *Mental
Health in the Workplace: Introduction.* International
Labour Office, http://www.ilo.org/wcmsp5/
groups/public/---ed_emp/---ifp_skills/
documents/publication/wcms_108221.pdf
(accessed October 15, 2016).

Gajalakshmi, C. K., and Peto, R. (1999) Tobacco epidemiology in the state of Tamil Nadu, India. Fifteenth
Asia Pacific Cancer Conference.

Giovino, G. A, Mirza, S. A., Samet, J. M., *et al.* (2012)
Tobacco use in 3 billion individuals from 16 countries: an analysis of nationally representative cross-
sectional household surveys. *The Lancet* **380**,
668–679.

Grucza, R. A., Norberg, K., Bucholz, K. K., and Bierut,
L. J. (2008) Correspondence between secular
changes in alcohol dependence and age of drinking onset among women in the United States.
Alcoholism: Clinical and Experimental Research
32(8), 1493–1501.

Hoang Anh, P. T., Thu, L. T., Ross, H., *et al.* (2016)
Direct and indirect costs of smoking in Vietnam.
Tobacco Control **25**, 96–100.

Jha, P. and Chaloupka, F. J. (2000) *Tobacco Control
in Developing Countries*, Oxford University Press,
Oxford.

Jha, P., Guindon, E., Joseph, R. A., *et al.* (2011)
A rational taxation system of bidis and cigarettes to
reduce smoking deaths in India. *Economic and
Political Weekly* **42**, 44–51.

John, R. M., Sung, H. Y., and Max, W. (2004) Economic
cost of tobacco use in India, 2004. *Tobacco Control*
18(21), 138–143.

Kaplan W. and Laing, R. (2004) *Priority Medicines
for Europe and the World*, http://apps.who.int/
iris/bitstream/10665/68769/1/WHO_EDM_
PAR_2004.7.pdf (accessed 15 October 2016).

Kraft, S. (2015) *What is Male Breast Cancer?* http://
www.medicalnewstoday.com/articles/179457.php
(accessed 15 October 2016).

Laramée, P., Kuse, J., Leonard, S., *et al.* (2013) The
economic burden of alcohol dependence in Europe.
Alcohol and Alcoholism **48**(3), 259–269.

Lin, H. H., Murray, M., Choen, T., *et al.* (2008) Effects
of smoking and solid-fuel use on COPD, lung cancer,
and tuberculosis in China: a time-based, multiple
risk factor, modeling study. *The Lancet* **372**(9648),
1473–1483.

Mackay, J., Jemal, A., Lee, N. C., and Parkin, D. M.
(2006) *The Cancer Atlas*, American Cancer Society,
Atlanta, GA.

Murray, C. J., and Lopez, A. D. (1997) Alternative
projections of mortality and disability by cause,
1990–2020: Global Burden of Disease Study. *The
Lancet* **349**, 1498–1504.

National Cancer Institute (2015) *What is Cancer?*
http://www.cancer.org/cancer/cancerbasics/
what-is-cancer (accessed October 19, 2016).

National Cancer Institute, National Institutes of
Health, and Department of Health and Human
Services (2015) *Cancer Trends Progress Report*, http://
progressreport.cancer.gov (accessed October 19, 2016).

Ng, M., Fleming, T., Robinson, M., *et al.* (2013) Global,
regional, and national prevalence of overweight
and obesity in children and adults during 1980–
2013: A systematic analysis for the Global Burden of
Disease Study. *The Lancet* **384**(9945), 766–781.

Non-Communicable Disease Alliance (n.d.) Tobacco:
A Major Risk Factor for Non-Communicable Diseases,
https://ncdalliance.org/sites/default/files/rfiles/
NCDA_Tobacco_and_Health.pdf (accessed October
20, 2016).

Nordqvist, C. (2016) *Breast Cancer: Causes and
Diagnosis*, http://www.medicalnewstoday.com/
articles/37136.php?page=2 (accessed 15 October
2016).

Peto, R., Lopez, A. D., Boreham, J., *et al.* (1994) *Mortality from Smoking in Developed Countries 1950–2000. Indirect Estimation from National Vital Statistics*, Oxford University Press, Oxford.

Peto, R., Lopez, A. D., Boreham, J. *et al.* (1996) Mortality from smoking worldwide. *British Medical Bulletin* **12**(1), 12–21.

Rehm, J., Baliunas, D., Brochu, S., *et al.* (2006) *The Costs of Substance Abuse in Canada 2002*, Canadian Centre on Substance Abuse, Ottawa.

Sacks, J. J., Gonzales, K. R., Bouchery, E. E., *et al.* (2015) 2010 National and state costs of excessive alcohol consumption. *American Journal of Preventive Medicine* **49**(5), 73–79.

Shafey, O., Eriksen, M., Ross, H., and Mackey, J. (2009) *The Tobacco Atlas* (3rd edn.). American Cancer Society, Atlanta, GA.

Sharecare (2016) *How Does Lung Cancer Usually Develop?* https://www.sharecare.com/health/lung-cancer/lung-cancer-usually-develop (accessed October 15, 2016).

World Health Organization (2001) *Mental Disorders Affect One in Four People*, http://www.who.int/whr/2001/media_centre/press_release/en/ (accessed October 20, 2016).

World Health Organization (2008) *WHO Report on the Global Tobacco Epidemic*, http://www.who.int/tobacco/mpower/mpower_report_full_2008.pdf (accessed October 20, 2016).

World Health Organization (2013a) *Global Action Plan for the Prevention and Control of NCDs 2013–2030*, http://apps.who.int/iris/bitstream/10665/94384/1/9789241506236_eng.pdf (accessed October 16, 2016).

World Health Organization (2013b) *Global Surveillance, Prevention and Control of Chronic Respiratory Diseases: A Comprehensive Approach*, World Health Organization, Geneva, http://www.who.int/gard/publications/GARD%20Book%202007.pdf (accessed October 15, 2016).

World Health Organization (2014) *Global Status Report on Alcohol and Health*, http://apps.who.int/iris/bitstream/10665/112736/1/9789240692763_eng.pdf?ua=1 (accessed October 15, 2016).

World Health Organization (2016a) *Obesity and Overweight*. Fact sheet no. 311, http://www.who.int/mediacentre/factsheets/fs311/en/ (accessed October 15, 2016).

World Health Organization (2016b) *World Pneumonia Day*, http://www.who.int/pmnch/media/events/2013/pneumonia_day/en/ (accessed October 5, 2016).

Zatoński, W. A., and Mańczuk, M. (2010) Tobacco smoking and tobacco-related harm in the European Union, with special attention to the new EU member states. In *Tobacco: Science, Policy, and Public Health* (ed. P. G. Boyle). Oxford University Press, Oxford, pp. 134–155.

FURTHER READING

American Cancer Society (2011) *Global Cancer Facts and Figures* (2nd edn). American Cancer Society, Atlanta, GA, http://www.cancer.org/acs/groups/content/@epidemiologysurveilance/documents/document/acspc-027766.pdf (accessed October 15, 2016).

Centers for Disease Control and Prevention (2011) *Taking On the Nation's Leading Killers*, https://www.cdc.gov/dhdsp/docs/dhdsp_factsheet.pdf (accessed October 25, 2016).

Cook, C.,Cole, G., Asaria, P., *et al.* (2014) The annual global economic burden of heart failure. *International Journal or Cardiology* **171**(3), 368–376.

Euromonitor International (2012) *Market Research for the Tobacco Industry: Cigarettes*, http://www.euromonitor.com/tobacco (accessed October 15, 2016).

Gøtzsche, P. C., and Jørgensen, K. J. (2013) Screening for breast cancer with mammography.*Cochrane Database of Systemic Reviews* **6** (Art. No.: cd001877).

John, R. and Ross, H. (2010) *The Global Economic Cost of Cancer*, American Cancer Society and the Livestrong Organization, http://news.cancerconnect.com/worldwide-cancer-has-biggest-economic-impact-of-any-cause-of-death/ (accessed 15 October 2016).

Keller, M. (n.d.) *Alcohol Consumption*, http://www.britannica.com/topic/alcohol-consumption (accessed 15 October 2016).

Mocumbi, A. O. (2013) Focus on non-communicable diseases: an important agenda for the African continent. *Cardiovascular Diagnosis and Therapy* **3**(4), 193–195.

Office for National Statistics (2001) *Psychiatric Morbidity Report*, ONS, London.

World Health Organization (2010) *Global Study to Reduce the Harmful Use of Alcohol*, http://www.who.int/substance_abuse/alcstratenglishfinal.pdf?ua=1 (accessed October 15, 2016).

4

Global burden of disease and measurement

Learning objectives

By the end of this chapter, you will be able to:

- ✔ List and explain at least two determinants of health;
- ✔ Explain at least two key health status indicators;
- ✔ Explain the significance of social determinants of health to global health;
- ✔ Identify and explain at least two indicators for measuring global burden of disease;
- ✔ Explain the rationale for measuring global burden of disease;
- ✔ Identify and explain at least two challenges associated with the measurement of global burden of disease;
- ✔ Describe least two strategies for addressing global burden of disease challenges.

Summary of key points

Establishing a shared understanding of the concepts of health and disease is fundamental to discussions about a population's health status. The ability to track and measure disease burden facilitates the assessment of changes in a population's health, provides the data needed to guide efforts towards the prevention, control, or treatment of ill health, and assists with the development and implementation of appropriate interventions to promote good health. While the absence of disease and infirmity determine health, so do the unequal distribution of wealth and access to resources within and between countries. This chapter focuses on the global burden of disease and how disease is measured. It begins by discussing the

definition of health and disease, and moves on to describe some key indicators of health, the social determinants that affect health, and the rationale and mechanisms for measuring the global burden of disease. This chapter concludes by discussing the global burden of disease challenges and global action and strategies in place to address them.

Health and disease

Following World War II, the World Health Organization (WHO) defined health in the preamble of its constitution, as a "state of complete physical, mental, and social wellbeing and not merely the absence of disease or infirmity" (World Health Organization, 1948). It also emphasized that "the enjoyment of the highest attainable

Global Health: Issues, Challenges, and Global Action Lecture Notes, First Edition. Elizabeth A. Armstrong-Mensah.
© 2017 John Wiley & Sons Ltd. Published 2017 by John Wiley & Sons Ltd.

standard of health is one of the fundamental rights of every human being without distinction of race, religion, political belief, economic or social condition" (World Health Organization, 1948).

Although praised for embracing a holistic viewpoint, WHO's definition of health has been criticized ever since its formulation. For some, the definition seems to have more to do with happiness than with health. The argument here is that, while having a serious disease is likely to negatively impact one's happiness, not having a serious disease will not necessarily result in happiness. To others, the definition is too inclusive and should focus primarily on the physical realm of health, as health issues are for the most part physical in nature. To others yet, the definition excludes the spiritual and ethical dimensions of health (Yach, n.d.) and does not indicate how the mental and social aspects of health should be measured. In the attempt to address the ambiguous connection between happiness and health, Rodolfo Saracci, an epidemiologist, suggested an alternative definition of health as "a condition of wellbeing free of disease or infirmity and a basic and universal human right" (World Health Organization, 1998). Regardless of the many criticisms, it must be noted that the WHO definition of health has not been modified since 1948.

Even though some of the criticisms levelled against WHO definition of health are justified, it is worthy of mention that, over the past several decades, the world has observed remarkable improvements in health as measured in physical terms; life expectancy at birth increased from 46 years in the 1950s to 89 years in 2016. The world has also witnessed a substantial decline in infant mortality rate along with improved access to healthcare, safe water, and improved sanitation. Regarding the mental aspect of the WHO definition of health, ageing, depression, and other sources of stress have been identified as indicators for measuring mental health, and poverty, education, income, and policies, have also been identified as social indicators for measuring health.

There is a link between health and disease. The malfunctioning of the mind or body can cause a departure from health, which may be attributable to a disease. A disease is a pathologic condition that impairs or disrupts the normal functioning of a living organism owing to environmental factors (such as malnutrition and climatic conditions), infective agents (including worms, bacteria, or viruses), or genetic anomalies, which result in extreme pain, dysfunction, distress, disability, disorders, infections, or death. A disease may be caused by a single factor (as is the case with malaria) or by a combination of factors (as is the case with cardiovascular disease). It may be airborne, communicable, noncommunicable, foodborne, or lifestyle related, and may affect a person's thoughts, emotions, memory, and personal and social behavior (Alzheimer's disease and schizophrenia).

Social determinants of health

Health, or the lack of it, was formerly attributed to biological or natural factors. Today, sociologists have added to, and expanded that notion. According to their observations, the attainment of good health or the contraction of disease is also influenced by a host of other factors, namely the socioeconomic status of individuals, culture, (White, 2002), the circumstances in which people are born, grow up, live, work and age, the physical environment, education, income level, social networks, unemployment and job security, housing, late childhood development, lifestyle, gender and power relations, policies, and political systems. Taken together, these factors and circumstances have been dubbed the social determinants of health (SDH).

Although listed as separate factors, the SDH are interrelated and are often shaped by the distribution of money, power, [geography], and resources in society (World Health Organization, 2008). Therefore, people who live in rural areas in developing countries are more likely to lack access to safe drinking water and adequate sanitation. These circumstances have the tendency to expose them to a variety of diseases, including guinea worm, elephantiasis, and malaria.

Women and girls in various parts of the world who cannot afford cooking stoves and thus, cook with fuel wood in poorly ventilated areas, are at risk of lower respiratory diseases, and people who live in geographic areas that do not have grocery shops that sell affordable and nutritious food within a reasonable distance, and who do not have automobiles, are at risk of diet-related health problems.

Being male or female has implications for one's health. Women by nature of their biological make up are at risk of cervical cancer and complications related to childbirth such as hemorrhaging and infection, and men by their constitution may experience prostate cancer or erectile dysfunction. Genetics may predispose people to disease. Mental illness, sickle cell disease, diabetes, hemophilia, cystic fibrosis, and cancer are diseases that may be genetically transferred from a parent to their child.

Unsafe working conditions may predispose people to disability, cause unproductivity, and bring about the loss of income. With high educational attainment, people are able to secure less hazardous jobs and thus, diminish their exposure to workplace injuries. They are likely to have an income, job security, and can therefore purchase health insurance. By virtue of their education, they have a better understanding of the relationship between pathogens, risk factors, and disease, can process health information, and administer medication.

Social networks give the sick something to live for. The knowledge that someone is rooting for them helps with their emotional state and desire to recuperate. People's way of life and perceptions determine their health-seeking behavior, their interpretation of health and disease, the type of healthcare personnel they will seek out, and the extent to which they will use a health facility in times of ill health. In certain societies, gender norms determine who has access to resources and who in the family can receive healthcare and when. The appropriateness of healthcare services, the cost of healthcare, transportation, and the availability of a well trained and geographically well distributed health workforce also determines one's health status. Politically, political decisions determine health resource allocation, the implementation of health policies and programs, the choice of technology, and the extent to which health services will be made available to different segments of society.

Key health status indicators

Health indicators are measureable characteristics that provide evidence about the health status of a population. Some key health indicators are discussed in this section.

Life expectancy

The average number of years a new born is expected to live, based on the year of their birth, sex, demographics, and trends of mortality, is referred to as life expectancy. Life expectancy increases, as people survive mortality associated with diseases. It varies from country to country and between women and men. In seventeenth-century England, life expectancy at birth was low; 35 years due to high infant and child mortality rates. In the twenty-first century, however,

people are living longer. In 2016 for example, Monaco, registered the highest life expectancy of 89.52 years (CIA, 2015).

Global variations in life expectancy can be said to stem from differences in public health investments and efforts, access to medical care, diet, ones sex, disease, lifestyle, and economic circumstances. Economically, life expectancy in wealthy countries tend to be higher than in poor countries. Regarding sex, women around the world tend to have higher life expectancy than men. The explanation provided for this variation is the general rule that, larger size individuals within a species tend to have on average, shorter lives (Samaras and Heigh, 1996), and the fact that women have more resistance to infections and degenerative diseases than men (Santrock, 2007).

Neonatal mortality rate

Neonatal mortality rate is the number of deaths of infants under 28 days of age per 1000 live births in a given year. Globally, neonatal mortality declined from 32% in 1990, to 22% in 2011; an average drop of 1.8%. The fastest reductions occurred in Eastern Asia (61%), followed by Latin America, the Caribbean, and then Northern Africa (55% respectively). The slowest reductions occurred in Oceania (23%), and sub-Saharan Africa (24%).

In 2013, neonatal mortality accounted for 42% of under-five child deaths compared with 37% in 1990. Globally, about 75% of all neonatal mortality occur within the first week of life, and 25% during the first 24 hours of life (Lawn *et al.*, 2005). In 2015, over 90% of all global neonatal mortality occurred in just ten countries in Asia and Africa, with India, Pakistan, and Nigeria ranking among the top three (see Figure 4.1).

During the Millennium Development Goals (MDG) era (1990–2015), neonatal mortality declined, but at a slower pace than child mortality: 47% compared with 58% globally. Consequently, the proportion of newborn deaths among all under-five deaths rose to 45% from 40% in 1990. This notwithstanding, global neonatal mortality has generally decreased from 5.1 million in 1990, to 2.7 million in 2015.

The main contributors to neonatal mortality worldwide are preterm birth complications – birth asphyxia, sepsis, neonatal pneumonia, congenital abnormalities, tetanus, and neonatal diarrhea. Between 2000 and 2013, prematurity, complications during childbirth, and neonatal infections were the main causes of death (see Figure 4.2).

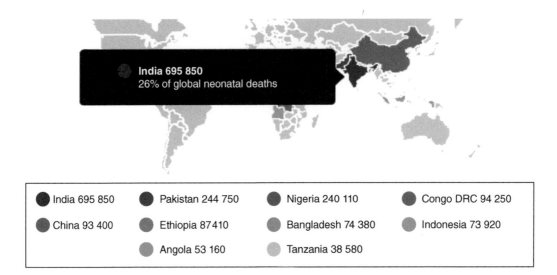

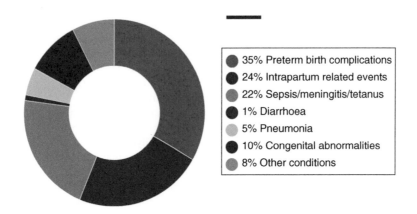

India 695 850	Pakistan 244 750	Nigeria 240 110	Congo DRC 94 250
China 93 400	Ethiopia 87 410	Bangladesh 74 380	Indonesia 73 920
	Angola 53 160	Tanzania 38 580	

Figure 4.1 Countries with the highest neonatal deaths in 2015.
Source: UN Interagency Group for Child Mortality Estimation (IGME) (2015) http://www.childmortality.org (accessed October 15, 2016), http://www.healthynewbornnetwork.org/numbers/ (accessed October 5, 2016), with permission.

- 35% Preterm birth complications
- 24% Intrapartum related events
- 22% Sepsis/meningitis/tetanus
- 1% Diarrhoea
- 5% Pneumonia
- 10% Congenital abnormalities
- 8% Other conditions

Figure 4.2 Global causes of neonatal deaths (2000–2013).
Source: Liu *et al.* (2014), with permission.

Infant mortality rate

Infant mortality rate is the number of deaths of infants under age 1 per 1000 live births in a given year. In developing countries, approximately 50% of all newborns do not receive skilled healthcare immediately after birth. In 2012, infant mortality rate was 2 per 1000 live births in Iceland and 117 per 1000 live births in Sierra Leone. In 2015, Afghanistan had the highest infant mortality rate of 115 per 1000 live births (see Table 4.1)

Also in 2015, infant mortality was higher in the WHO African region (55 per 1000 live births) than in the WHO European region (10 per 1000 live births). Universally, infant mortality rate decreased from an estimated 63 deaths per 1000 live births in 1990, to 32 deaths per 1000 live births in 2015. Annual infant mortality declined from 8.9 million in 1990 to 4.5 million in 2015 (Global Health Observatory, 2016).

Child mortality rate

Also known as the under-five mortality rate, child mortality rate is the probability that a new born baby will die before reaching age five, per 1000 live births in a given year. Child mortality rate is a leading indicator of child

Table 4.1 Global infant mortality rate by country in 2015.

Rank	Country	(Deaths/1000 live births)	Date of information
1	Afghanistan	115.08	2015 est.
2	Mali	102.23	2015 est.
3	Somalia	98.39	2015 est.
4	Central African Republic	90.63	2015 est.
5	Guinea-Bissau	89.21	2015 est.
6	Chad	88.69	2015 est.
7	Niger	84.59	2015 est.
8	Angola	78.26	2015 est.
9	Burkina Faso	75.32	2015 est.
10	Nigeria	72.70	2015 est.
215	Hong Kong	2.73	2015 est.
216	Czech Republic	2.63	2015 est.
217	Sweden	2.60	2015 est.
218	Finland	2.52	2015 est.
219	Bermuda	2.48	2015 est.
220	Norway	2.48	2015 est.
221	Singapore	2.48	2015 est.
222	Japan	2.08	2015 est.
223	Iceland	2.06	2015 est.
224	Monaco	1.82	2015 est.

Source: CIA, *The World Fact Book 2015.*

health globally. Child mortality rates are highest in sub-Saharan Africa and South-East Asia, with about 50% of under-five deaths occurring in India, Nigeria, Democratic Republic of the Congo, Pakistan, and China. Combined, child mortality rates in these countries account for more than a third of global under-five deaths.

In 2015, 5.9 million children under the age of five died. Over 50% of these early child deaths were due to preventable or treatable conditions specifically, diarrhea, malaria, pneumonia, preterm birth complications, birth asphyxia, sepsis, neonatal pneumonia, congenital abnormalities, and tetanus (see Figure 4.3). In South-East Asia, acute respiratory infections and diarrhea are the main killers. Nutrition-related conditions also account for about 45% of under-five deaths. Wide gaps in child mortality have been documented across subgroups and within countries. Children born in rural areas and in poor households, or to mothers without basic education, are at a higher risk of not making it to their fifth birthday.

Worldwide, significant progress has been made toward reducing child mortality. Indeed, under-five mortality dropped from 12.7 million in 1990 to 5.9 million in 2015, and from 91 deaths per 1000 live births in 1990, to 43 per 1000 in 2015. Sub-Saharan Africa, the region with the highest under-five mortality rate in the world, made considerable strides by reducing its annual child mortality rate from 1.6% in the 1990s, to 4.1% between 2000 and 2015. Countries in Eastern Asia, Northern Africa, Latin America, the Caribbean, and Western Asia have reduced their under-five mortality rates beyond 50%.

Maternal mortality ratio (MMR)

Maternal mortality ratio (MMR) is the number of women who die as a result of pregnancy and child birth complications per 100000 live births in a given year. Globally, there were an estimated 287000 maternal deaths in 2010. That same year, developing countries accounted for 99% of those deaths, with sub-Saharan Africa and South Asia accounting for 85% of the total number of deaths (World Health Organization, Western Pacific Region, 2016). In 2015, the MMR in

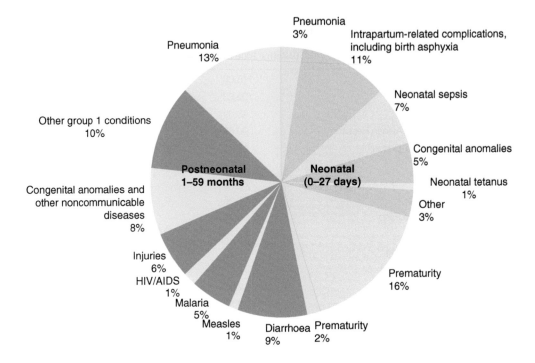

Figure 4.3 Causes of death among children under five years, 2015.
Source: World Health Organization, http://www.who.int/gho/child_health/mortality/causes/en/ (accessed October 15, 2016), with permission.

developing countries was 239 per 100 000 live births and 12 per 100 000 live births in developed countries (World Health Organization, 2015).

All around the world, pregnant women tend to die from pre-existing conditions, severe bleeding, pregnancy-induced high blood pressure, infections after birth, obstructed labor, abortion complications, blood clot, and existing medical conditions (see Figure 4.4).

Global maternal mortality dropped by 44% between 1990 and 2015. During this period, sub-Saharan Africa halved its maternal mortality and other regions of the world, including Asia and North Africa, made even greater strides. Certain countries experienced over a 5.5% reduction in maternal mortality between 2000 and 2010, the rate needed to achieve the MDGs.

The concept of global burden of disease

Health status has implications for the global burden of disease, in that, it can increase or decrease the collective level of ill health in a country, or negatively impact the quality of life. Until recently, the quality of a society's health was measured by the death rate per population, or by death rate by age per population. With the launch of the global burden of disease studies, the focus shifted to comparing diseases, disabilities, and injuries across populations.

Global burden of disease is a comprehensive regional and global assessment of the comparative magnitude of health lost, mortality, and disability from major diseases, injuries, and risk factors by age, sex, and geography for specific points in time through systematic and scientific efforts. It is also the gap between existing health status created by premature mortality, disability, and exposure to certain risk factors that contribute to illness, and a desired end state in which populations live long, free of disease and disability.

Global burden of disease studies

In 1993, WHO and the World Bank published a report (World Development Report) on a global burden of disease study they had jointly sponsored.

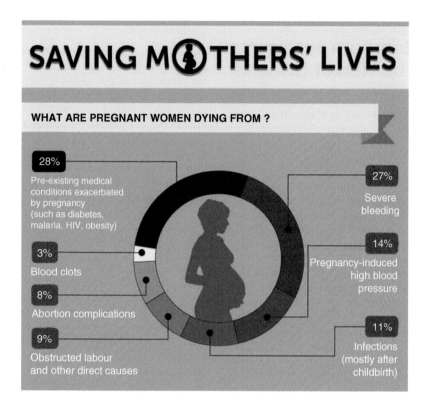

Figure 4.4 Causes of maternal deaths.
Source: World Health Organization (2014), http://www.thedailystar.net/sites/default/files/upload-2014/gallery/image/online/meternal-deaths-who.jpg (accessed October 15, 2016).

The study measured the total loss of health arising from diseases and injuries. Reconducted in 1996, and yet again in 2000, the study produced a comprehensive and reliable set of estimates of mortality and morbidity by age, sex, and region. The original report revealed that infectious diseases accounted for 43% of the global burden of disease.

In 2010, Bill and Melinda Gates funded yet another global burden of disease study spearheaded by Christopher Murray and Alan Lopez. The study spanned 1990, 2005, and 2010, and focused on 291 diseases and injuries, 67 risk factors, 1160 nonfatal health consequences, 21 regions, 20 age groups, and 187 countries. The purpose of the study was to estimate annual deaths and their causes between 1990 and 2010, by age and sex. The study was a collaborative effort between 488 researchers from 303 institutions in 50 countries and a host of institutions including Harvard University, Imperial College London, Johns Hopkins University, University of Queensland, University of Tokyo, and WHO (Murray and Lopez, 2013).

Study findings showed that people were living longer and that life expectancy had increased in 19 of 21 regions owing to reductions in child and maternal mortality rates among other factors. The study also established that global disability was on the rise, as people with disabilities (mental health disorders, diabetes, vision loss, and chronic respiratory diseases) were living longer. It pointed out that risk factors such as unsafe water and sanitation and micronutrient deficiencies, which were the main causes of communicable diseases in children, had dropped. Findings from the study further indicated that there were major differences in disease burden between regions. Risk factors assessed by the study and attributable to the burden of disease in 2010 were high blood pressure (ranked first), tobacco smoking including second-hand smoke (ranked second), household air pollution (ranked third), and childhood underweight (ranked eighth).

Indicators for measuring global burden of disease

A set of indicators are used to measure global injury, disability, and premature mortality. This segment provides an overview of some of these indicators.

Morbidity and mortality

The occurrence of poor health and the consequence of disease in a population is known as morbidity. A person may suffer several morbidities at the same time. Morbidity is measured by incidence and prevalence and ranges from parasitic infections and diabetes to tuberculosis.

Mortality refers to the death of people in a population owing to a disease divided by the total population. It is calculated by mortality rate, which is the number of deaths per thousand people in a given year. Crude mortality rate, maternal mortality rate, and infant mortality rate are some examples of mortality rate. Each rate relates to number of deaths across a section of a population.

Incidence

Epidemiologically, incidence is the measure of the probability of the occurrence of a specific medical condition in a population at risk for developing a disease within a specified period. Incidence is a risk measure that can assess risk in a population by age, sex, demographic characteristics, or other causal factors. Incidence rate is measured by the number of new cases per population at risk in a given time period.

Prevalence

Most often, people confuse the term "incidence" with "prevalence." Unlike incidence, prevalence is the proportion of the total number of cases of a medical condition or disease prevalent in a population at a given time. It focuses on the incidence of a disease that occurred in the past and continues to prevail at present or to a specified time. Prevalence measures the burden of disease on society with no focus on time of exposure to a possible risk factor. Prevalence shows how widespread a disease is within a population.

Disability-adjusted life years (DALY)

Disability-adjusted life years (DALY) is an internationally accepted time-based measure developed in 1990 by WHO and other organizations involved with public health, to facilitate the consistent measurement of disease burden across diseases, risk factors, age, and regions (see Figure 4.5). It combines years of life lost to premature mortality and the number of productive years lost to disability within a particular population based on the assumption that everyone has a right to the best life expectancy in the world. One DALY is equivalent to one year of healthy life lost.

Disability-adjusted life years attempt to show the effect of nonfatal diseases and disability on health, and overall disease burden as a result of ill health, disability, or premature death over a period. They help to inform decision making on health-service delivery, research and planning, compare the health status of populations within and across countries, and to identify health inequalities.

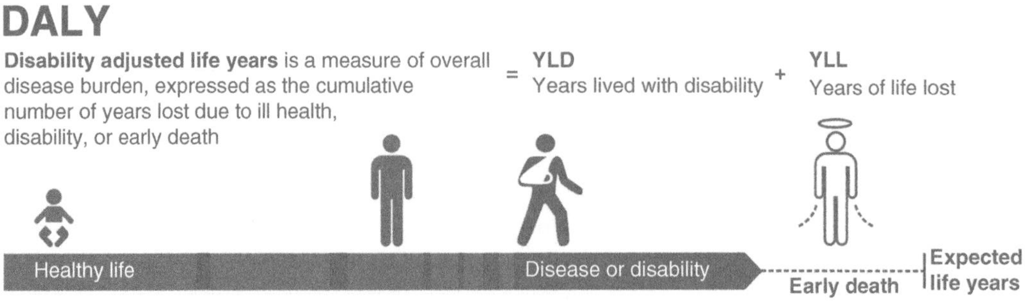

DALY

Disability adjusted life years is a measure of overall disease burden, expressed as the cumulative number of years lost due to ill health, disability, or early death

= **YLD** Years lived with disability + **YLL** Years of life lost

Healthy life   Disease or disability   Early death   Expected life years

Figure 4.5 Explanation and computation of DALY.
Sources: Commons.wikimedia.org., and *The World Health Organization and Metrics: Disability-Adjusted Life Year (DALY)*, https://en.wikipedia.org/wiki/Disability-adjusted_life_year (accessed October 15, 2016).

Rationale for measuring global burden of disease

Global burden of disease is measured to obtain reliable and accurate information about the amount of disease, disability, and death among populations in the world, and to promote health decision making based on evidence. Measuring disease burden helps countries to set priorities for healthcare, informs health resource and budget allocation and unearths the potential cost and benefits of public health interventions. Measuring global disease burden also facilitates the comparison of health outcomes within and between countries, provides information on the leading causes of morbidity and mortality, sets the stage for dialogue on health policies, and helps with the identification of high-risk populations and planning for future health initiatives.

Patterns of global disease distribution

Different disease patterns exist in high-income, middle-income, and low-income countries. The general diseases associated with high-income countries are primarily chronic noncommunicable diseases, such as heart disease and cancer, and those associated with middle- and low-income countries are communicable diseases including cholera and malaria. While disease burden by country income level (see Figure 4.6) was exclusive several years ago, the situation has changed, as noncommunicable diseases are now present in middle-income and low-income countries, and infectious diseases, in high-income countries, although at varying rates.

Customarily associated with developed countries, cardiovascular disease-related deaths now occur in low- and middle-income countries. In 2000, 67% of the estimated 171 million people with diabetes were living in developing countries. That year, the worst affected countries were China and India, where there were 20.8 million and 31.7 million cases of diabetes, respectively (Marshall, 2004). In 1996, yellow fever was introduced into the United States and Switzerland by tourists who had travelled to yellow fever endemic countries without being vaccinated against the disease. That same year, about 10 000 cases of malaria were imported into Europe, with about 25% of those cases occurring in the United Kingdom. In 1991, cholera re-emerged in Peru through poor sanitation and water systems, leaving more than 3000 people dead. Consequently, seafood exports from Peru were embargoed and tourism declined, costing the

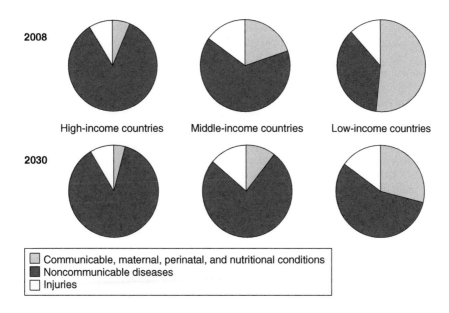

Figure 4.6 Burden of disease by country income level.
Source: World Health Organization, *Projections of Mortality and Burden of Disease, 2004–2030*, http://www.who.int/healthinfo/global_burden_disease/projections/en/index.html (accessed October 15, 2016), with permission.

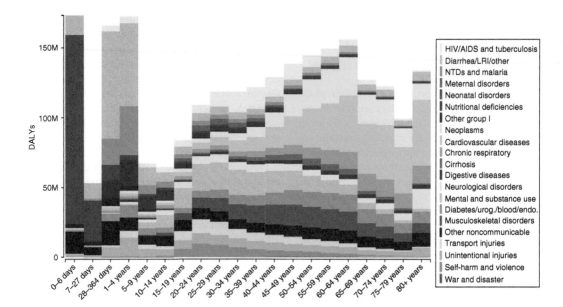

Figure 4.7 Global burden of disease distributed by age for both sexes, 2013.
Source: Institute for Health Metrics and Evaluation (IHME) (2015) *GBD Compare*. IHME, University of Washington, Seattle, WA, http://vizhub.healthdata.org/gbd-compare/ (accessed October 15, 2016), with permission.

Peruvian government an estimated $770 million in economic losses (World Health Organization, 2016).

Some diseases are age occurring and affect certain populations more than others. Globally, in 2013, diarrhea, neonatal disorders, nutritional deficiencies and certain noncommunicable and infectious diseases occurred more in younger children aged zero to four years, whilst musculoskeletal disorders, cardiovascular disease, chronic respiratory diseases and neurological disorders occurred more in adults aged 40 to 80 years and above (see Figure 4.7). In 2013, people aged 1 to 4 and 80 years and above, accounted for the world's most unintentionally injured.

Women and girls accounted for more cases of musculoskeletal and neurological disorders in 2013 than men. That same year, men on the other hand, accounted for more disease burden associated with cardiovascular diseases, unintentional injuries, war, and disaster compared to women (see Figure 4.8).

disease burden have relied on assumptions rather than on precise numbers. This is especially the case in countries where official health statistics are incomplete (Cliff and Haggett, 2004), inaccurate, unavailable, or out of date, and where civil registration of births and deaths is limited. When deaths and their causes are not accounted for, governments are unable to put in place effective public health policies or to measure their impact. Information on births and deaths by age, sex, and cause are crucial to public health and by extension, to global health planning (World Health Organization, 2004).

Disability-adjusted life years calculations require numerical information about the specific incidence of disease, the proportion of disease incidence leading to disability, the average age of disability onset, the duration of disability, and the distribution of disability across six levels of severity. Unfortunately, such information is often not available in all countries (Pleis and Lethbridge-Çejku, 2007).

Global burden of disease measurement challenges

Underreporting and the underascertainment of diseases in certain countries create challenges for the accurate estimation of the global burden of disease. On occasion, the methods used in the calculation of

Global action and strategies

The World Bank initiated an Integrated Disease Surveillance Project (IDSP) in India in 2004, to provide guidelines for integrated disease surveillance

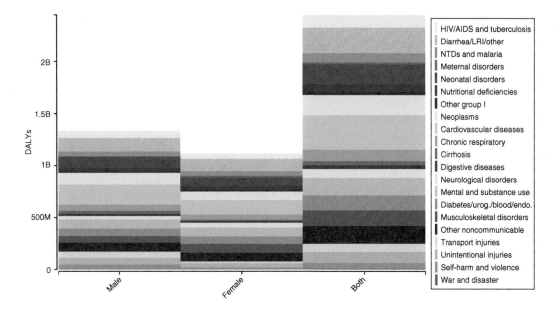

Figure 4.8 Global burden of disease distributed by sex, 2013.
Source: Institute for Health Metrics and Evaluation (IHME) (2015), with permission.

and response, as well as to provide technical assistance for strengthening national communicable disease surveillance systems through the implementation of the Regional Strategy for Integrated Disease Surveillance and the International Health Regulations. The IDSP creates links with national centers of excellence, regional, and global networks for disease surveillance in an effort to monitor disease trends and outbreaks.

In 2005, WHO established the Commission on Social Determinants of Health (CSDH) to provide support to countries and global health partners to address the social factors leading to ill health and health inequities. The goal of the Commission was to draw the attention of governments and societies to the ills of the SDH and to create improved social conditions for health, particularly among the most vulnerable populations in the world.

To aid the coordination of activities, WHO established the SDH Unit with a mandate to work with countries to support, guide, and strengthen their capacities to develop, implement, monitor, and evaluate initiatives that address SDH inequities. Based on its 2008 report, WHO CSDH identified two broad areas of SDH that need to be addressed. The first area focuses on daily living conditions including healthy physical environments, fair employment, decent work, social protection across one's lifespan, and access to healthcare. The second area focuses on the distribution of power, money, and resources, equity in health programs, removal of economic inequalities, healthy working conditions, gender equity, political empowerment, and a balance of power and prosperity of nations (World Health Organization, 2008).

Discussion points

1 What is health? How do you reconcile your definition with WHO's definition of health?
2 What are some of the factors that determine health?
3 What are some key indicators that show the health status of a population? Describe the indicators.
4 What is global burden of disease?
5 What is the rationale for measuring global disease burden?
6 Describe four methods for measuring disease burden.
7 How useful is the 2010 Global Burden of Disease Study?
8 What can countries do to improve upon disease surveillance?
9 What are some of the challenges associated with the measurement of global disease burden?
10 What actions and strategies have been established to handle the issues related to global burden of disease measurement? How useful are these strategies and actions?

REFERENCES

CIA (2015) *World Factbook, 2015. Life Expectancy for Countries* http://www.infoplease.com/world/statistics/life-expectancy-country.html (accessed October 15, 2016).

Cliff, F. A. and Haggett, P. (2004) Time, travel and infection. *British Medical Bulletin* **69**, 87–99.

Global Health Observatory (2016) *Infant Mortality: Situation and Trends* http://www.who.int/gho/child_health/mortality/neonatal_infant_text/en/ (accessed October 15, 2016).

Institute for Health Metrics and Evaluation (IHME) (2015) *GBD Compare*. IHME, University of Washington, Seattle, WA, http://vizhub.healthdata.org/gbd-compare/ (accessed October 15, 2016).

Lawn, J. E., Cousens, S., and Zupan, J. (2005) 4 million neonatal deaths: When? Where? Why? *The Lancet* **365**, 891–900.

Liu, L. Oza, S., Hogan, D., *et al.* (2014) Global, regional, and national causes of child mortality in 2000–2013: an updated systematic analysis. *The Lancet* **385**(9966), 430–440.

Marshall, S. J. (2004) Developing countries face double burden of disease. *Bulletin of the World Health Organization* **82**(7), 556.

Murray, C. J. L. and Lopez, A. D. (2013) Measuring the global burden of disease. *New England Journal of Medicine* **369**, 448–457.

Pleis, J. R. and Lethbridge-Çejku, M. (2007) Summary health statistics for US adults: National health interview survey. National Center for Health Statistics. *Vital Health Statistics* **10**, 235.

Samaras, T. T. and Heigh, G. H. (1996) How human size affects longevity and mortality from degenerative diseases. *Townsend Letter for Doctors and Patients* **159**, 78–85, 133–139.

Santrock, J. (2007) *Life Expectancy. A Topical Approach to: Life-Span Development* McGraw-Hill, New York, NY.

Saracci, R. (1997) The World Health Organization needs to reconsider its definition of health. *British Medical Journal* **314**(7091), 1409–1410.

White, K. (2002) *An Introduction to the Sociology of Health and Illness*, SAGE Publishing, London. http://apps.who.int/iris/bitstream/10665/69832/1/WHO_IER_CSDH_08.1_eng.pdf (accessed October 16, 2016).

World Health Organization (1948) *World Health Organization Constitution*, http://who.int/about/mission/en/ (accessed October 15, 2016).

World Health Organization (1998) *The World Health Report. Life in the 21st Century: A Vision for All*, http://www.who.int/whr/1998/en/whr98_en.pdf?ua=1 (accessed October 15, 2016).

World Health Organization (2004) *Civil Registration: Why Counting Births and Deaths is Important* Fact sheet no. 324, http://www.who.int/mediacentre/factsheets/fs324/en/ (accessed October 15, 2016).

World Health Organization (2015) *Maternal Mortality*. Fact sheet no. 348, http://www.who.int/mediacentre/factsheets/fs348/en/ (accessed October 15, 2016).

World Health Organization. (2016) *Global Infectious Disease Surveillance* http://www.who.int/mediacentre/factsheets/fs200/en/ (accessed October 15, 2016).

World Health Organization (2008) *Health Equity Through Action on the Social Determinants of Health*, Commission on Social Determinants of Health Final Report, http://apps.who.int/iris/bitstream/10665/43943/1/9789241563703_eng.pdf (accessed October 25, 2016).

World Health Organization, Western Pacific Region (2016) Maternal Health. Retrieved October 17, 2016, http://www.wpro.who.int/laos/topics/maternal_health/en/ (accessed October 20, 2016).

Yach, R. (n.d.) *Health and Illness: The Definition of the World Health Organization* http://www.medizin-ethik.ch/publik/health_illness.htm (accessed October 15, 2016).

FURTHER READING

Hoy, D., Roth, A., Viney, K., *et al.* (2014) Findings and implications of the global burden of disease 2010 Study for the Pacific Islands. *Preventing Chronic Disease* **11**(130344).

6

Water, sanitation, and global health

Learning objectives

By the end of this chapter, you will be able to:

✔ List and explain at least two water and sanitation-related diseases;

✔ Discuss the role of women in water and sanitation;

✔ Explain the effects of unsafe water and inadequate sanitation on global health;

✔ Discuss global water and sanitation coverage;

✔ List and explain at least two challenges to achieving the sanitation MDG target;

✔ Discuss at least two global water supply and sanitation initiatives.

Summary of key points

Access to safe drinking water and improved sanitation are basic human rights, yet not everyone in the world has access to them. Although the Millennium Development Goal (MDG) target for access to safe drinking water was achieved recently, about 750 million people, that is, one in nine people still rely on unimproved water sources to meet their water needs. The sanitation situation is not any better; about 2.5 billion or one in three people lack access to improved sanitation globally. The lack of access to safe water and improved sanitation not only predispose people to diseases and disability – it also reduces productivity, creates poverty, and brings about poor socioeconomic development. In the developing world, women and girls bear a disproportionate burden when it comes to water and sanitation. They are responsible for collecting and managing water, as well as maintaining family hygiene. Carrying out these tasks often negatively impacts their health, increases their workload unduly, and leaves them little to no room for the pursuit of economic activities or leisure. In this chapter, select commonly used water and sanitation terms are defined. Next, diseases related to water and sanitation are discussed, followed by a presentation on the role of women in water and sanitation. The effects, benefits, coverage, challenges, and strategies for safe water and improved sanitation are also discussed.

Global Health: Issues, Challenges, and Global Action Lecture Notes, First Edition. Elizabeth A. Armstrong-Mensah.
© 2017 John Wiley & Sons Ltd. Published 2017 by John Wiley & Sons Ltd.

Key water and sanitation terms

Certain terms are frequently used in the water and sanitation subsector. An understanding of these terms creates a better appreciation of the sector. In this section, select key terms are defined.

Key water terms

Safe Water

Water that is free from chemical substances, microorganisms, and radiological hazards that constitute a threat to a person's health. Safe water is usually determined by national or local standards and therefore, differs from place to place.

Sufficient water

Continuous availability of enough water for personal and domestic use, such as drinking, food preparation, and washing of clothes. According to World Health Organization (WHO) and the United Nations Children Fund (Unicef), people need a minimum of 20 liters of water per capita per day to take care of their water needs.

Acceptable water

Water for personal or domestic use that is without color, odor, and taste.

Physically accessible water

Water sources that are physically within, or in the immediate vicinity of the household, educational institution, workplace, or health institution. According to WHO, water sources should be between 100 and 1000 meters from the home, and collection time should not exceed 5 to 30 minutes.

Affordable water

Reasonably priced water that does not disproportionately affect the utilization of water services by the poor. According to the United Nations Development Fund (UNDP), water costs should not exceed 3% of household income.

Improved drinking water sources

Water sources that, by nature of their construction, are protected from outside contamination (see Figure 6.1). They include boreholes fitted with hand pumps, public and private piped systems, rain catchment systems, and spring catchment systems.

Unimproved drinking water sources

These are water sources that, by nature of their construction, are not protected from outside contamination (see Figure 6.2). Common examples are shallow wells, unprotected hand-dug wells, and surface water like dams, ponds, streams, and rivers. These sources are often used by humans and animals for their water-related activities, making them highly unsafe for human consumption.

Key sanitation terms

Sanitation

The management and safe disposal of domestic waste water, feces, human urine, and solid waste in and around communities and households. The most dangerous waste product, and thus the focus of many global health efforts, is feces.

Latrine

A small and very simple outdoor toilet, usually just a pit or trench for defecation.

Open defecation

Defecation in bushes, bodies of water, fields, forests, or other open spaces.

Improved sanitation facilities

These are sanitation facilities that provide barriers and hygienically separate human feces and urine from human contact, so as to prevent the transmission of disease (see Figure 6.3). They comprise water closets, pour-flush systems, and ventilated improved pit latrines.

Unimproved sanitation facilities

Sanitation facilities that do not hygienically separate excreta and waste from human contact (see Figure 6.4). They include latrines.

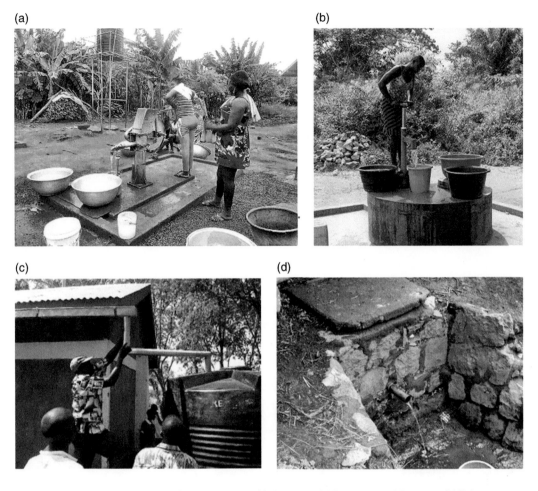

Figure 6.1 Improved water sources. (a) Bore hole with Afridev pump. (b) Borehole with Nira pump. (c) Rainwater catchment system. (d) Spring system.
Sources: Himalayan Institute (2011); Tanira Ltd., http://www.tanira-pumps.com/products/af-85-well-pump (accessed October 21, 2016); Water Charity (2012, 2016), with permission.

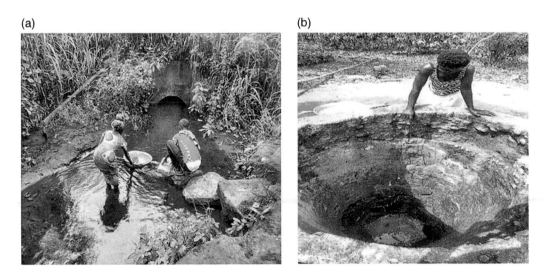

Figure 6.2 Unimproved water sources. (a) Pond and (b) well with no cover.
Source: Water Charity (2016), with permission.

(a)   (b)   (c)

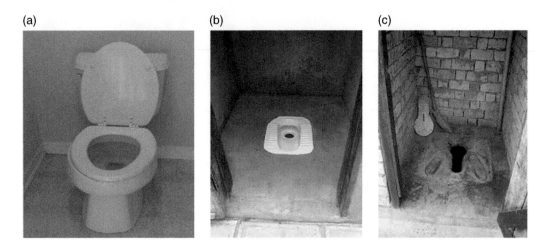

Figure 6.3 Improved sanitation facilities. (a) Water closet. (b) Pour-flush system. (c) Improved pit latrine.
Sources: Parker (2014); Sustainable Sanitation Alliance (SuSanA) Secretariat (n.d.), with permission.

(a)   (b)

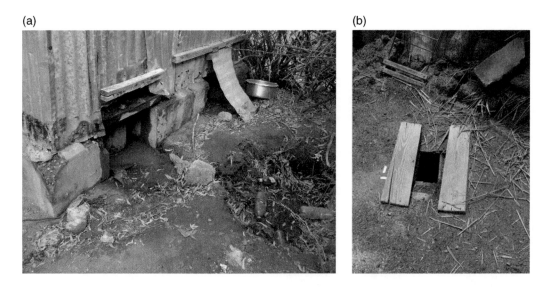

Figure 6.4 Unimproved sanitation facilities. (a) Bucket latrine. (b) Pit latrine.
Sources: Sustainable Sanitation Alliance (SuSanA) Secretariat: https://www.flickr.com/photos/gtzecosan/6394968051/ (accessed October 21, 2016), and https://www.flickr.com/photos/gtzecosan/5014325656 (accessed October 21, 2016), with permission.

Water and sanitation-related diseases

Safe water and improved sanitation are essential for human health, economic growth, and the development of any country. The lack of access to safe water and improved sanitation are environmental risk factors that predispose populations all over the world to a myriad of diseases, which cause not only ill health and disability, but sometimes death. Globally, the lack of access to safe water and improved sanitation causes about 1.9 million deaths per annum and accounts for 4.2% of the global burden of disease (Carlton *et al.*, 2012).

Water

Water-related diseases are preventable diseases that are caused by the lack of access to clean water. They are mostly prevalent in developing countries and disproportionately affect the poor and children. There are four main types of water-related diseases: water-based, waterborne, water-washed, and water-related insect vector diseases.

Water-based diseases emerge when pathogens are transmitted to humans through contact with aquatic intermediate hosts such as worms. These worms penetrate the skin if unclean water is used for washing or bathing. Examples of water-based diseases are schistosomiasis and dracunculiasis (guinea-worm disease). Globally, about 200 million people have schistosomiasis and around 20 million of these are severe cases. Schistosomiasis is a common disease in rural areas in sub-Saharan Africa, where four out of every five people are infected. Dracunculiasis is a debilitating disease, which leaves its victims incapacitated. In some people, it leads to arthritis, and even permanent stiffness of the limbs. Due to WHO-backed eradication campaign, and the tireless efforts of the Carter Center, the global incidence of guinea worm has significantly dropped to only five cases. In 2015, the disease was prevalent in only two countries: Chad (four cases) and Ethiopia (one case) (National Academy of Sciences, 2007).

Waterborne diseases occur as a result of ingesting water or food contaminated with human or animal feces. They cause diarrheal diseases such as cholera, dysentery, gastroenteritis, and typhoid, which can be life threatening to children, the elderly, and people who may have compromised immune systems. Cholera is prevalent in much of the developing world, especially in Asia and Africa, and typhoid affects about 17 million people globally each year.

Water-washed diseases are infections that arise when pathogens spread from person to person as a result of lack of adequate water for personal hygiene and domestic use. Leprosy, scabies, trachoma, and yaws are examples of water-washed diseases. An estimated 300 million people contract scabies annually, and over 6 million people worldwide become blind as a result of trachoma.

Water-related insect vector diseases occur when humans become infected with pathogens transmitted by insects that breed in inadequately managed surface water. These insects include black flies and mosquitoes, which breed in stagnant water. Dengue fever, filiariasis, malaria, river blindness, trypanosomiasis, and yellow fever are vector-borne diseases. Malaria is a killer disease in the tropical and subtropical regions of Asia, Africa, and South America, and is especially deadly among children under the age of five. Worldwide, an estimated 300 to 500 million people contract malaria each year, and about 1 million of this number dies from the disease.

Sanitation

Sanitation-related diseases are diseases caused by human contact with human feces in places where improved sanitation facilities are absent. Cholera, diarrhea, dysentery, hookworms, water- and soil-transmitted helminthic infections are examples of sanitation-related diseases. Hookworm is a tropical disease that affects about 1 billion people around the globe annually – that is, one in every six people on earth. Sanitation-related diseases account for about 4% and 5.7% of global mortality and morbidity, respectively.

The F diagram (see Figure 6.5) shows how improperly disposed fecal matter in the environment can lead to the transmission of disease directly to hosts, and indirectly to food, through fingers, flies, fluids, fields, or floods via the fecal-oral route. It is referred to as the F diagram because the pathways through which fecal matter is transmitted to humans all begin with the letter "F".

Through the water pathway, germs in feces on the ground can contaminate drinking water (fluids). Through fingers or unwashed hands after defecating, germs can be transmitted to foods and eaten. Through the fly's pathway, germs can be transferred from feces into food. Through fields, germs can enter produce and other sources of food, and through floods, germs in feces can seep into water sources during a flood. The F diagram also provides information on actions to be taken to prevent exposure to sanitation-related diseases.

Table 6.1 shows a few examples of water- and sanitation-related diseases, their microbial agent, mode of transmission, and symptoms.

Women, water, and sanitation

In the rural areas of developing countries, water and sanitation are at the core of women and girls' traditional roles. They collect, store, and manage water, in addition to maintaining household sanitation and hygiene. In performing these tasks, women and girls are exposed to numerous health, environmental, and social risks.

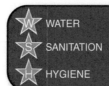

WATER

SANITATION

HYGIENE

Barriers can stop the transmission of disease; these can be primary (preventing the initial contact with the feces) or secondary (preventing it being ingested by a new person). They can be controlled by water, sanitation and hygiene interventions.

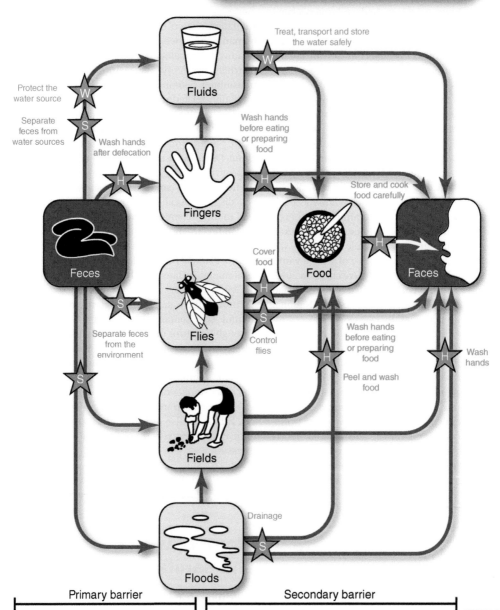

Note: The diagram is a summary of pathways: other associated routes may be important. Drinking water may be contaminated by a dirty water container, for example, or food may be infected by dirty cooking utensils.

WEDC

Figure 6.5 The "F" diagram.
Source: Reed *et al.* (2012), with permission.

Table 6.1 Water- and sanitation-related diseases.

Disease	Microbial agent	Mode of transmission	Symptoms
Cholera	*Vibrio cholerae*	Ingestion of water or food contaminated with the bacterium *Vibrio cholerae*.	Extremely watery diarrhea, nausea, cramps, nosebleed, rapid pulse, and vomiting. Bacteria manifests in feces, 7–14 days after infection.
Dracunculiasis (guinea-worm disease)	*Dracunculus medinensis*	Ingestion of water from stagnant sources contaminated with parasites (tiny water fleas) that carry infective guinea-worm larvae.	Allergic reaction, rash, nausea, vomiting, and diarrhea. Symptoms usually appear a year after infection. Shortly before worm emerges, one may develop a fever and have swelling and pain in the infected area. Over 90% of worms appear on legs and feet, but may occur anywhere on the body.
Schistosomiasis (bilharzia or snail fever)	*Schistosoma*	Contact with contaminated fresh water (e.g., lakes, ponds, rivers, dams) inhabited by snails infected with one of the five varieties of the *Schistosoma* parasite, through daily chores and activities such as bathing, doing laundry, farming, fishing, fetching water, herding animals, and swimming.	Blood in urine (depending on the type of parasite and its location), bloody diarrhea, anemia, fever, chills, cough, inflammation and muscle aches. Infected persons may develop a rash or itchy skin days after being infected.
Typhoid fever	*Salmonella typhi*	Ingestion of food or water contaminated with the feces or urine of infected people.	Fever up to 40 °C (104 °F), profuse sweating, diarrhea malaise, headache, constipation or diarrhea, rose-colored spots on chest, and enlarged spleen and liver. Usually develops 1–3 weeks after exposure, and may be mild or severe.

Sources: Carter Center (2016). World Health Organization (2015c, 2016, n.d.).

On a daily basis, women and girls head out at dawn and at dusk to collect water to meet their family's water needs. This routine makes them easy targets for assault, harassment, and rape by men who sometimes ambush them. As women and girls usually travel long distances to collect water, they end up spending a greater part of their day and time on the journey and therefore miss opportunities for education, productive economic activities, or leisure. In Egypt, for example, an estimated 30% of women walk over an hour a day to meet their family's water needs. According to studies conducted by WHO, women in developing countries cumulatively spend 40 billion hours annually collecting and carrying water from unimproved sources to their homes. In some mountainous regions of East Africa, women use up to 27% of their caloric intake just collecting water (World Health Organization, 2012).

On average, water weighs about 8.35 pounds per gallon, and many women in developing countries carry up to 5 gallons of water per trip. This, however, does not include the weight of the babies they carry on their backs on those trips. Carrying heavy containers of water on their head often leaves women and girls with musculoskeletal disorders, which often impairs their ability to function normally. According to WHO, an estimated $24 billion in economic value is lost each year due to the time spent collecting water.

Women and girls in rural areas in the developing world bear the most burden where there are no sanitation facilities. The lack of sanitation facilities at institutions of learning affects girls' menstrual hygiene management, and consequently, their school attendance and performance. Defecating in open spaces compromises the safety and dignity of women and girls, and especially pregnant women. In communities where some type of sanitation facility exists, its cleaning and maintenance is often the responsibility of women and girls.

Even though women are the main collectors and transporters of water and the custodians of family hygiene, they often tend to be left out of the planning and implementation of rural water supply and sanitation projects. Thus, it is not surprising that many rural water supply and sanitation projects implemented in the past failed. A study conducted by the International Water and Sanitation Center of community water and sanitation projects in 88 communities in 2008, found that projects designed and implemented with the involvement of women were more effective, successful, and sustainable than those that did not. Presently, the trend is shifting towards increased women involvement in rural water and sanitation projects. Women are not only performing manual tasks, but are also actively involved in discussions around the selection and siting of communal water and sanitation facilities.

Effects of unsafe water and poor sanitation on global health

Unsafe water and poor sanitation trap people and entire communities in a cycle of ill health and unproductivity. They suppress economic growth, put undue pressure on already overwhelmed health systems, cause disability and premature death, and have negative social consequences for populations.

Health effects

In developing countries, the poor, and especially children in poorer households, suffer disproportionately from water and sanitation-related diseases (Prüss et al., 2002). They experience diarrheal diseases, dehydration, nausea, vomiting, and sometimes underweight, which in turn predisposes them to acute respiratory infections, malaria, and sometimes even death. Globally, diarrhea is the fourth leading cause of child mortality. Every year, it claims the lives of about 1.8 billion people, 90% of which are children under the age of five. Every 2.5 minutes, diarrhea claims the life of a child.

Cholera is a highly infectious water- and sanitation-related disease that causes acute, watery diarrhea, dehydration, low blood pressure, vomiting, muscle cramps, and rapid heart rate. In severe cases it causes acute renal failure, severe electrolyte imbalances, and coma. If left untreated, the dehydration that cholera causes can lead to shock and death hours after infection. Cholera is endemic in Africa, the Americas, Asia, and Oceania. Worldwide, it causes about 1.4 to 4.3 million cases of disease and 28 000 to 142 000 deaths per year. In 2013, 47 countries reported a total of 129 064 cases of cholera to WHO. Of these cases, 43% were reported from Africa and more than 47% were reported from the Americas. This included the outbreak that occurred in Haiti at the end of October 2010, which later spread to the Dominican Republic (Global Health Observatory, 2015).

Malaria is also a water-related disease that is endemic in 97 countries and territories. As mentioned earlier, it is the leading cause of illness and death in children under the age of five and pregnant women in developing countries. In 2013, 198 million cases of malaria were reported worldwide. Ninety percent of the cases were in sub-Saharan Africa and among children under the age of five.

Economic effects

The economic costs associated with water and sanitation-related diseases cannot be overlooked. In addition to national costs and medical costs (direct and indirect), there are also losses in productive time, high outpatient and inpatient costs, patient travel expenditures, and medication costs.

National costs

According to WHO estimates, unsafe water and poor sanitation result in $260 billion in economic losses annually in developing countries (United Nations, 2014). In 18 sub-Saharan African countries including Central African Republic, Ghana, Kenya, Liberia, Madagascar, Nigeria, Rwanda, and Zambia, inadequate sanitation accounts for $5.5 billion and between 1% and 2.5% of GDP in economic losses annually. These losses affect about 554 million people, which is more than 50% of the entire population of Africa. Poor sanitation also negatively impacts between 0.5% and

7.2% of GDP in some Asian countries: $448 million or 7.2% of GDP in Cambodia, $53.8 billion or 6.4% of GDP in India, $6.3 billion or 2.3% of GDP in Indonesia, and $1 billion or 6.3% of GDP in Pakistan (Sanitation Drive, 2016).

In Bangladesh, the estimated annual economic impact of inadequate sanitation in 2007 was Tk. 295.48 billion ($4.23 billion), about 6.3% of the country's GDP. Health losses due to inadequate sanitation and hygiene had the most impact on the Bangladeshi economy. Financial losses owing to ill health and unsafe water was approximately TK. 34 554 million ($494 million) and premature deaths from diarrhea accounted for 70% of economic losses (Tk. 110 489 million) (Water and Sanitation Program, 2012a). In India, inadequate sanitation caused economic losses of about $53.8 billion, accounting for 6.4% of the country's GDP in 2006 alone (Water and Sanitation Program, 2016a).

Medical costs

Medical costs associated with water and sanitation-related diseases in the developing world are huge. The direct medical cost of diarrhea for families and households in developing countries ranges from $2.63 per episode in Gambia, to $4.11 in Mali, and $6.24 in Kenya (Rheingans, 2012). The cost of consultation, medication, user fees, and in some cases, hospitalization, puts a heavy burden on already over stretched household incomes. Indirect medical costs such as transport expenditures and indebtedness also further economic losses (Water and Sanitation Program, 2016b).

Productive time losses

Financial losses brought about by reduced productivity in Bangladesh in 2007 was Tk. 29 030 million due to diarrhea, Tk. 714 million due to helminthes or intestinal worms, and Tk. 0.24 million due to malaria. In Tanzania, losses in productivity brought about by sick visits to health clinics or hospitals, absenteeism from work or school, and the time spent caring for children under the age of five due to diarrheal diseases, cost the country $1.6 million each year (Water and Sanitation Program, 2012b).

The productivity costs associated with open defecation are higher than those associated with other types of unimproved sanitation. In Tanzania, time spent finding a suitable place to defecate in the open results in a loss of $14 million per annum. The losses in access time impact women more than men

as they are the caregivers and the one's who accompany young children, the sick, and elderly relatives to defecation sites (Water and Sanitation Program, 2012b).

Social effects

According to the UNDP and Unicef, children miss approximately 443 million days of school every year due to water-related illnesses, and an estimated 10% of girls of school-going age in Africa, do not attend school during menstruation, or drop out at puberty due to the absence of safe and separate sanitation facilities in schools (United Nations Children's Fund, 2003). In Uganda, malaria negatively affects the ability of about 60% of schoolchildren to learn. Open defecation brings about considerable social costs. In addition to the loss of dignity and privacy, it creates a security issue, in that, it puts people at risk of physical attack and sexual violence.

Investing in safe water supply and sanitation

Investments in safe water supply and improved sanitation are essential, as the benefits to be derived mostly outstrip their cost. Access to safe water facilities located within reasonable distances of beneficiary communities reduces water collection time and thus, increases school attendance rates for girls, as they no longer have to walk long distances to collect water. A study conducted in 2011, on water hauling and girls' school attendance in Ghana, found that the proportion of girls attending school increased from 8 to 12% when water collection time was reduced by 15 minutes. Another water haulage study conducted in Morocco, Pakistan, and Yemen found that a 1 hour reduction in water-collection time increased girls' school attendance by 11%, 18% and 8%, respectively (Nauges and Strand, 2013). In Bangladesh, the provision of separate sanitation facilities for boys and girls boosted girls' school attendance rates by 11% annually from 1992 to 1999.

Investing in safe water supply and improved sanitation can reduce the incidence of diseases by approximately 28%, prevent ill health, reduce healthcare costs, and boost workforce productivity. It can also result in about $32 billion in economic gain globally per year (World Health Organization, 2015a). Investing in safe water and improved sanitation can attract foreign direct investments, and positively impact economic growth and development. According to the World Bank, for every dollar invested in safe water and the elimination of open defecation, there is a $4 and $6 economic return respectively, and, per WHO, investments in water supply, sanitation, and hygiene can reduce global burden of disease by 10%.

Global water and sanitation coverage and progress

Global water and sanitation coverage and progress have not been identical. The score card shows greater improvements in water coverage than in sanitation, with certain regions and countries doing better than others.

Water

At the end of 2010, the world had met and exceeded by 1%, the MDG target (89%) of halving the proportion of people without access to safe drinking water. This was well in advance of the 2015 deadline. To date, 147 countries in the regions of Eastern Asia, Latin America and the Caribbean, Southern Asia, South-Eastern Asia, and the Western Pacific have met their water MDG targets (see Figure 6.6), but those in the Caucasus and Central Asia, Northern Africa, Oceania, and sub-Saharan Africa regions have not.

Presently, 4.2 billion people worldwide have access to piped connections and 2.4 billion have access to other improved sources, such as public taps, protected wells, and boreholes (World Health Organization, 2015b). Although global water coverage thus far has been impressive, 663 million people around the world still lack access to safe drinking water and 159 million of this population, depends on surface water.

Between 1990 and 2015, water coverage in rural areas improved significantly (see Figure 6.6). This upsurge can be attributed to the increased implementation of rural water supply projects sponsored by bilateral development agencies, such as the Canadian International Development Agency (CIDA), the Danish International Development Agency (DANIDA), and the Japanese International Cooperation Agency (JICA). By 2015, 96% of people living in urban areas and 84% of the people living in rural areas had gained access to improved drinking water sources.

The reliance on surface water in rural areas in the developing world dropped from 10% to 5% between 1990 and 2010. The number of people who relied on tanker trucks and small vendors for their water supply needs increased from 44 million to 85 million, and the number of people using boreholes increased from 1 billion to 1.3 billion.

Sanitation

In contrast to the situation regarding water, the world did not achieve the MDG sanitation target of 75% coverage by the end of 2015. Global sanitation coverage lags behind. Although between 1990 and 2015, 68%, or 2.1 billion of the world's population, gained access to improved sanitation facilities, 2.5 billion people still lack access to improved sanitation facilities and about 946 million of that population practices open defecation in water bodies, behind bushes, or in street gutters. A significant proportion of people who practice open defecation live in just three regions of the world (Southern Asia, sub-Saharan Africa, and Eastern Asia), and 40% of that population lives in Southern Asia (United Nations Children's Fund and World Health Organization, 2015).

Sanitation coverage in rural and urban areas is varied. Globally, about 82% of urban populations and 51% of rural populations have access to improved sanitation facilities. Indeed, more people in urban (398 million) areas use shared sanitation facilities than people in the rural areas (240 million). Presently, 95 countries in the regions of the Caucasus and Central Asia, Eastern Asia, Northern Africa, and Western Asia have met their MDG sanitation target (see Figure 6.7)

Global water and sanitation challenges

Population growth

Population growth has implications for a country's ability to meet the water and sanitation needs of its citizens. In the developing world, the provision of safe water and improved sanitation facilities have not kept up with population growth. In 2015 for example, the population of sub-Saharan Africa and Oceania grew by 94% and 68%, respectively but, unfortunately, only 36% of the added population in these regions gained access to improved sanitation.

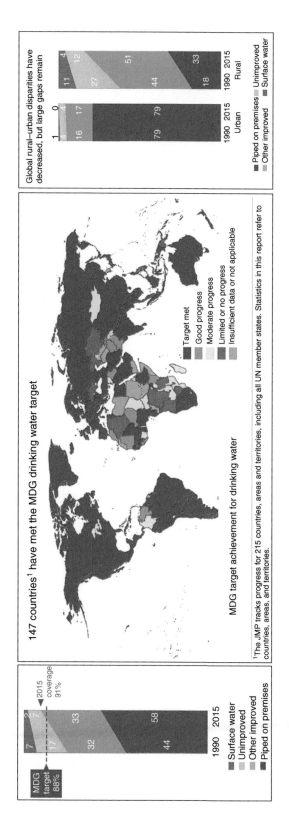

Figure 6.6 Global water coverage, 1990–2015.

Source: United Nations Children's Fund and World Health Organization (2015), with permission.

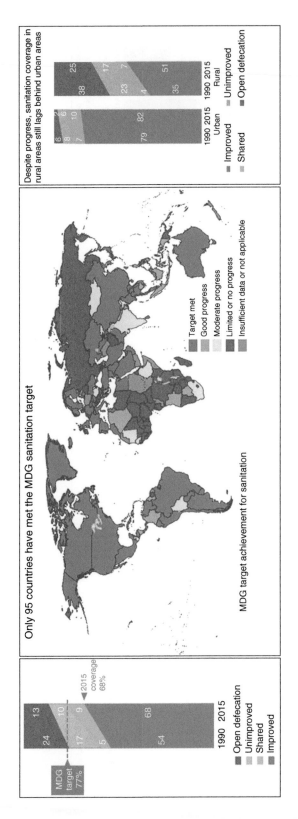

Figure 6.7 Global sanitation coverage, 1990–2015.

Source: United Nations Children's Fund and World Health Organization (2015), with permission.

Financial support

In most developing countries, international financial flows in the form of overseas development assistance (ODA) fall short of what is needed for the provision of universal water and sanitation coverage. Compared to other major social sectors, the water and sanitation sector appears to receive relatively low ODA funding. This is especially true of developing countries that have progressed from a low income status, to a relatively higher income status. In 1997, over 8% of ODA was allocated for water and sanitation in developing countries, exceeding what was allocated to other sectors, such as education and health. However, in 2008, things changed; the proportion of ODA allocated to water and sanitation dropped from 8% to 5%, while what was allocated to health increased from 7% to 11.5%, and that for education remained steady at around 7% (United Nations Children's Fund and World Health Organization, 2015).

Political will

The political will to allocate increased national funds to improve sanitation and hygiene is low in developing countries. Current national investments in sanitation in many developing countries is less than 0.1% of GDP. In Africa, only a few countries have made efforts to invest between 0.1% and 0.5% of their GDP in sanitation, despite commitments made by Ministers and Heads of Delegations responsible for sanitation and hygiene from 32 countries, to increase budgetary allocations for sanitation to no less than 0.5% of GDP at the AfricaSan + 5 conference held in Durban, South Africa in 2008 (Water and Sanitation Program, 2016b).

In Uganda, investments in sanitation and hygiene have been historically low, with coverage in some districts, dropping to below 20%. This state of affairs can be attributed to the reduction of national funds for water, sanitation, and hygiene by more than 50% between 2004 and 2012 (Williams and Kyomuhangi, 2015). Current investments in sanitation in Tanzania are also low: less than 0.1% of GDP. Reduced investments prevent the realization of health, welfare, and economic benefits associated with improved sanitation.

The breakdown of expenditure between sanitation and drinking water in many developing countries shows that funding for drinking water is about three or more times higher than that for sanitation. According to WHO estimates, about

$9.5 billion would have been needed per annum to meet the MDG sanitation target of reducing by 50%, the proportion of people without access to basic sanitation.

Sustainability

To be sustainable, sanitation systems must be economically viable, accessible, and socially acceptable. In Ghana, access to improved sanitation in rural areas is progressing, but is not where it should be. Budgetary allocation for rural sanitation is about 0.1% of the national budget. This is inadequate, as over 60% of the Ghanaian population lives in rural areas.

The provision of improved communal latrines in rural areas in Ghana is demand driven and based on household subsidies (from national budgetary allocations) and on bilateral and multilateral donor support. While this approach promotes the acquisition of communal and household latrines, it has been found to be unsustainable, as funding from external donors is not guaranteed, and can only be made available when donors choose to provide. Although the provision of household subsidies for latrine construction is laudable, the inability of households to come up with supplemental funds or in-kind contributions to finance facilities, defeats the purpose. Affordability and ability to pay for latrines is crucial and necessary if sanitation behavior change is to be achieved and sustained in the long term.

Global action and strategies

The global community has embarked on several initiatives to accelerate progress towards a world where people have universal access to safe drinking water and improved sanitation.

Following the United Nations Water Conference at Mar del Plata in 1977, the International Decade for Clean Drinking Water (1981–1990) was launched. The aim of the decade was to encourage developing countries to prioritize and make access to clean water and sanitary waste disposal available to their populations by 1990. Thanks to the decade, 1.3 billion people in developing countries gained access to safe drinking water and almost 770 million to improved sanitation. However, the provision of services during the decade could not keep up with increasing population size and rapid urbanization. Thus, in 2000, United Nations Member States adopted a set of eight MDGs aimed at reducing poverty and improving human health among other things. The seventh MDG focused on ensuring environmental sustainability and target 7c of that goal sought to halve by 2015, the proportion of the global population without sustainable access to safe drinking water and basic sanitation.

The world met its water MDG target in 2010. This notwithstanding, almost 700 million people still lack access to safe drinking water globally. The world did not achieve its MDG target for sanitation by 2015. Although more than a quarter of the world's population gained access to improved sanitation since 1990, 2.5 billion people still lack access to improved sanitation and about 1 billion people practice open defecation.

In 2003, 15 years after the International Decade for Clean Drinking Water was launched, the United Nations General Assembly launched a second International Water Decade dubbed the International Decade for Action "Water for Life" for the period 2005–2015. The aim of this decade was to promote efforts towards the attainment of the water-related MDG by 2015.

Recognizing the world's sanitation crises and the need to draw global attention to the situation, the United Nations General Assembly in December 2006, declared 2008 the International Year of Sanitation (IYS). The central focus of the IYS was to accelerate global progress towards the attainment of the sanitation-related MDG. Focusing on five key messages (sanitation is vital for health, contributes to social development, is a good economic investment, helps the environment, and is achievable), the IYS sought to generate new resources to address the crisis at the international, national and community levels, increase global sanitation awareness and commitment, and to encourage demand-driven, sustainable, and traditional solutions to sanitation, to mention a few of its aims.

From October 9 to 14, 2011, the landmark Global Forum on Sanitation and Hygiene was held in Mumbai, India. Although the forum did not result in an official declaration, statement, or manifesto, it provided participants with a platform for dialogue on sanitation and created global energy around hygiene and sanitation. As the deadline for achieving the United Nations MDGs loomed, and as progress towards global attainment of the MDG target on sanitation remained elusive, Jan Eliasson, the UN Deputy Secretary-General, on behalf of the United Nations Secretary General, initiated a Call to Action on Sanitation in 2014 in an attempt to renew global efforts towards sanitation progress by 2015 and beyond. His intent was to start a global campaign to encourage increased national government discussions on the taboo or unpopular topic of sanitation, to break the silence, and spur on action to tackle the global issue of poor sanitation and open defecation in particular.

Discussion points

1 Of what importance are safe water and improved sanitation to global health?
2 What are some types of improved water supply systems? Describe them.
3 What are some types of unsafe sanitation facilities? Describe them.
4 How significant is the role of women in water and sanitation?
5 What are the water-related diseases? How are they transmitted?
6 What are the health, social, and economic effects of unsafe water and poor sanitation on populations?
7 Describe global progress made towards safe water and improved sanitation.
8 What national benefits are there to be derived from investing in safe water and improved sanitation?
9 What are the main challenges of poor sanitation?
10 How relevant were the two United Nations Decades to the improvement of global water and sanitation?

REFERENCES

Carlton, E. J., Liang, S., McDowell, J. Z. *et al.* (2012). Regional disparities in the burden of disease attributable to unsafe water and poor sanitation in China. *Bulletin of the World Health Organization* **90**, 578–587.

Carter Center (2016) *Schistosomiasis*, http://www.cartercenter.org/health/schistosomiasis/index.html (accessed 21 October, 2016).

Global Health Observatory (2015) *Number of Reported Cholera Cases*, http://www.who.int/gho/epidemic_diseases/cholera/cases_text/en/ (accessed October 22, 2016).

Himalayan Institute (2011) *Clean Water for Takui, Cameroon*, https://www.himalayaninstitute.org/2011/06/06/clean-water-for-takui-cameroon/ (accessed 21 October, 2016).

National Academy of Sciences (2007) *Safe Drinking Water is Essential*, https://www.koshland-science-museum.org/water/html/en/Treatment/Water-based.html (accessed October 22, 2016).

Nauges, C. and Strand, J. (2013) *Water Hauling and Girls' School Attendance: Some New Evidence from Ghana*. Policy research working paper no. WPS 6443. World Bank, Washington DC, http://documents.worldbank.org/curated/en/2013/05/17714533/water-hauling-girls-school-attendance-some-new-evidence-ghana (accessed October 22, 2016).

Parker, A. (2014) *A Pit Latrine in Madagascar*, http://blogs.egu.eu/network/gfgd/2014/01/06/3364/ (accessed October 22, 2016)

Prüss, A., Kay, D., Fewtrell, L. and Bartram, J. (2002). Estimating the burden of disease from water, sanitation, and hygiene at a global level. *Environmental Health Perspectives* **110**, 537–554.

Reed, B. J., Skinner, B. H., Scott, R. E., and Shaw, R. J. (2012) *The "F" Diagram*, WEDC, Loughborough University, Loughborough, http://wedc.lboro.ac.uk/resources/factsheets/FS009_FDI_Pages_Poster.pdf (accessed October 21, 2016).

Rheingans, R. K. (2012) Exploring household economic impacts of childhood diarrheal illnesses in three African settings. *Clinical Infectious Diseases* **55**(Suppl 4), S317–S326.

Sanitation Drive (2016) *Fast Facts*, http://sanitationdrive2015.org/resources-2/fast-facts/ (accessed October 22, 2016).

Sustainable Sanitation Alliance (SuSanA) Secretariat (2009) *Unimproved Sanitation Facilities*, https://www.flickr.com/photos/gtzecosan/5014325656 (accessed October 21, 2016).

Sustainable Sanitation Alliance (SuSanA) Secretariat (2010) *Prefabricated Pour Flush Toilet Connected to Soak Pit*, https://www.flickr.com/photos/gtzecosan/5277540655/ (accessed October 21, 2016).

Sustainable Sanitation Alliance (SuSanA) Secretariat (n.d.) *Prefabricated Pour Flush Toilet Connected to Soak Pit*, https://www.flickr.com/photos/gtzecosan/5277540655/ (accessed October 21, 2016).

United Nations (2014) *End Open Defecation*, http://www.un.org/millenniumgoals/endopendefecation.shtml (accessed October 22, 2016).

United Nations Children's Fund (2003) *WASH and Women*, http://www.unicef.org/wash/index_womenandgirls.html (accessed October 22, 2016).

United Nations Children's Fund and World Health Organization (2015) *Progress on Sanitation and Drinking Water – 2015 Update and MDG Assessment*, http://files.unicef.org/publications/files/Progress_on_Sanitation_and_Drinking_Water_2015_Update_.pdf, with permission (accessed October 22, 2016).

Water Charity (2012) *Small Mountains*, http://www.water4everyone.org/author/jack/ (accessed October 21, 2016).

Water Charity (2016) *Bonkwae Well Rehab and Water System Project, Ghana*, http://watercharity.com/country/ghana (accessed October 21, 2016).

Water and Sanitation Program (2012a) *Economic Impacts of Inadequate Sanitation in Bangladesh*, https://openknowledge.worldbank.org/bitstream/handle/10986/17349/717330WP0Box370SI0Bangladesh0Report.pdf;sequence=1 (accessed October 22, 2016).

Water and Sanitation Program (2012b). *Economic Impacts of Poor Sanitation in Africa, Tanzania*, https://www.wsp.org/sites/wsp.org/files/publications/WSP-Econ-San-TZ1.pdf (accessed October 22, 2016).

Water and Sanitation Program (2016a) *Inadequate Sanitataion Costs India the Equivalent of 6.4% of GDP*, https://www.wsp.org/featuresevents/features/inadequate-sanitation-costs-india-equivalent-64-cent-gdp (accessed October 22, 2016).

Water and Sanitation Program (2016b) *Inadequate Sanitataion Costs 18 African Countries around US$5.5 Billion Every Year*, https://www.wsp.org/FeaturesEvents/Features/inadequate-sanitation-costs-18-african-countries-around-us55-billion-each-ye (accessed October 22, 2016).

Williams, C. W. and Kyomuhangi, J. (2015) *Silent Emergency*, http://web.unep.org/ourplanet/may-2015/articles/silent-emergency (accessed October 22, 2016).

World Health Organization (2012) *Global Costs and Benefits of Drinking-Water Supply and Sanitation Interventions to Reach the MDG Target and Universal Coverage*, http://www.who.int/water_sanitation_health/publications/2012/globalcosts.pdf (accessed October 22, 2016).

World Health Organization (2015a) *Global Costs and Benefits of Drinking-Water Supply and Sanitation Interventions to Reach the MDG Target and Universal Coverage*, http://www.who.int/water_sanitation_health/publications/2012/globalcosts.pdf (accessed October 22, 2016).

World Health Organization (2015b) *Drinking Water*. Fact sheet no. 391, http://www.who.int/mediacentre/factsheets/fs391/en/ets/fs391/en/ (accessed October 22, 2016).

World Health Organization. (2015c) *Cholera*. Fact sheet, http://www.who.int/mediacentre/factsheets/fs107/en/ (accessed October 21, 2016).

World Health Organization (2016) *Typhoid Fever*, http://www.who.int/topics/typhoid_fever/en/ (accessed October 21, 2016).

World Health Organization (n.d.). *Ten Facts on Guinea Worm Disease*, http://www.who.int/features/factfiles/guinea_worm/facts/en/ (accessed October 21, 2016).

FURTHER READING

Inter-agency Task Force on Gender and Water (2006) G*ender, Water and Sanitation: A Policy Brief*, http://www.un.org/waterforlifedecade/pdf/un_water_policy_brief_2_gender.pdf (accessed October 22, 2016).

King, C. F. (2011). Schistosomiasis: challenges and opportunities, in: *The Causes and Impacts of Neglected Tropical and Zoonotic Diseases: Opportunities for Integrated Intervention Strategies* (ed. Institute of Medicine Forum on Microbial Threats). National Academic Press, Washington DC, pp. 323–341.

King, C. H. (2010) Parasites and poverty: The case of schistosomiasis. *Acta Tropica* **113**(2), 95–104.

King, C. H. and Dangerfield-Cha, M. (2008) The unacknowledged impact of chronic schistosomiasis. *Chronic Illness* **4**, 65–79.

King, C. H, Dickman, K., and Tisch, D. J. (2005) Reassessment of the cost of chronic helminthic infection: A meta-analysis of disability-related outcomes in endemic schistosomiasis. *The Lancet* **365**, 1561–1569.

King C. H, Sturrock, R. F., Karuiki, H. C., and Hamburger, J. (2006) Transmission control for schistosomiasis – why it matters now. *Trends in Parasitology* **22**(12), 575–582.

Lozano, R., Naghavi, M., Foreman, K., *et al.* (2012). Global and regional mortality from 235 causes of death for 20 age groups in 1990 and 2010: a systematic analysis for the Global Burden of Disease Study. *The Lancet* **9859**, 2095–2128.

Organization for Economic Corporation and Development (2013. *Financing Water and Sanitation in Developing Countries: The Contribution of External Aid*, http://www.oecd.org/dac/stats/Brochure_water_2013.pdf (accessed October 22, 2016).

Prüss-Ustin, A., Bartram, J., Clasen, T., *et al.* (2014) Burden of disease from inadequate water, sanitation and hygiene in low- and middle-income settings: a retrospective analysis of data from 145 countries. *Tropical Medicine and International Health* **19**(8), 894–905.

Water-related Disease Facts (2016), http://water.org/water-crisis/water-facts/disease/ (accessed October 22, 2016).

What is the Economic Impact of Malaria. (2016) https://www.k4health.org/sites/default/files/What%20is%20the%20Economic%20Impact%20of%20Malaria.pdf (accessed October 22, 2016).

7

Global hunger, nutrition, and food security

Learning objectives

By the end of this chapter, you will be able to:

✔ Discuss the difference between hunger and malnutrition;

✔ Describe the global burden of hunger and malnutrition;

✔ Discuss the effects of global food insecurity;

✔ Describe global challenges related to hunger, malnutrition, and food insecurity;

✔ List and explain at least two global strategies to reduce hunger and malnutrition.

Summary of key points

Issues related to hunger, nutrition, and food security are global concerns, hence their inclusion in the recently expired Millennium Development Goals (MDGs) and the recently adopted Sustainable Development Goals (SDGs). In 2000, MDG 1 sought to halve, between 1990 and 2015, the proportion of people who suffer from hunger. Launched in 2015, SDG 2 seeks to by 2030, end hunger and ensure access by all people, particularly the poor and vulnerable including infants, to safe, nutritious and sufficient food all year round. It also seeks to end all forms of malnutrition, double agricultural productivity and incomes of small-scale food producers, and ensure sustainable food production systems through the implementation of resilient agricultural practices. This chapter focuses on hunger, malnutrition, and food security. Specifically, it discusses the global burden of hunger and malnutrition, the causes of food insecurity, how to measure hunger and nutritional status, as well as micronutrient deficiencies. It also discusses some challenges associated with hunger, malnutrition and food insecurity, and global action and strategies to address them.

Global hunger and malnutrition

Studies indicate that the world produces enough food to feed the over 7 billion people who inhabit the Earth, so the questions are: why do one in eight people go hungry every day, why are some people malnourished, and why are there food shortages in certain parts of the world? The reasons are myriad.

Global Health: Issues, Challenges, and Global Action Lecture Notes, First Edition. Elizabeth A. Armstrong-Mensah.
© 2017 John Wiley & Sons Ltd. Published 2017 by John Wiley & Sons Ltd.

Hunger and its causes

Hunger is the uneasy or painful sensation caused by the want of food (*Oxford English Dictionary*). It is not having enough food to eat to meet one's energy requirements. According to the World Food Program (WFP), hunger is one of the world's greatest health risks. While hunger over a sustained period may lead to malnutrition, the absence of hunger does not necessarily suggest the absence of malnutrition in a population. Globally, poverty makes it difficult for families to meet their food and nutrition needs. Without income, farmers are unable to buy seed for planting, and where the existence is one of subsistence, they are unable to feed their families. Poverty undermines health, and the ability of people to obtain an education and thus, seek gainful employment. As of 2015, there were just over 1 billion poor people in the world living on $1.25 a day or less, a reduction from 1.91 billion in 1990 (World Bank, 2015, 2016).

Inadequate agricultural infrastructure, manifested in the form of unreliable water supply, the lack of adequate storage facilities, and inconsistent, undependable and expensive transportation, have a deleterious impact on crop yield, food availability, and food prices. Adverse weather conditions due to climate change affect soil fertility and can cause soil salination when irrigation systems dry up and leave toxic levels of salt in the soil. The outcome is decreased osmotic potential of the soil, and the inability of plants to take up water from the soil. Salinization is a global issue especially in the semi-arid areas of the Middle East, China's North Plain, Central Asia, the San Joaquin Valley of California, and in the Colorado River Basin; areas where the soil profile is never (or rarely) well flushed. Famine, floods, tropical storms, and long periods of drought also cause hunger. In 2011, the recurrent drought in certain parts of Ethiopia and Kenya resulted in enormous crop failure and in the loss of livestock.

Improper land-use practices by humans such as deforestation and its concomitant erosion of fertile farmlands affect food production. Armed conflicts, such as those which occurred in Liberia (1989–2003) and Sudan (2003–2004) disrupt farming activities and cause hunger, as they leave people without a means of producing food to feed themselves. In times of war, feuding factions sometimes use food as a weapon of war. In this situation they may seize or destroy farms and livestock of the opponent, raze down local markets, mine fields with land mines, or contaminate water sources as a means of securing subjugation. Joseph Stalin of the Soviet Union and Adolf Hitler of Germany both used access to food to destroy internal opposition, reward accomplishment, punish failure, and to establish the class distinctions of their "new orders."

Malnutrition

Referred to as a nutrition disorder, malnutrition is a health condition that results from eating a diet that is deficient or too high in nutrients (protein, carbohydrates, vitamins or minerals) (cf. *Dorland's Illustrated Medical Dictionary*), starvation due to food shortages, eating disorders, or the inability of the human body to absorb, assimilate, or adequately utilize food consumed. Some diseases and health conditions prevent the human body from digesting or absorbing food properly. For example, untreated celiac disease, an intestinal condition triggered by eating foods with gluten, a protein found in wheat, rye and barley, can damage the intestinal villi, rendering them ineffective to absorb nutrients. Cystic fibrosis also prevents the absorption of nutrients by the body, as the disease affects the pancreas, the organ responsible for producing enzymes needed for food digestion.

Many consider malnutrition as only associated with undernutrition or insufficient nutrient intake. This is an inaccurate view, as it also has to do with the overconsumption of nutrients and food to the extent that they adversely affect one's health. Sustained overnutrition can develop into obesity, which increases the risk of serious health conditions, such as cardiovascular disease and type 2 diabetes. Until recently, overnutrition was considered a health condition that pertained to only developed countries. Recent studies, however, point to the fact that it is also now widespread in developing countries where hunger is prevalent. Capturing this reality, the World Health Organization (WHO) stated:

> In the poorest countries, even though infectious diseases and undernutrition dominate their current disease burden, the major risk factors for chronic diseases are spreading. The prevalence of overweight and obesity is increasing in developing countries, and even in low-income groups in richer countries (World Health Organization, 2004: 2).

In 2002, WHO reported that the number of overweight and obese women in the Eastern Mediterranean region and North Africa surpassed that in the United States, while the number of overweight and obese women in Eastern Europe and Latin America were comparable to those in the United States (Chopra *et al.*, 2002).

Malnutrition may be mild with no symptoms, or very severe, causing irreversible damage to the body. Health conditions related to malnutrition are beriberi, bulimia, kwashiorkor, pellagra, rickets, scurvy, and vitamin deficiencies. Children under the age of five, pregnant and lactating women, people with disability, the elderly, and the poor are the most vulnerable groups for malnutrition. In children, diarrhea, malaria, HIV/AIDS, pneumonia, the lack of optimal breastfeeding, and inappropriate complementary feeding can cause undernutrition.

In pregnant women, malnutrition can result in low birth weight babies who due to their health condition, become susceptible to a variety of infectious diseases, or premature death. The symptoms of malnutrition vary and depend on its cause. General symptoms include fatigue, dizziness, and weight loss (Blössner and de Onis, 2005). According to WHO, majority of the world's underweight children live in Southern Asia.

Key concepts related to hunger and malnutrition

To aid the understanding of issues related to hunger and malnutrition, some frequently used terms are described.

Wasting

Sometimes referred to as moderate acute malnutrition, wasting occurs when the body consumes its own muscle and body fat tissues as it searches for nutrients and energy it needs to survive after using up its energy reserves. Wasting may be caused by exceptionally low energy intake, the loss of nutrients due to infection, or by both factors. Wasting slows down the body's metabolism, disrupts thermal regulation, impairs kidney function, and diminishes the capacity of the immune system (Action Against Hunger, 2009).

If left untreated, moderately malnourished children may experience severe acute malnutrition (edema), severe stunting, or death. Children with severe wasting look elderly and have extremely thin and skeletal bodies. Wasting differs from stunting in the sense that it has a shorter duration than the latter.

In children, wasting is measured by a weight for height indicator between minus two and minus three standard deviations from the median weight for height of the standard reference population (United Nations Children's Fund, n.d., a).

It is computed as follows, and the less than 80% (close to –2 Z-score) cutoff is frequently used:

$$WFH = \frac{\text{weight of a given child}}{\text{median weight for a given child at that weight}} \times 100$$

In adults, a person with a body mass index less than 18.5 is regarded as wasting.

Stunting

Defined by WHO as weight for height below minus three standard deviations from the median weight for height of the standard reference population (World Health Organization, 2016b), stunting is also reduced growth rate in human development over time. Children who are stunted or chronically malnourished are normally proportional, but are shorter for their age. Stunting may occur before birth in the fetus due to poor maternal nutrition, or due to poor feeding practices, poor food quality, and frequent exposure to infections such as diarrhea and helminthiasis in children. Stunted children are at greater risk for delayed mental development, poor academic performance, reduced cognitive ability, infection, and premature death. Stunted women may suffer childbirth complications as a result of smaller pelvis and may pass the condition on to their next generation, creating an intergenerational cycle of malnutrition.

Stunting in children is irreversible after 18 months. Thus, interventions to improve child nutritional status must target women during pregnancy and children from birth to 18 months of age. This is the critical window of opportunity. A 2006 World Bank study of children under the age of five across several regions of the world confirmed this fact. From Figure 7.1, it can be observed that the largest decline in nutritional status occurred in the first 18 months of life, despite the region.

Micronutrient deficiencies

The nonconsumption of foods with adequate quantities of essential micronutrients can create a nutritional deficiency in the body, which in turn may cause serious health problems. Unlike macronutrients, such as carbohydrates, proteins, and fats, micronutrients are permanently required by the body in very small amounts. Micronutrients are primarily vitamins and minerals. They are essential for the healthy functioning of the body's systems for a range of physiological functions, from bone growth to brain function. The adult human body needs dietary trace minerals (copper, chromium, fluoride, iodine, iron, molybdenum, manganese, selenium, and zinc) of less than 100 mg/day, as opposed to macrominerals (sodium,

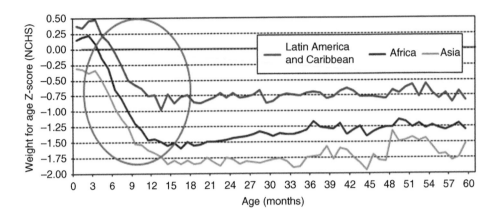

Figure 7.1 Chronic malnutrition: The window of opportunity.
Source: United Nations Children Fund (n.d., b).

chloride, potassium, phosphorus, magnesium, and calcium), which are needed in larger quantities. Vitamins are needed by the human body in different quantities and are classified into A, B, C, D, E, and K by their biological and chemical activities. Deficiencies in iron, iodine, vitamin A, and zinc cause serious health consequences for people all over the world.

Iron

Iron deficiency is the most widespread form of malnutrition globally, affecting millions of people. It is caused by insufficient amounts of iron in the body due to inadequate iron intake or reduced iron absorption by the body. Iron produces red blood cells in the body, and helps to carry oxygen in the blood from the lungs to the rest of the body. It also helps to maintain healthy cells, skin and hair, enhances muscle formation, and provides the oxygen necessary for muscle contraction. Without iron, muscles lose their tone and elasticity.

Iron deficiency is particularly prevalent among women who have heavy menstrual periods, people who loose blood during major surgery or physical trauma, and people who have gastrointestinal diseases such as celiac disease (sprue), inflammatory bowel diseases (such as ulcerative colitis), or Crohn's disease. Vegetarians, vegans, and other people whose diets do not include iron-rich foods may be deficient in iron.

Symptoms of iron deficiency are reduced cognitive development, fatigue, lethargy, pale coloring, feeling cold, restless leg syndrome, decreased productivity, difficulty maintaining body temperature, decreased immune function, hair loss, irritability, Plummer–Vinson syndrome, and glossitis (an inflamed tongue).

Iron deficiency affects the cognitive development of 40–60% of children aged 6–24 months in developing countries. It also causes anemia, excessive menstrual bleeding or nonmenstrual bleeding, and rheumatoid arthritis. Indeed, over 30% of the world's population is anemic and about 20% of all maternal deaths are due to anemia. Eating read meat, poultry, pork, seafood, beans, dark leafy vegetables, iron fortified cereals, and peas may help to reduce iron deficiency. Consuming high-iron foods with citrus juices or foods rich in vitamin C increases iron absorption.

Iodine

Iodine deficiency affects about 780 million people worldwide. Iodine is a vital dietary element for the synthesis of the thyroid hormones, thyroxine (T_4), and triiodothyronine (T_3). These hormones control cellular oxidation and therefore affect calorigenesis, thermoregulation, and intermediary metabolism. A healthy human body should contain 15–20 mg of iodine, 70 to 80% of which will be found in the thyroid gland (Kapil, 2007a; Stanbury, 1987).

Iodine deficiency causes goiter (swelling of the thyroid gland), brain damage, and mental retardation. In pregnant women, iodine deficiency may cause retarded fetal growth, fetal death in the womb, infant death within a week of birth, and fetal wastage such as abortion, still birth, and congenital abnormalities, however, firm evidence to support the aforementioned is limited (Hetzel, 1997). According to a United Nations Children Fund (Unicef) report, nearly 20 million children are born mentally impaired because their mothers did not consume enough iodine during pregnancy.

The severely impacted suffer cretinism, a condition associated with severe mental retardation and physical stunting.

Approximately 90% of iodine can be obtained from food, and the remaining 10%, from water. Seaweeds, spongy shells, sea fish, green vegetables and leaves grown in iodine rich soil, milk, meat, cereals, and common salt fortified with small quantities of potassium iodate are rich sources of iodine.

Zinc

Zinc is a trace mineral that supports the body's immune system from pathogens, infections, and disease. It helps with the breakdown of carbohydrates, which produces energy, growth, the division and reproduction of cells, the healing of wounds, tissue repair, and the stabilization of cellular components and membranes. An estimated 60% of zinc in the human body is found in the skeletal muscle and 30% in bone mass (United Nations Food and Agriculture Organization and World Health Organization, 2001).

Zinc deficiency is caused by insufficient dietary consumption or absorption, augmented zinc excretion, or increased bodily need for zinc. Zinc deficiency is associated with growth failure, hair loss, impotence, eye and skin conditions, loss of appetite, weakened immunity, diarrhea, pneumonia, weight loss, delayed wound healing, taste changes, and mental slowness (United Nations World Food Program, 2016b).

Red meat, poultry, oyster, crab, lobster, pulses, nuts and legumes, wholegrain cereals, fortified breakfast cereal, and dairy products like cheese are good dietary sources of zinc (Office of Dietary Supplements, National Institutes of Health, 2013). Increasing zinc levels in the soil and thus crops, is an effective preventative measure of zinc deficiency.

Vitamin A

Vitamin A is a group of related nutrients that provide different health benefits. There are two forms of vitamin A: retinoids (which are found in animal foods) and carotenoids (which are found in plant foods). These two forms of vitamin A are chemically different (World's Healthiest Foods, 2006). Retinoid forms of vitamin A help with pregnancy and childbirth, infancy, growth, night vision, red blood cell production, and resistance to infectious disease. Carotenoid forms of vitamin A function as antioxidant and anti-inflammatory nutrients.

Vitamin A deficiency causes blindness in children, night blindness and increased mortality rates in pregnant women, weak immune systems, increased child vulnerability to diseases, and the risk of mortality from diarrhea, measles, and malaria. Worldwide, about 250 000 to 500 000 children become blind every year as a consequence of vitamin A deficiency. Around 50% of these children die within a year of losing their sight (Boyd, 2012).

Foods rich in the retinoid form of vitamin A include cow milk, shrimp, eggs, salmon, halibut, cheese, yogurt, scallops, sardines, tuna, cod, and chicken, and foods rich in the carotenoid form of vitamin A are fruits and vegetables.

Global burden of hunger and malnutrition

Hunger

An estimated 795 million people in the world lack access to enough food, and approximately 75% of this number live in Asia. Although the percentage of hungry people in Southern Asia dropped in recent times, the same cannot be said of Western Asia (United Nations World Food Program, 2016b). Per available statistics, Southern Asia has the highest hunger burden, with a total of about 281 million undernourished people.

Sub-Saharan Africa has been reported to have a high *prevalence* (percentage of population) of hunger – one in four people on that continent is undernourished. About 66 million children in developing countries of primary (elementary) school age, go to school on an empty stomach. According to the WFP, $3.2 billion is needed per year to meet the food needs of these 66 million children.

Malnutrition

Women and young children in developing countries usually bear the brunt of diseases associated with malnutrition. In Africa and South Asia, about 27 to 51% of women of reproductive age are underweight. Approximately 10% of adolescent girls in Indonesia aged 15 to 19 are either mothers with their first child or are pregnant. Most of the pregnant girls have poor nutritional status. This has implications for the weight and health of their babies (United Nations World Food Program, 2014).

Poor nutrition accounts for 45% of deaths in children under the age of five. That is about 3.1 million child deaths per year. In spite of the steady progress made after the 2012 crisis in Mali, 2.5 million

Table 7.1 Number of children under age five who are moderately or severely wasted.

Ranked by burden (2011)	Country	Year	Wasting (%, moderate or severe)	Wasting (%, severe)	Number of wasted children, 2011 (moderate or severe, thousands)
1	India	2005–2006	20	6	25 461
2	Nigeria	2008	14	7	3783
3	Pakistan	2011	15	6	3339
4	Indonesia	2010	13	6	2820
5	Bangladesh	2011	16	4	2251
6	China	2010	3	–	1891
7	Ethiopia	2011	10	3	1156
8	Democratic Republic of the Congo	2010	9	3	1024
9	Sudan	2010	16	5	817
10	Philippines	2008	7	–	769

Source: United Nations Children Fund. (2013).

Malians still struggle to feed themselves and their families. Consequently, about 30% of children under the age of two in Mali are chronically malnourished. Through its nutrition programs, the WFP in 2015 provided food assistance to 1.1 million people across Mali in an attempt to address the hunger issue in the country (United Nations World Food Program, 2015c).

In El Salvador, 17% of children under the age of five also suffer from chronic malnutrition. In 2008, 1% of this population suffered from acute malnutrition, and in 2013, 37 of the 262 municipalities in the country were identified as having acute malnutrition rates above 2.5%. In Indonesia, malnutrition costs the government more than $5 billion annually in the form of lost productivity and diminished physical capability (United Nations World Food Program, 2014). Overweight and obesity in adults in Indonesia has almost doubled in the last decade and is causing a quick rise in overnutrition. In 2011, there were about 52 million wasted children under the age of five worldwide, with about 70% of that population living in South-Central Asia (United Nations Children's Fund, World Health Organization, and World Bank, 2012). Sixty percent of the entire world's children under the age of five with moderate and severe wasting live in ten countries, and over 10% of those children live in Africa and Asia. Between 2008 and 2011, wasting rates in children were high (10% or more) in countries with large populations including India, Bangladesh, Pakistan, Nigeria, Indonesia, and Ethiopia (see Table 7.1). In 2013, about 51 million children under the age of five were wasted globally and 17 million were severely wasted. Global prevalence of wasting in 2013 was estimated at almost 8%.

Globally, in 2013, an estimated 161 million children under the age of five were stunted. Between 2000 and 2013, stunting prevalence declined from 33% to 25%, respectively, and in 2013, about 50% of all stunted children lived in Asia and over 30% in Africa (United Nations Children Fund, World Health Organization, and World Bank. 2014). Stunting rates in the Northern, Upper East, and Upper West regions of Ghana are 32, 36, and 25%, respectively, well above the national average of 28% (United Nations World Food Program, 2016a), and in Indonesia, which ranks fifth in the number of stunted children in the world, 37% of the population is stunted.

Food security

After the shock of the almost empty grain bin in 1974, thinking around food security came to focus on the volume and stability of food supply in national and international grain reserves (Gilmore and Huddleston, 1983). For this reason, at the 1974 United Nations Food and Agriculture Organization (FAO) World Food Conference held in Rome, food security was defined as "availability at all times of adequate world food supplies of basic foodstuffs to sustain a steady expansion of food consumption and to offset fluctuations in production and prices" (United Nations, 1975). As global food shortage began to diminish in the 1980s, and as the number of hungry people remained high, the focus of food security shifted from concerns over national food supplies to hungry people, and came to be defined as "access by all people at all times to enough food for an active, healthy life" (Reutlinger *et al.*, 1986). By concentrating on people, there was a shift in focus from global hunger issues related to food production, to the ability of families at risk for undernutrition to buy adequate food.

Shortly after, debates on food security suggested that the issue with undernutrition was not insufficient food, but poor distribution, and the fact that levels of food production did not meet food needs. Therefore, in 1983, the FAO expanded the concept of food security to embrace securing access by vulnerable people to available supplies, underscoring the fact that attention needed to be balanced between the demand and supply side of the food security equation. In this vein, food security came to be understood as ensuring that all people at all times have both physical and economic access to the basic food that they need (United Nations Food and Agriculture Organization, 1983).

Arising from concerns with food composition and micronutrient requirements for an active and healthy life, the concept of food security was further broadened in the mid-1990s to include food safety and nutritional balance. Thus, at the 1996 World Food Summit convened in Rome, under the auspices of the FAO, food security was defined from the individual, household, national, regional, and global levels as existing "when all people at all times have access to sufficient, safe, nutritious food to maintain a healthy and active life." This definition of food security includes both physical and economic access to food that meets people's dietary needs as well as their food preferences and is founded on four main pillars: food availability (the regular availability of food in sufficient quantities through production, distribution, and exchange); food access (the affordability, allocation of food, and individuals' and households' preferences), food use (safety of food ingestion and in quantities that meet the physiological requirements of people), and stability (the ability to obtain food over time).

Causes of food insecurity

For the most part, food insecurity around the world is triggered by conflict, drought, climate change, disaster, agricultural problems, rapid population growth, and income among others.

Politically, armed conflicts contribute to the creation of food insecurity in certain parts of the world. In South Sudan for example, about 2.84 million people are facing emergency food security conditions, and in Iraq, about 1.5 million people, including internally displaced persons, refugees, host communities, and returnees affected by the ongoing conflict, require food assistance. In Yemen, where there has been enduring fighting between Houthi fighters and the Yemeni military since 2014, over 50% of the population is food insecure.

As a result of the civil war in Syria, which began in 2011 between the forces of President Bashar al-Assad and other factions, an estimated 6.3 million people have become food insecure. Food production in Syria has dropped by 40% compared to preconflict levels (United Nations World Food Program, 2015c).

Drought and extreme weather conditions have resulted in poor or failed harvests in certain parts of the world, creating food scarcity and driving the price of available food up. Pests such as desert locusts, cattle and livestock diseases, and other agricultural problems including erosion and land degradation, soil infertility, water scarcity, and pollution, also contribute to food insecurity (Harvest Help African Food Issues, 2012). Rapid population growth puts populations at risk for increased food crises, as food production often does not keep pace with population increase.

Food price volatility affects access to quantity and quality of food (Johnson, 2013). In 2012, global corn and soybean prices in the United States and Europe reached all-time highs because of the summer drought. As grains were mostly consumed by livestock in those parts of the world, and as grain prices were high, it impacted the price consumers had to pay for dairy products and meat.

Measuring hunger and nutritional status

Counting or gauging global hunger is not an easy task as it requires tracking who is eating what, where. To measure annual estimates of undernourished populations, the FAO utilizes population data from United Nations agencies (Weeks, 2013). These data are made available by individual countries based on their own calculations of the quantity of major food commodities they produce, import, and export. National surveys are also used in many countries to capture information about the amount of food households acquire. Based on all these information, the FAO is able to calculate how many people in a country lack access to a minimum calorie threshold. A challenge posed by this approach is the inability of FAO to obtain up-to-date data on a country's grain inventories, as well as the issue of surveys not containing accurate information.

Another tool used to measure malnutrition across countries, regions, and the world, is the Global Hunger Index (GHI), developed by the International Food Policy Research Institute (IFPRI). Based on FAO's measure of undernourishment, WHO's data on underweight among children under the age of five and Unicef's data on mortality among children under the age of five, the GHI not only reflects calorie deficits, but a wide range of aspects and consequences related to food insecurity. The GHI attempts to measure food insecurity and its consequences for countries by focusing on loss of lives and nutrition, and on the potential of children in the future. Using three indicators (the proportion of the population who are food-energy deficient as compiled by the FAO, the prevalence of children under the age of five who are underweight as estimated by WHO, and children under the age of five mortality rates as compiled by Unicef), the GHI ranks countries on a 100-point scale, with zero being the desired score (no hunger) and 100 being the worst, and facilitates country comparison on efforts towards addressing hunger. Whilst the GHI provides a multidimensional view of food insecurity, the information it makes available is only as accurate and current as the data on which it is based.

Action Aid, an international nongovernmental organization that seeks to work to reduce poverty and injustice worldwide, developed an index, the HungerFREE Scorecard to measure nutrition outcomes, as well as a country's political commitment to combating undernutrition. The score card assesses four categories: outcomes of hunger and undernutrition, the country's legal commitment to provide its people with the right to food, investments in agriculture, and investments in social protection (Action Aid, 2011).

Countries receive a letter grade for each of the four categories based on hunger and malnutrition statistics obtained from the FAO and WHO. The primary purpose of the scorecard is to encourage governments in both developed and developing countries to commit to hunger eradication. To date, there are 29 developing countries and 22 developed countries with scorecards available. Scorecards are prepared only for countries where reliable data is available and where HungerFREE campaigns are present. Action Aid's nutrition scorecard provides a means for monitoring and evaluating hunger outcomes and some of their political determi-

nants. It assesses the nutritional status of a country and provides information for policy formation and advocacy (Masset, 2011).

Global challenges of hunger, malnutrition, and food security

Nutrition has no clear institutional or sector home. In some countries, it is handled by several ministries or departments. This hinders the effective planning and management of nutrition-related programs and interventions. The prevalence of high levels of malnutrition has the tendency to predispose countries to poverty, economic crises, and even conflict.

Politically, addressing issues related to malnutrition is not high on national development agendas. This is because returns on investments take a long time to manifest and are for that matter' not readily visible.

Food insecurity has health, social, and economic consequences for adults and children, but more especially for the latter owing to their increased susceptibility to illness and the likelihood of long-term effects. Regarding health, children in food-insecure households often experience poor health and stunted growth in the first two years of life. They may also be hospitalized for chronic health conditions (such as anemia), have oral health issues, or poor quality of life, which may hamper their involvement in daily activities at school and social interaction with their peers. Expectant women who experience food insecurity are likely to have birth complications and low birth weight babies.

Socially, food insecurity puts children at a greater risk for emotional problems, truancy, school tardiness, and behavioral issues manifested in the form of aggression, anxiety, bullying, fighting, hyperactivity, mood swings, stealing, and vandalism. It may also cause them to experience delayed development, poor emotional attachment, and learning difficulties.

Economically, the high price of certain nutrient-rich foods cause food available for domestic consumption to be diverted and exported for economic gain. In 2012, Peru, the world's second-largest exporter of quinoa after Bolivia, tripled its exports to 23 000 tonnes since 2007, accounting for nearly half of the global supply. Export activities caused, domestic prices of quinoa to rise to PEN10 ($3.77) per kg, four times more than the price of rice (Oxford Business Group, 2016).

Within countries, domestic food producers who are unable to compete with external crop producers often stop food production, hence reducing domestic food supplies and creating negative multiplier food availability effects on populations. Through international trade in agricultural products, countries become exposed to, and more vulnerable to sudden changes in global agricultural markets. The sudden increase in the volume of agricultural imports from one year to the next often creates a sudden disruption of domestic food production. This has disastrous effects on local farmers and workers, creates the loss of jobs, reduced income, and negative consequences for food security. From 1984 to 2013, China, Ecuador, India, Kenya, Nigeria, Pakistan, Uganda, the United Republic of Tanzania, and Zimbabwe were negatively affected by increases in agricultural imports – their imports exceeded the average of the previous three years by more than 30% (Dawe and Krivonos, 2014).

Global action and strategies

In 1998, WHO together with Unicef, the Canadian International Development Agency, the United States Agency for International Development, and the Micronutrient Initiative, launched the Vitamin A Global Initiative. Through this initiative, they provide children in developing countries with vitamin A capsules twice a year or food (sugar or flour) fortified with vitamin A with the aim of helping countries to eliminate vitamin A deficiency (World Health Organization, 2016c).

The End Child Hunger and Undernutrition Initiative (ECHUI) led by the WFP and Unicef is a partnership to address the hunger and nutrition issues related to MDG 1. Its aim is to mobilize attention and catalyze action on the causes, extent, and impact of child hunger and undernutrition and the approaches and remedies available to tackle them. Specifically, the objectives of the Initiative are to mobilize political support, secure financial resources, develop capacity, and establish partnerships, so as to radically reduce child hunger and undernutrition within a generation.

Ready-to-Use Therapeutic Food (RUTF), the recently developed home-based treatment for severe acute malnutrition, is improving the weight and health conditions of hundreds of thousands of malnourished children globally. Made from peanut butter mixed with dried skimmed milk, vitamins, and minerals, RUTF can be consumed directly. It does not need to be mixed with water, hence avoiding potential contamination. It can be stored for three to four months without refrigeration, even at tropical temperatures. The production of RUTF paste is ongoing in several countries including Congo, Ethiopia, Malawi, and Niger (World Health Organization, 2016a; World Health Organization, n.d.).

Through Project *Nutrimos El Salvador* (Nourishing El Salvador), the WFP, focusing on the first 1000 days of life, works with the government of El Salvador to prevent chronic malnutrition in children. In the past few years, the health condition of over 54 807 children who participated in the nutrition project improved (United Nations World Food Program, 2015a). The WFP is helping to improve food security in Mali by supporting local farmers' organizations; in 2014, WFP bought 6000 metric tons of food from smallholder farmers in Mali (United Nations World Food Program, 2015b).

Discussion points

1 Why are the issues of hunger and malnutrition important components of the Sustainable Development Goals?
2 What is malnutrition? How different is it from hunger?
3 Discuss the causes and symptoms of wasting and stunting.
4 What are micronutrients and how relevant are they to health?
5 Discuss the global burden of hunger and malnutrition.
6 What is food security and what are its implications for health globally?
7 What is the utility of measuring global hunger and nutrition status?
8 What tools are used to measure hunger and nutritional status?
9 What are some of the challenges associated with hunger, malnutrition, and food security?
10 To what extent are issues related to hunger, malnutrition, and food security being addressed globally?

REFERENCES

Action Against Hunger (2009) *Acute Malnutrition: A Preventable Pandemic*, http://www.actionagainst hunger.org/sites/default/files/publications/Acute_Malnutrition_A_Preventable_Pandemic_01.2009. pdf (accessed October 22, 2016).
Action Aid (2011) *Who's Really Fighting Hunger?* http://www.uniteforsight.org/nutrition/module9 (accessed October 22, 2016).

Blössner, M. and de Onis, M. (2005) *Malnutrition: Quantifying the Health Impact at National and Local Levels*. WHO Environmental Burden of Disease Series, 12. World Health Organization, Geneva, http://www.who.int/quantifying_ehimpacts/publications/MalnutritionEBD12.pdf?ua=1 (accessed October 22, 2016).

Boyd, K. (2012) *What Is Vitamin A Deficiency?* http://www.aao.org/eye-health/diseases/vitamin-deficiency (accessed October 22, 2016).

Chopra, M., Galbraith, S., and Darnton-Hill, I. (2002) A global response to a global problem: the epidemic of overnutrition. *Bulletin of the World Health Organization* **80**, 952–958.

Dawe, D. and Krivonos, R. (2014) *Policy Responses to High Food Prices in Latin America and the Caribbean: Country Case Studies*, FAO, Rome.

Gilmore, R. and Huddleston, B. (1983) The food security challenge. *Food Policy* **8**, 31–45.

Harvest Help African Food Issues (2012) *Causes of Food Insecurity in African and Other Third World Countries*, http://www.harvesthelp.org.uk/causes-of-food-insecurity-in-african-and-other-third-world-countries.html (accessed October 22, 2016).

Hetzel, B. S. (1997) SOS for a billion – the nature and magnitude of iodine deficiency disorders. In: *SOS for a Billion – The Conquest of Iodine Deficiency Disorders* (eds B. S. Hetzel and C.V. Pandav) (2nd edn.). Oxford University Press, New Delhi.

Johnson, T. (2013) *Food Price Volatility and Insecurity*, http://www.cfr.org/food-security/food-price-volatility-insecurity/p16662 (accessed October 26, 2016).

Kapil, U. (2007a) Health consequences of iodine deficiency. *Sultan Qaboos University Medical Journal* **7**(3), 267–272.

Masset, E. (2011) A review of hunger indices and methods to monitor country commitment to fighting hunger. *Food Policy* **36**, S102–108.

Office of Dietary Supplements, National Institutes of Health (2013) *Zinc*. Fact Sheet for Health Professionals, https://ods.od.nih.gov/factsheets/Zinc-HealthProfessional/ (accessed October 22, 2016).

Oxford Business Group (2016) *Going with the Grain: Quinoa Exports are Rising at a Rapid Pace*, http://www.oxfordbusinessgroup.com/analysis/going-grain-quinoa-exports-are-rising-rapid-pace (accessed October 22, 2016).

Reutlinger, S., van Holst, J. P., Lissner, C., *et al.* (1986) *Poverty and Hunger-Issues and Options for Food Security in Developing Countries*, World Bank: Washington DC.

Stanbury, J. B. (1987) Vitamin and mineral deficiency, a global damage assessment repo. The iodine deficiency disorders: Introduction and general aspects, in *The Prevention and Control of Iodine Deficiency Disorders* (eds. B. S. Hetzel, J. T. Dunn, and J. B. Stanbury), Elsevier Science, Amsterdam.

United Nations (1975) *Report of the World Food Conference, Rome*, United Nations, New York, NY.

United Nations Children Fund (2013) *Improving Child Nutrition: The Achievable Imperative for Global Progress*, http://www.unicef.org/gambia/Improving_Child_Nutrition_-_the_achievable_imperative_for_global_progress.pdf (accessed October 26, 2016).

United Nations Children's Fund (n.d., a) *Chronic Malnutrition: Stunting*, http://www.unicef.org/publications/files/Tracking_Progress_on_Child_and_Maternal_Nutrition_EN_110309.pd (accessed October 22, 2016).

United Nations Children's Fund (n.d., b) *Harmonized Training Package: Resource Material for Training on Nutrition in Emergencies*, http://www.unicef.org/nutrition/training/2.3/23.html (accessed October 22, 2016).

United Nations Children's Fund, World Health Organization, and World Bank (2012) *Joint Child Malnutrition Estimates*, http://www.who.int/nutgrowthdb/jme_unicef_who_wb.pdf (accessed October 22, 2016).

United Nations Children's Fund, World Health Organization, and World Bank (2014) *Summary of Key Facts about the 2013 Joint Malnutrition Estimates*, http://www.who.int/entity/nutgrowthdb/summary_jme_2013.pdf?ua=1 (accessed October 22, 2016).

United Nations Food and Agriculture Organization (1983) *World Food Security: A Reappraisal of the Concepts and Approaches. Director General's Report*, United Nations Food and Agricultural Organization, Rome.

United Nations Food and Agriculture Organization and World Health Organization (2001) *Human Vitamin and Mineral Requirements*, Chapter 16, http://www.fao.org/docrep/004/y2809e/y2809e0m.htm (accessed October 26, 2016).

United Nations World Food Program (2014) *Ten Facts about Malnutrition in Indonesia*, http://www.wfp.org/stories/10-facts-about-malnutrition-indonesia (accessed October 22, 2016).

United Nations World Food Program (2015a) *Ten Facts about Hunger in El Salvador*, http://www.wfp.org/stories/10-facts-about-hunger-el-salvador (accessed October 22, 2016).

United Nations World Food Program (2015b) *Ten Things Everyone Should Know about Hunger in*

Mali, http://www.wfp.org/stories/10-things-everyone-should-know-about-hunger-mali (accessed October 22, 2016).

United Nations World Food Program (2015c) *Eight Facts on Disasters, Hunger and Nutrition*, http://www.wfp.org/stories/8-facts-disasters-hunger-and-nutrition (accessed October 22, 2016).

United Nations World Food Program (2016a) *Ten Things Everyone Should Know about Hunger in Ghana*, http://www.wfp.org/stories/10-facts-about-hunger-ghana (accessed October 22, 2016).

United Nations World Food Program (2016b) *Hunger Statistics*, https://www.wfp.org/hunger/stats (accessed October 22, 2016).

United Nations World Food Program (2016c) *Types of Malnutrition*, https://www.wfp.org/hunger/malnutrition/types (accessed October 22, 2016).

Weeks, J. (2013) *Measuring Hunger*, http://insights.ifpri.info/2013/04/measuring-hunger/(accessed October 22, 2016).

World Bank (2015) *Poverty*, http://www.worldbank.org/en/topic/poverty (accessed October 22, 2016).

World Bank (2016) *Overview*, http://www.worldbank.org/en/topic/poverty/overview (accessed October 22, 2016).

World Health Organization (2004) *Global Strategy on Diet, Physical Activity and Health*, http://www.who.int/dietphysicalactivity/strategy/eb11344/strategy_english_web.pdf (accessed October 22, 2016).

World Health Organization (2016a) *Malnutrition*, http://www.who.int/maternal_child_adolescent/topics/child/malnutrition/en/(accessed October 22, 2016).

World Health Organization (2016b) *Moderate Malnutrition*, http://www.who.int/nutrition/topics/moderate_malnutrition/en/(accessed October 22, 2016).

World Health Organization (2016c) *Micronutrient Deficiency: Vitamin A Deficiency,The Challenge*, http://www.who.int/nutrition/topics/vad/en/(accessed October 22, 2016).

World Health Organization (n.d.) *Global Database on the Implementation of Nutrition Action: An interactive Platform and Mapping Tool on Nutrition Policies and Action*, http://www.who.int/nutrition/GINA_presentation.pdf?ua=1 (accessed October 22, 2016).

World's Healthiest Foods (2006) *Vitamin A*, http://www.whfoods.com/genpage.php?tname=nutrient&dbid=106 (accessed October 22, 2016).

FURTHER READING

Kapil, U. (2007b) Vitamin and mineral deficiency, a global damage assessment. Health consequences of iodine deficiency. *Sultan Qaboos University Medical Journal* **7**(3), 267–272.

United Nations Children's Fund (2010) *Facts for Life* (4 edn.). United Nations Children's Fund, New York, NY.

United Nations Children Fund (n.d., c) *Accelerating Disease Control*, http://www.unicef.org/immunization/index_control.html (accessed October 22, 2016).

8

Global health and human rights

Learning objectives

By the end of this chapter, you will be able to:

✔ Describe the relevance of human rights to health;

✔ List and explain the international instruments that safeguard the rights of special populations;

✔ Describe global and national obligations to the right to health;

✔ List and explain at least two challenges associated with the right to health;

✔ Describe global action to address health and human rights issues.

Summary of key points

In its definition of health, the World Health Organization (WHO) emphasized that "The right to the highest attainable standard of health...is a fundamental right of every human being," yet, some marginalized groups around the world do not enjoy this right. Minorities, the aged, children, women, prisoners, migrants, and persons with disability especially tend to lack access to adequate healthcare due to a variety of reasons. This chapter provides an overview of human rights and select international and regional human rights instruments. It discusses the right to health, focusing on key human rights standards, the right to health of special populations, and global and national obligations towards the right to health. It wraps up by sharing some challenges related to a rights-based approach to health, and actions and strategies used by the global community to address health and human rights issues.

The concept of human rights

All people, by virtue of being human beings, are entitled to certain inalienable basic rights and freedoms, regardless of their nationality, ethnic origin, sex, religion, race, or any other status (Office of the High Commissioner of Human Rights, 2014). These rights, which describe certain standards of human behavior, are upheld in municipal and international law, require the rule of law, and impose a responsibility on persons to respect the human rights of others (Bass, 2010; Nickel, 2010).

The doctrine of human rights is strongly debated, especially its content, nature, and justifications. While there are ongoing debates about what the term "right" really means, there appears to be some consensus on the fact that human rights cover a wide variety of rights including the right to a fair trial, prohibition of genocide, free speech, and education. This

Global Health: Issues, Challenges, and Global Action Lecture Notes, First Edition. Elizabeth A. Armstrong-Mensah.
© 2017 John Wiley & Sons Ltd. Published 2017 by John Wiley & Sons Ltd.

notwithstanding, there are still differences in opinion about which particular rights should be contained within the general framework of human rights. To some scholars, human rights should be a minimum requirement to avoid extreme abuses, but to others, they should be a higher standard.

International and regional human rights instruments

International human rights instruments comprise global instruments to which any country in the world can be a party, while regional instruments comprise those that are limited to only countries in a particular region of the world. International human rights instruments are treaties and international documents that protect human rights. They can be classified into declarations (which are not legally binding) and conventions (which are legally binding). There are 9 core instruments including the International Bill of Human Rights, which consists of two international treaties – the Universal Declaration of Human Rights (adopted in 1948) and the International Covenant on Civil and Political Rights (adopted in 1966) with its two Optional Protocols – and the International Covenant on Economic, Social and Cultural Rights (also adopted in 1966). These covenants entered into force in 1976, after ratification by a majority of United Nations Member States.

Regional human rights instruments include the African Charter on Human and Peoples' Rights adopted by the African Union, the American Convention on Human Rights adopted by the Organization of American States, the Charter of Fundamental Rights of the European Union adopted by the Council of Europe and the European Union, the Arab Charter of Human Rights adopted by Arab states in the Middle East and North Africa, the ASEAN Human Rights Declaration adopted by Asian nations, and the Commonwealth of Independent States Convention on Human Rights and Fundamental Freedoms adopted by member countries.

The Universal Declaration of Human Rights (UDHR) forms the basis for the international protection of human rights. It was adopted by the United Nations General Assembly in 1948. Comprising 30 articles, the UDHR establishes the civil, political, economic, social, and cultural rights of all people, and is a vision for human dignity that surpasses political boundaries and authority, obligating governments to defend the fundamental rights of their citizens (Amnesty USA, 2016).

Article 25 of the UDHR, article 12 of the International Covenant on Economic, Social and Cultural Rights (ICESCR), article 24 of the Convention on the Rights of the Child (CRC), article 5 of the International Convention on the Elimination of All Forms of Racial Discrimination (ICERD), articles 12 and 14 of the Convention on the Elimination of All Forms of Discrimination Against Women (CEDAW), and article 25 of the Convention on the Rights of Persons with Disabilities (CRPD), all protect human rights to health.

The right to health

The right to health is a vital part of human rights. It encompasses the economic, social, and cultural right to a general minimum standard of health to which all people in the world are entitled without discrimination. However, there are international differences regarding what the term means and how it should be applied. Particular discrepancies exist around the concept of health, the minimum entitlements that a right to health should encompass, and which institutions should be responsible for ensuring a right to health for citizens.

The human right to healthcare requires that all people have access to good quality and acceptable medicines, services, and care from all doctors, hospitals, and clinics, on an equitable basis, as and when needed. For this to be achieved, health systems need to acquaint themselves with and operate under certain key minimum human rights standards. Specifically, they need to ensure that access to healthcare is universal, assured for all on an equitable basis, is affordable, comprehensive, and physically accessible by all. They also need to have in place adequate healthcare infrastructure and resources (hospitals, healthcare centers, trained professional health workforce, medicines, and equipment) in all geographical areas; both rural and urban, and ensure that care is provided with respect and in an environment that is culturally appropriate, responsive to the age, language, and gender of patients while maintaining medical ethics and protecting patient confidentiality during consultations. Care provided must be medically appropriate, timely, safe, patient-centered, and guided by quality standards and control mechanisms.

With regards to procedures, the human right to healthcare necessitates the provision of care that does not discriminate against patients based on their health status, race, ethnicity, age, sex, sexuality, disability, language, religion, national origin, income, or social status. It also emphasizes easy access to health information, the enforcing of standards that hold entities accountable for protecting patients' right to healthcare, as well as meaningful public participation in all decisions that affect a patient's right to healthcare.

The right to health and special populations

Children, adolescents, women, migrants, and people with disability often experience discrimination when it comes to exercising their right to health and healthcare.

Children and adolescents

Like adults, children and adolescents also have the right to enjoy freedoms related to access to healthcare, nutrition, adequate standards of living, and education on health and healthcare, but unfortunately, their rights are often violated by the very people whose responsibility it is to protect and care for them. Generally, children and adolescents are discriminated against because of their lack of maturity, dependence on guardians, sex, status in society, and membership to minority groups or indigenous communities. Though boys and girls both suffer discrimination related to access to healthcare, the latter group usually suffers it the most (Harvard School of Public Health, 2016).

At present, many children and adolescents in certain parts of the world experience poverty, homelessness, abuse and neglect, are forced to work long hours under perilous conditions, are the subject of targeted violent attacks at school, lack equal access to education, suffer inhumane treatment in institutions and detention facilities, suffer from harmful traditional practices or are exposed to preventable diseases. All of these situations adversely affect their health. In 2011, an estimated 7.6 million children under the age of five (United Nations Children's Fund, 2012) died from preventable diseases including diarrhea, pneumonia, and malnutrition. Owing to poverty, nutritional deficiencies, and inadequate opportunities for learning, about 200 million children also under the age of five, failed to realize their full developmental potential (Walker *et al.*, 2011).

It has been reported that adolescents experience a high burden of neuropsychiatric disorders (including depression and substance abuse), violence, accidents, maternal-related conditions, and infectious diseases (Gore *et al.*, 2011; Sawyer *et al.*, 2012). Curtailing child and adolescent morbidity and mortality is crucial to their health and existence, and has consequently become a major priority of the international community. Thus, in 1989, the United Nations adopted the CRC, which entered into force in 1990.

The CRC is an agreement that is legally binding on over 192 United Nations Member States. It defines a child as "every human being below the age of eighteen years" (United Nations General Assembly, 1989) and seeks to protect the civil, political, economic, social, health, and cultural rights of children. Article 24 of the CRC (see Box 8.1) indicates that children are entitled to the highest attainable standard of health as well as to facilities for the treatment of illness and rehabilitation of health. This right is all inclusive, thus, it not only encompasses the protection of children from violations such as limited access to healthcare, but also a range of freedoms including the right to nondiscrimination, access to health-related education and information, freedom from harmful traditional practices (Office of the High Commissioner of Human Rights and World Health Organization, n.d.), and access to "safe water and adequate sanitation, adequate nutritious food and housing, [and] healthy occupational and environmental conditions" (United Nations Committee on Economic, Social and Cultural Rights, 1994, n.d.). Also promoting of the health rights of children is the International Covenant on Economic, Social and Cultural Rights. Like the CRC, this Convention obligates countries to reduce infant and child mortality, and to combat disease and malnutrition.

Women

Women and girls make up over 50% of the world's population, yet they are discriminated against in some countries, and their human rights and right to healthcare are not upheld. Owing to poverty, sociocultural, and economic factors, women tend to experience gender-based discrimination, limited power over their sexual and reproductive lives, and nonparticipation in health decision making, all of which negatively affect their health.

Ideally, women and men should have equal access to healthcare, but in reality, men tend to have more access than women. This is because men wield more power in the home, as they are usually the providers and controllers of family finances. In situations where men and women both have access to healthcare and suffer from the same illness, men still tend to receive

---

Box 8.1 Article 24 of the Convention on the Rights of the Child.

1 States Parties recognize the right of the child to the enjoyment of the highest attainable standard of health and to facilities for the treatment of illness and rehabilitation of health. States Parties shall strive to ensure that no child is deprived of his or her right of access to such healthcare services.

2 States Parties shall pursue full implementation of this right and, in particular, shall take appropriate measures:

  a To diminish infant and child mortality;

  b To ensure the provision of necessary medical assistance and healthcare to all children with emphasis on the development of primary healthcare;

  c To combat disease and malnutrition, including within the framework of primary healthcare, through, inter alia, the application of readily available technology and through the provision of adequate nutritious foods and clean drinking water, taking into consideration the dangers and risks of environmental pollution;

  d To ensure appropriate prenatal and post-natal healthcare for mothers;

  e To ensure that all segments of society, in particular parents and children, are informed, have access to education and are supported in the use of basic knowledge of child health and nutrition, the advantages of breastfeeding, hygiene and environmental sanitation and the prevention of accidents;

  f To develop preventive healthcare, guidance for parents and family planning education and services.

3 States Parties shall take all effective and appropriate measures with a view to abolishing traditional practices prejudicial to the health of children.

4 States Parties undertake to promote and encourage international cooperation with a view to achieving progressively the full realization of the right recognized in the present article. In this regard, particular account shall be taken of the needs of developing countries.

Source: United Nations Human Rights Office of the High Commissioner.

---

better care than women. Indeed, a study conducted on eczema and psoriasis in an outpatient clinic in Sweden revealed that men received more intensive treatment than women (Osika *et al.*, 2005).

The reproductive rights of women include the right to birth control and contraception, freedom from forced sterilization, access to health information and good-quality reproductive healthcare, the right to receive education about sexually transmitted infections and other aspects of sexuality, and protection from harmful cultural practices such as female genital mutilation (FGM) (Cook and Fathalla, 1996; Freedman and Isaacs, 1993). However, in 2012, an estimated 63.2 million women did not have access to modern contraception resulting in increased rates of unintended pregnancies. Per a recent study published in The *Lancet,* the lives of over 100 000 women could have been saved from maternal death annually if they had access to effective contraceptive methods (Partners in Health, 2013).

Lack of access to health education and information creates a gap for women when it comes to their right to health and healthcare. Owing to poverty and their over dependence on men for financial resources, many women are unable to negotiate safe sex or the number of children they want to have. This puts them at an increased risk for frequent pregnancies, pregnancy-related health issues, and maternal death. As noted by Amnesty International, over 350 000 women die each year from pregnancy-related issues, the majority of which could have been prevented if those women had access to education or information on how to handle their pregnancy, or had access to trained antenatal caregivers and skilled attendants at birth.

Women generally face certain forms of discrimination related to their right to health and healthcare, but some group of women, including refugee or internally displaced women, women in slums and suburban settings, indigenous and rural women, and women with disabilities or living with HIV/AIDS, experience manifold and greater forms of discrimination.

The CEDAW and ICESCR emphasize the elimination of discrimination against women in healthcare and promote equal access to healthcare for women and men. Article 14 (see Box 8.2) of CEDAW calls on "State Parties," or national governments, to "take into account the particular problems faced by rural women and the significant roles which rural women play in the economic survival of their families…(and to) take all appropriate measures to eliminate discrimination against women in rural areas in order to ensure, on a basis of equality of men and women, that they participate in and benefit from rural development and, in particular, have access to adequate healthcare facilities, including information, counselling, and services in family planning.

The Committee on the Elimination of Discrimination against Women in addition requires national

---

Box 8.2 Article 14 of the Convention on the Elimination of All Forms of Discrimination against Women.

1 States Parties shall take into account the particular problems faced by rural women and the significant roles which rural women play in the economic survival of their families, including their work in the non-monetized sectors of the economy, and shall take all appropriate measures to ensure the application of the provisions of the present Convention to women in rural areas.

2 States Parties shall take all appropriate measures to eliminate discrimination against women in rural areas in order to ensure, on a basis of equality of men and women, that they participate in and benefit from rural development and, in particular, shall ensure to such women the right:

a To participate in the elaboration and implementation of development planning at all levels;

b To have access to adequate healthcare facilities, including information, counselling and services in family planning;

c To benefit directly from social security program;

d To obtain all types of training and education, formal and non-formal, including that relating to functional literacy, as well as, inter alia, the benefit of all community and extension services, in order to increase their technical proficiency;

e To organize self-help groups and co-operatives in order to obtain equal access to economic opportunities through employment or self-employment;

f To participate in all community activities;

g To have access to agricultural credit and loans, marketing facilities, appropriate technology and equal treatment in land and agrarian reform as well as in land resettlement schemes;

h To enjoy adequate living conditions, particularly in relation to housing, sanitation, electricity and water supply, transport and communications.

Source: United Nations Human Rights Office of the High Commissioner.

---

governments to ensure that women have access to appropriate pregnancy, childbirth and postnatal services, including family planning and emergency obstetric care, in order to ensure safe motherhood and reduce maternal morbidity and mortality. The Committee further requires national governments to permit women to have control over their own bodies, and to make decisions about their sexual and reproductive health, free from lack of information, discrimination, and violence.

The Program of Action of the International Conference on Population and Development and the Beijing Platform for Action, among other things, emphasize that women and men should have the right to be informed, have access to safe, effective, affordable and acceptable methods of family planning of their choice, and have access to appropriate healthcare services that will ensure safe pregnancies and childbirth.

Migrants

Migration affects every region of the world, as many countries are either countries of origin, destination, or transition (Office of the High Commissioner of Human Rights, 2016). Globally, a large number of people live in countries other than their own for a variety of reasons ranging from searching for refuge to securing better opportunities in life.

According to the International Organization for Migration, there are currently around 200 million international migrants worldwide, and 90 million of this population, as confirmed by the International Labor Organization, are migrant workers. As a social and economic phenomenon, global migration has implications for the right to health, especially for host countries. Migrants in foreign countries are often denied their right to health because of their legal status, inability to communicate in the language of the host country, or because of cultural barriers.

In some situations, host countries are only willing to provide migrants with "essential or emergency healthcare." The issue with this is that, health personnel around the world interpret what constitutes essential or emergency healthcare differently. To safeguard the right to health by migrants and to address the differences in interpretation, Article 28 of the International Convention on the Protection of the Rights of All Migrant Workers and Members of their Families specifies that, all migrant workers and their families are entitled to emergency medical care to save their lives and to prevent them from suffering irreversible damage to their health. This service, the Convention indicates, shall be provided to migrants regardless of their legal status or job situation. On the issue of safety and health at the work place, Article 25 of the Convention stipulates that migrant workers are to receive the same treatment as citizens of the employing country (see Box 8.3).

> **Box 8.3 International Convention on the Protection of the Rights of All Migrant Workers and Members of their Families.**
>
> 1 Migrant workers shall enjoy treatment not less favorable than that which applies to nationals of the State of employment in respect of remuneration and:
>
>   a Other conditions of work, that is to say, overtime, hours of work, weekly rest, holidays with pay, safety, health, termination of the employment relationship and any other conditions of work which, according to national law and practice, are covered by these terms;
>
>   b Other terms of employment, that is to say, minimum age of employment, restriction on work and any other matters which, according to national law and practice, are considered a term of employment.
>
> 2 It shall not be lawful to derogate in private contracts of employment from the principle of equality of treatment referred to in paragraph 1 of the present article.
>
> 3 States Parties shall take all appropriate measures to ensure that migrant workers are not deprived of any rights derived from this principle by reason of any irregularity in their stay or employment. In particular, employers shall not be relieved of any legal or contractual obligations, nor shall their obligations be limited in any manner by reason of such irregularity.
>
> *Source:* United Nations Human Rights Office of the High Commissioner.

General comment number 30 (2004) of the Committee on the Elimination of Racial Discrimination on noncitizens and general recommendation number 14 of the Committee on Economic, Social and Cultural Rights, emphasize the right of migrants to the highest attainable standard of health, including access to adequate standard of physical and mental health, preventive, curative, and palliative health services.

Persons with disabilities

Over a billion people worldwide have some kind of disability, yet, it was only in 2006 that the human rights and the right to health of this population were formally recognized by the global community.

People with disabilities experience a number of challenges that reduce their enjoyment of the right to health. In rural areas, slums, and suburban settings, this population often has difficulties accessing healthcare, and in certain parts of the world, those with psychosocial disabilities are often neglected or provided with inadequate medical care. A recent survey of people with serious mental disorders revealed that 35–50% and 76–85% of people with mental disabilities in developed and developing countries, respectively did not receive treatment in the year preceding the study. In situations where people with physical disabilities receive care, their consent for treatment is not often sought by medical practitioners.

Defining people with disabilities as "those who have long-term physical, mental, intellectual, or sensory impairments which in interaction with various barriers may hinder their full and effective participation in society on an equal basis with others," Article 1 of the CRPD, requires States to "promote, protect and ensure the full and equal enjoyment of all human rights and fundamental freedoms by persons with disabilities, including their right to health, and to promote respect for their inherent dignity." Article 25 of the Convention additionally requires people with disabilities to have the "right to the enjoyment of the highest attainable standard of health without discrimination."

The CRPD thus, obligates national governments to ensure that people with disabilities have access to medical and social services in order to diminish and avoid further disabilities, and to locate health services and centers in close proximity to where people with disabilities live. To address the issue of discrimination, the CRPD states that people with disabilities are further to be afforded access to the same range, quality, and standard of healthcare as those provided to other persons.

Global and national obligations towards the right to health

Countries have a primary obligation to protect and promote the human rights and right to health of their citizens. These obligations are defined and guaranteed by international customary law and international human rights treaties, which are binding on countries who are signatories to those agreements. Global and national obligations towards the right to health take the form of progressive realization, mechanisms to realize the right to health, and the provision of core minimum obligations.

Progressive realization

Article 2 (1) of the ICESCR underscores the need for countries, at a minimum, to show that they are doing all they can, within available resources, both internally and externally, to better protect and promote all rights with the recognition that some countries may have resource constraints.

Mechanisms to realize the right to health

As the steps to realize human rights and the right to health will vary from country to country, the Covenant does not prescribe a particular mechanism for implementation. The Covenant, however, allows for the development of legislative measures and country strategies to safeguard the enjoyment of the right to health by all, based on human rights principles defined in the objectives of those strategies. Indicators and benchmarks of the strategies need to be identified so as to monitor progress towards the right to health.

Core minimum obligations

According to the Committee on Economic, Social, and Cultural Rights, countries have a core minimum obligation towards their citizens with respect to the right to health. At a minimum, they must ensure access to health facilities, goods and services on a nondiscriminatory basis for all, including vulnerable or marginalized groups, minimum nutritionally essential food that is adequate and safe, shelter, housing, sanitation, and adequate and safe drinking water, and the equitable distribution of essential drugs to all health facilities.

Challenges to the right to health

The discriminatory treatment of women, children, adolescents, people with disabilities, and migrants prevents them from enjoying their right to health. The actions or inactions of governments, and their policies, also affect the right to health of their citizens. According to the United Nations Children Fund (Unicef), almost every government sector policy (education and public health among others) affects children, especially the short-sighted policies that fail to consider children.

Young and adolescent girls are subjected to inhumane acts including FGM, early marriage, child trafficking, the preference of male children over female children, and the preferential feeding and care of boys. All of these acts compromise the health of young females and reduce their access to a wide range of healthcare services.

Regardless of the adoption and enforcement of CRPD, people with disabilities still face a number of challenges in accessing and utilizing essential health services (Becker *et al.*, 1997). Attitudinal biases of health and social service providers, physical barriers in clinical settings, and poor dissemination of information affect their quality of life (Gilmour, 2006). Studies on healthcare disparities between immigrants and citizens show an especially marked impact on children. Even where born in the United States, children of noncitizens tend to have poorer health not only because of the likelihood of not being insured, but also because they have less access to medical and dental care (Fremstad and Cox, 2004; Huang *et al.*, 2006) due to the immigrant status of their parents.

Global action and strategies

A global commitment has been made by WHO to incorporate mainstream human rights into healthcare programs and policies as part of its comprehensive approach to health and human rights. The organization has also taken steps to strengthen its capacity and role in the provision of technical, intellectual, and political leadership on the right to health by strengthening the capacity of Member States to integrate a human rights-based approach to health into their health strategies. Additionally, WHO promotes the right to health in international law and international development processes, and advocates for health-related human rights, including the right to health (World Health Organization, 2015).

To improve access to health services for people with disabilities, WHO specifically guides and supports Member States to increase awareness of disability issues within their countries, and promotes the inclusion of disability as a crucial aspect of national health policies and programs. The WHO achieves this by facilitating, collecting, and disseminating disability-related data and by promoting strategies that create awareness among people with disabilities about their health conditions.

Human rights mechanisms, such as the Special Rapporteur on the Human Rights of Migrants and the Committee on Migrant Workers state that, although countries are sovereign entities and therefore have the right to determine circumstances of entry and stay within their territories, they also have an obligation to respect, protect, and fulfill the human rights of all individuals under their jurisdiction, regardless of their nationality or origin and regardless of their immigration status.

Discussion points

1 What instruments safeguard the right to health?
2 Why should health and access to healthcare be a right?
3 What is the difference between international and regional human rights instruments?
4 Why should the right to heath of children and adolescents be safeguarded? Describe the instruments that safeguard their health.
5 Identify and describe the instrument(s) that protects the rights of migrants.
6 What difficulties might persons with disabilities experience if their right to health is not protected?
7 What factors affect women's right to health? Which instruments protect women's right to health? Describe each instrument.
8 What challenges do special populations experience with regards to their health?
9 What strategies is WHO implementing to address the challenges associated with the right to health?
10 What should national governments do to safeguard the right to health of their citizens?

REFERENCES

Amnesty USA (2016) *Human Rights Basics*, https://www.amnestyusa.org/research/human-rights-basics (accessed October 23, 2016).

Bass, G. J. (2010) The old new thing. *The New Republic*, https://newrepublic.com/article/78542/the-old-new-thing-human-rights (accessed October 23, 2016).

Becker, H., Stuifbergen, A., and Tinkle, M. (1997) Reproductive health care experiences of women with physical disabilities: a qualitative study. *Archives of Physical Medicine and Rehabilitation* **78** (12 Suppl 5), S26–33.

Cook, R. J. and Fathalla, M. F. (1996) Advancing reproductive rights beyond Cairo and Beijing. *International Family Planning Perspectives* **22**(3), 115–121.

Freedman, L. P. and Isaacs, S. L. (1993) Human rights and reproductive choice. *Studies in Family Planning* **24**(1), 18–30.

Fremstad, S. and Cox, L. (2004) *Covering New Americans: A Review of Federal and State Policies Related to Immigrants' Eligibility and Access to Publicly Funded Health Insurance*, http://kff.org/medicaid/report/covering-new-americans-a-review-of-federal/ (accessed October 23, 2016).

Gilmour, J. M., Mykitiuk, R., and Frazee, C. (2006) *Now You See Her, Now You Don't: How Law Shapes Disabled Women's Experience of Exposure, Surveillance and Assessment in the Clinical Encounter. Clinical Disability Theory: Essays in Philosophy, Politics and Law*, University of British Columbia Press, Vancouver.

Gore, F. M., Bloem, P. J., Patton, G. C. *et al.* (2011) Global burden of disease in young people aged 10–24 years: a systematic analysis. *The Lancet* **377**, 2093–102.

Havard School of Public Health. (2016) *How is Children's Health a Human Rights Issue?* https://www.hhrguide.org/2014/03/16/how-is-childrens-health-a-human-rights-issue/ (accessed October 23, 2016).

Huang, Z. J., Yu, S.M., and Ledsky, R. (2006) Health status and health service access and use among children in US immigrant families. *American Journal of Public Health* **96**(4), 634–640.

Nickel, J. (2010). Human Rights. *In Stanford Encyclopedia of Philosophy*, http://plato.stanford.edu/archives/fall2010/entries/rights-human/ (accessed October 30, 2016).

Office of the High Commissioner of Human Rights (1979) *Convention on the Elimination of All Forms of Discrimination against Women*, http://www.ohchr.org/EN/ProfessionalInterest/Pages/CEDAW.aspx (accessed October 23, 2016).

Office of the High Commissioner of Human Rights. (2014) *What are Human Rights?* http://www.ohchr.org/EN/Issues/Pages/WhatareHumanRights.aspx (accessed October 23, 2016).

Office of the High Commissioner of Human Rights (2016) *Migration and Human Rights*, http://www.ohchr.org/EN/Issues/Migration/Pages/MigrationAndHumanRightsIndex.aspx (accessed October 23, 2016).

Office of the High Commissioner of Human Rights and World Health Organization (n.d.) *The Right to*

Health. Fact sheet, http://www.ohchr.org/Documents/Publications/Factsheet31.pdf (accessed October 23, 2016).

Osika, I., Evengard, B., Waernulf, L., and Nyberg, F. (2005) The laundry-basket project--gender differences to the very skin. Different treatment of some common skin diseases in men and women. *Lakartidningen* **102**(40), 2846–2848.

Partners in Health (2013) *Women Still Face Big Gaps in Access to Health Care*, http://www.pih.org/blog/women-still-face-big-gaps-in-access-to-health-care (accessed October 23, 2016).

Sawyer, S. M., Afifi, R. A., Bearinger, L. H., *et al.* (2012) Adolescence: a foundation for future health. *The Lancet* **379**, 1630–1640.

United Nations Children's Fund (2012) *State of the World's Children 2012: Children in an Urban World*, United Nations Publications, New York, NY.

United Nations Committee on Economic, Social and Cultural Rights (1994) *General Comment No. 5: Persons with Disabilities*, http://www.refworld.org/docid/4538838f0.html (accessed October 23, 2016).

United Nations Committee on Economic, Social and Cultural Rights (n.d.) *General Comment No. 14*, para. 45, in *Submission on the Content of a Future General Comment on the Right of the Child to the Enjoyment of the Highest Attainable Standard of Healt*h (art. 24) (OHCHR) (A. Nolan, A. E. Yamin, and B. M. Meier), http://www2.ohchr.org/english/bodies/crc/callsubmissionsCRC_received.htm (accessed October 28, 2016).

United Nations General Assembly (1989) *Convention on the Rights of the Child (CRC)*, http://www.ohchr.org/en/professionalinterest/pages/crc.aspx (accessed October 23, 2016).

Walker, S. P, Wachs, T. D., Grantham-McGregor, S., *et al.* (2011) Inequality in early childhood: Risk and protective factors for early child development. *The Lancet* **378**(9799), 1325–1338.

World Health Organization. (2015) *Health and Human Rights.*Fact sheet, http://www.who.int/mediacentre/factsheets/fs323/en/(accessed October 23, 2016).

FURTHER READING

Nielsen, C. K., Nielsen, S. M., and Lazarus, J. (2012) Key barriers to the use of modern contraceptives among women in Albania: A qualitative study. *Reproductive Health Matters* **20**(40), 158–165.

Office of the High Commission on Human Rights (1948) *The International Bill of Human Rights*, http://www.ohchr.org/Documents/Publications/Compilation1.1en.pdf (accessed October 23, 2016).

Shaw, M. (2008) *International Law* (6th ed.). Cambridge University Press, Leiden.

United Nations Children's Fund (2014) *Addressing the Needs of Children*, http://www.unicef.org/crc/index_30167.html (accessed October 23, 2016).

United Nations Children's Fund (2016) *Millennium Development Goals 4: Reduce Child Mortality*, http://www.un.org/millenniumgoals/childhealth.shtml (accessed October 23, 2016).

World Health Organization (2001) *The Second Decade:Improving Adolescent Health and Development*, http://apps.who.int/iris/bitstream/10665/64320/1/WHO_FRH_ADH_98.18_Rev.1.pdf (accessed October 23, 2016).

9

Natural disasters and complex humanitarian emergencies

Learning objectives

By the end of this chapter, you will be able to:

✔ Distinguish between natural disasters and complex humanitarian emergencies;

✔ Describe the importance of disasters to global health;

✔ Describe the management of disasters;

✔ Identify at least two challenges of disaster management;

✔ Describe global disaster risk reduction and management strategies and action.

Summary of key points

Disasters wreak significant devastation in society, are costly, and negatively affect global health. They cause increased morbidity, mortality, disability, and economic loss in populations affected. The hazards that cause disasters may be natural or manmade. The ability of countries and the international community to respond to and manage disasters are crucial to human survival and reconstruction. This chapter reviews natural disasters and complex humanitarian emergencies (CHEs). It focuses on key terms, describes some natural and CHEs and their impact on global health, presents a disaster-management cycle, discusses disaster management challenges, and global disaster strategies and action.

The concept of disaster

Disasters are events or activities that seriously disrupt the functioning of a society and cause widespread damage to humans, physical infrastructure, the economy, and the environment. The disruptions usually exceed the ability of affected populations to recover with their own resources and therefore require external assistance. The occurrence of disasters is associated with the improper management of risk, the existence of vulnerabilities, as well as human failure to put in place appropriate disaster-prevention and management measures (Blaikie *et al.*, 2003). According to disaster researchers, areas with low vulnerability are less likely to experience a disaster when hazards strike and vice versa (Quarantelli, 1998).

Global Health: Issues, Challenges, and Global Action Lecture Notes, First Edition. Elizabeth A. Armstrong-Mensah.
© 2017 John Wiley & Sons Ltd. Published 2017 by John Wiley & Sons Ltd.

Key disaster-related terms

Hazard

A hazard is a potentially damaging physical event, phenomenon, human activity, or situation that may threaten life, health, and property, and cause social and economic disruption, or environmental degradation. Hazards may be dormant (a theoretical risk of harm) or active (actually occur creating accidents, disasters, emergencies, or incidents).

Hazards may be of natural origins or induced by man-made processes (United Nations International Strategy for Disaster Reduction, 2007). They may be physical, chemical, biological, or psychological in nature. Physical hazards cause intense physical harm and stress to the human body with or without contact. They include ergonomic hazards, radiation, heat and cold stress, vibration hazards, and noise hazards.

Chemical hazards cause harm or damage to the human body, property, or the environment by exposure to chemical substances through inhalation of fumes, ingestion, poisoning, or explosion. Just like physical hazards, chemical hazards may be caused by natural elements, or by human activity. The 1984 Bhopal gas leak at the Union Carbide pesticide plant in India is one of the worst industrial chemical disasters in history. Occurring without warning, a gas leak caused by mechanical and human failures released lethal methyl isocyanate over the city while people were asleep, killing about 1000 people instantly and 8000 at a later time.

As its name suggests, biological hazards are caused by biological agents, such as viruses, parasites, bacteria, food, fungi, and foreign toxins, which cause harm to the human body. Psychological hazards are the result of work-related stress, or stressful environments. They may be triggered by shift patterns, the influence of alcohol, illness, and the lack of training to perform tasks.

Internally displaced person

Internally displaced persons (IDPs) are people who have remained in their home countries and have not crossed an international border to find sanctuary in the event of a disaster. These people remain under the protection of their country governments and retain their human rights and protections under international humanitarian law, even though those same governments may be the cause of their flight.

By the end of 2011, an estimated 26.4 million people were internally displaced globally, and by the end of 2014, a record 38 million people were internally displaced. An estimated 11 million of this population were newly uprooted in 2014 alone. As indicated by the Norwegian Refugee Council's Geneva-based Internal Displacement Monitoring Centre (IDMC), the surge in new displacements was the outcome of long drawn-out crises in five countries (the Democratic Republic of the Congo, Iraq, Nigeria, South Sudan and Syria), and accounted for 60% of the new displacements worldwide.

Refugee

A refugee, according to the United Nations High Commission for Refugees (UNHCR), is someone who has been forced to flee his or her country "owing to a well-founded fear of being persecuted for reasons of race, religion, nationality, membership of a particular social group or political opinion, is outside the country of his nationality, and is unable to, or owing to such fear, is unwilling to avail himself of the protection of that country." Wars are the leading cause of refugee situations.

According to UNHCR, approximately 1 million men, women, and children were reported to have fled their homes in the Central African Republic to mosques and churches in neighboring Cameroon, Democratic Republic of the Congo, and Chad, in search of refuge after walking for days without adequate food and water.

Humanitarian assistance

Generally, humanitarian assistance is referred to as aid and actions designed to save lives, alleviate suffering, and maintain and protect human dignity during and after a disaster. It may be material or logistical and is usually short-term. While also targeted at populations in need, it differs from other forms of aid, in that it focuses primarily on saving lives based on a pressing need, without discrimination between or within affected populations, and without being subject to the autonomy of any government during implementation. Humanitarian assistance takes a variety of forms including food aid, healthcare, protection, in-kind goods, cash, and vouchers (Overseas Development Institute, n.d.). The United States Agency for International Development (USAID) provides humanitarian assistance to meet humanitarian and food assistance needs of conflict- and disaster-affected populations in Afghanistan.

Risk assessment

Risk assessment is the process of identifying potential hazards, analyzing, or evaluating the risk associated with that hazard, and coming up with

---

Box 9.1 Conducting a comprehensive risk assessment from the United Nations Development Fund (UNDP) is a seven-step process.

1 Gaining an understanding of the situation at hand, as well as needs and gaps, so as to avoid duplication of efforts, and to build on existing information and capacities.

2 Conducting an assessment of hazards to identify their nature, location, and intensity and the likelihood of major hazards prevailing in a community or society.

3 Conducting an exposure assessment to identify populations and assets at risk and demarcating disaster-prone areas.

4 Conducting vulnerability analysis to determine the capability (or lack of it) of elements at risk to withstand the given hazard situation.

5 Performing a loss/impact analysis to estimate potential losses of exposed population, property, services, livelihoods and environment, and assessing their potential impacts on society.

6 Undertaking risk profiling and evaluation to identify cost-effective risk reduction options in terms of the socio-economic concerns of a society and its capacity for risk reduction.

7 Formulating or revising disaster risk reduction strategies and action plans that include priority setting, the allocation of resources (financial or human), and the initiation of disaster risk reduction programs.

Source: United Nations Development Fund Bureau for Crisis Prevention and Recovery (2010).

---

appropriate measures to eliminate or control them. Risk assessments help to create awareness of hazards and risks, determine who may be at risk and the adequacy of existing control mechanisms, and prioritize hazards and their control measures. Risk assessments are integral to decision and policy-making and are most effective when done in collaboration with appropriate sectors of society (see Box 9.1).

Vulnerability

Vulnerability is the state of being open to suffer injury or damage due to external events. It applies not only to individuals, groups of individuals, communities, or societies, but also to structures. People of low socio-economic status are usually more vulnerable during and after disasters.

the loss of life, and displacement. The occurrence, timing, and location of some natural disasters can be predicted, but the extent of their damage cannot. Although primarily caused by nature, disasters labeled as "natural" may also be caused by humans. Natural disasters may be triggered by biological, geophysical, or climatic factors.

Manmade disasters, also referred to as CHEs, are events that occur intentionally or unintentionally as a result of human activity related to technology failure such as engineering or structural failures, chemical or nuclear accidents, or sociological factors initiated by human motives, such as attacks and workplace violence. They are typically characterized by extensive violence, mortality, internal and external displacement of populations, extensive harm to societies and economies, and large-scale multifaceted humanitarian assistance.

Natural disasters and complex humanitarian emergencies

The hazards that cause disasters may be classified as either natural or manmade. Natural disasters are major adverse events that occur from natural processes including avalanches, droughts, earthquakes, extreme temperatures, mudslides, floods, volcanic eruptions, tropical storms and tornadoes, tsunamis, typhoons, wildfires, and other similar processes. They can cause major damage to physical infrastructure,

Global instances of natural disasters and complex humanitarian emergencies

Throughout history, populations in different parts of the world have experienced natural disasters or CHEs. The impact of these events has varied depending on their severity and the level of preparedness, geographic location, and economic standing of the affected countries and populations.

Natural disasters

Droughts

Some countries around the world experience deficiencies in precipitation that extend over long periods, creating water shortages (ground or surface) that adversely impact the environment, animal and human life, and economies. Environmentally, droughts may damage terrestrial, aquatic, and wildlife habitats, cause dust bowls, and parched land. These circumstances affect crop production and bring about famine, hunger, malnutrition, dehydration, and drought-related diseases. Chronic droughts and desertification in East Africa created severe ecological catastrophes and consequent food shortages in 2006 and 2011. Between 1980 and 2005, the United States (US) experienced nine drought events, which caused about $1 billion in damages. The most costly of these droughts occurred in the central and eastern US from 1988 to 1989, resulting in severe losses to agriculture and related industries (National Weather Service, 2008).

In Australia, the Millennium Drought, which lasted from 1997 to 2009, caused a water supply crisis across much of the country, causing state governments to create desalination plants in Perth (the Kwinana plant in 2006) and Sydney (the Kurnell Desalination Plant in 2010) to purify seawater using reverse osmosis technology (*Sydney Morning Herald,* 2010).

In 2006, Sichuan Province in China experienced its worst drought, which caused severe water shortages for about 8 million people and over 7 million cattle. The Darfur conflict in Sudan, which began in 2003, was fueled by land and water access disputes between semi-nomadic livestock farmers and sedentary farmers following decades of drought in the country (Wachman, 2007). Between 2006 and 2011, Syria experienced severe drought and crop failure. The decrease in water availability, coupled with water mismanagement, agricultural failures, and associated economic decline, contributed to population displacements, the migration of people in rural communities to nearby cities, urban unemployment, and food insecurity for over a million people (Iceland, 2015).

Earthquakes

Also known as quakes or tremors, earthquakes are naturally occurring events mostly caused by the rupture of geological faults, volcanic activity, landslides, mine blasts, and nuclear tests. They often damage buildings and solid infrastructure and cause soil liquefaction, which results in buildings sinking into the ground and eventually imploding, as was the case with the 1964 Alaska earthquake (United States Geological Survey, 2016).

In 2015, Nepal witnessed one of history's worst earthquakes. It claimed the lives of more than 5000 people and damaged several historical sites. The Haiti earthquake in Port au Prince in 2010, left 316 000 people dead, 300 000 injured, destroyed an estimated 250 000 houses and 30 000 commercial buildings, and caused 1 000 000 people to be homeless. The estimated economic cost of that earthquake was $14.1 billion (Balkhi, 2015). In 2011, a 9.03 magnitude earthquake struck the east coast of Tohoku in Japan, claiming 15 878 lives, leaving 6126 people injured, rendering an estimated 2173 people missing in 20 prefectures, and causing great damage to four major nuclear power stations (Balkhi, 2015).

Tsunamis

Caused by large undersea earthquakes, underwater landslides, or volcanic eruptions, tsunamis are a series of ocean waves that deposit a rush of water onto land, resulting in extensive destruction. Tsunami waves can rise to over 100 feet (30.5 m) and can travel at about 500 miles (805 km) per hour. About 80% of tsunamis occur in the Pacific Ocean's "Ring of Fire" (National Geographic, 2016). In 2004, an earthquake in the Indian Ocean set off a chain of devastating tsunamis that killed 230 000 people in 14 countries and submerged communities along the coast. Indonesia was the hardest-hit by the tsunami followed by Sri Lanka, India, and Thailand. This tsunami was one of the most lethal natural disasters in history. In 2011, a series of tsunamis caused the death of hundreds of people in the north-eastern part of Japan. The devastating effects of the waves from the tsunamis were felt as far away as in California. The tsunami killed 16 273 people, injured 27 074 people, and caused 3061 people to go missing. The total economic loss to Japan was $275 billion with a direct cost of $65 billion in damages to the Fukushima power plant.

Volcanic eruptions

Volcanoes cause a lot of distraction in various ways. The hot, dangerous gases, ash, lava, and rock they emit are very destructive. Volcanic eruptions may cause rocks to tumble down and the intense heat from lava can destroy buildings, plants, and animals in its path. Volcanic eruptions may contaminate water sources, cause floods, mudslides, power outages, wildfires, disease outbreaks, respiratory illness, suffocation, burns, injuries from falls, and vehicle accidents due to the slippery, hazy conditions created by cooled ash. Cooled ashes from volcanoes have the tendency to settle thickly on nearby locations and in sufficient quantities, can cause roofs to collapse.

In 2010, a volcano erupted in southern Iceland, forcing about 600 people to evacuate the area and causing flights to be diverted. Also in 2010, volcanic ash in Iceland travelled to North Africa and over Turkey, and forced authorities to shut down the air space over Turkey and airports in Casablanca, Morocco, and Spain.

Complex humanitarian emergencies

Complex humanitarian emergencies in the form of armed conflict may occur at the national level between armed factions within a country, or may manifest in the form of war between the armies of two or more feuding countries. Regardless of what form they take, CHEs culminate in the outbreak of communicable diseases, disability, hunger, displacement of people and families, refugee situations, lack of access to shelter, disruption of water supply, sewer systems, physical and utility infrastructure, and death. Complex humanitarian emergencies are brought about either by a single factor or combination of factors, namely ethnic hostility, inequality, unemployment, and low income.

Civil wars

The multisided civil war in Syria has been labeled the worst humanitarian crisis of recent times. Sparked by violent crackdowns on anti-government demonstrators by government forces in 2011, the civil war had claimed the lives of over 220 000 people by 2016 (50% of which were civilians), caused 4.7 million people to flee to neighboring Egypt, Jordan, Lebanon, Turkey, and northern Iraq in search of refuge, and rendered about 6.6 million Syrians internally displaced within Syria. Shelling by feuding factions has destroyed cities and infrastructure, and caused basic necessities like food and medical care to be in short supply (MercyCorps, 2016).

Social life in Syria has been disrupted and refugees have become susceptible to diseases, chronic malnutrition and exploitation by human traffickers. With the hope of finding a better future in Europe, hundreds of thousands of Syrian refugees have attempted dangerous trips across the ocean to Greece from Turkey, with huge casualties. Refugees who managed to make it to Greece, faced serious challenges, as the government of Greece lacked the financial wherewithal to cater to them. To address the humanitarian needs of people within Syria, the UN appealed to the global community for $7.4 billion in financial assistance and received 50% of that amount. The economic loss as a result of the civil war is estimated at $202 billion (World Vision, 2015).

The civil war in South Sudan, which broke out in 2013, began as a political squabble between President Salva Kiir and soldiers loyal to his former vice-president, Riek Machar, whom he removed from office on suspicion of spearheading an attempted coup against him. As the civil war intensified, 1.66 million people fled their homes to UN protected camps and 640 000 became refugees in neighboring countries. The civil war created untold economic hardship, in that, it disrupted farming activities, caused families to lose their livestock, and much-needed income. Hunger, malnutrition, and disease set in, threatening the lives of children. Humanitarian agencies responding to the crisis in South Sudan indicated that, 6.4 million people needed humanitarian assistance, 3.9 million of that population were experiencing severe food shortages, and about 250 000 children were severely malnourished (World Vision, 2015).

Terrorist attacks

The four coordinated terrorist attacks against symbolic US landmarks in 2001 by the Islamic terrorist group Al-Qaeda, as the result of a *fatwā* signed by Osama bin Laden, destroyed property and claimed lives. In Manhattan, New York, the 110-floor Twin Towers of the World Trade Center complex, World Trade Center buildings 3 through 7, and the St. Nicholas Greek Orthodox Church were destroyed. The US Customs House and the pedestrian bridges connecting buildings were also severely damaged (Summers and Robbyn, 2011). The Deutsche Bank Building on 130 Liberty Street in Manhattan and the two buildings of the World Financial Center were partially damaged. In Arlington, Virginia, the western side of the Pentagon was severely damaged by the impact of American Airlines Flight 77. The fire it created caused a section of the building to collapse.

The terrorist attacks significantly affected global markets, as they closed Wall Street for six days and civilian airspace in the US and Canada for two days. The attacks caused the death of 2996 people and over 6000 nonfatal injuries to people. The death toll included all the 265 people aboard the four planes used in the attacks, 2606 people in the World Trade Center and surrounding areas, and 125 people at the Pentagon. Those who perished included thousands of civilians, 343 firefighters, 72 law-enforcement officers, 55 military personnel, and the 19 terrorists who orchestrated the attacks (Stone, 2002). By way of response, relief funds were immediately set up by the US government to provide financial assistance to the survivors of the attacks and to the families of victims. By 2003, 2833 applications had been received from the families of those who were killed.

Global impact of natural disasters and complex humanitarian emergencies

Globally, natural disasters and CHEs create human, health, social, and economic problems. Every year, millions of people are affected by natural disasters,

which have catastrophic impact; from the destruction of buildings to the spread of disease, and the devastation of countries or societies within a short time. Droughts, earthquakes, tsunamis, typhoons, and volcanic eruptions do not just wreak havoc on the land, they also disrupt people's lives and livelihoods in both densely populated cities and remote villages.

The extent of harm wreaked by natural disasters depends on the level of vulnerability, exposure, susceptibility, coping, and adaptive capacities of countries or regions. Exposure to natural disasters is beyond human control, but susceptibility, coping, and adaptive capacities are within human control and can be worsened by poverty. Approximately 325 million of the world's extremely poor are anticipated to live in the 49 most hazard-prone countries by 2030.

Between 2005 and 2014, 1.7 billion people were affected by natural disasters worldwide, 7 million were killed, and damages totaled $1.3 trillion (see Figure 9.1 and Figure 9.2). In 2010 alone, the earthquake that occurred in Haiti killed more than 200 000 people in seconds, and that same year the floods in Pakistan affected 20 million people and left 20% of Pakistan

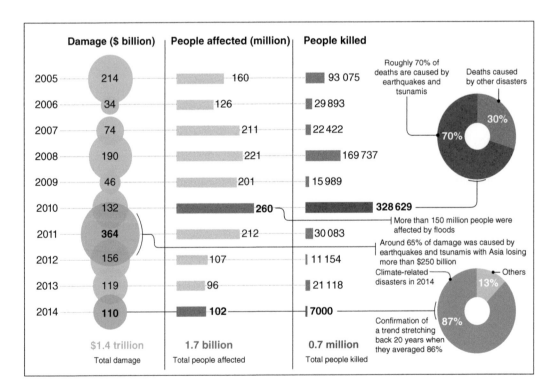

Figure 9.1 The economic and human impact of disasters from 2005 to 2014.
Source: UNISDR with data from EM-DAT database, Centre for Research on the Epidemiology of Disasters (CRED) and Munich Re, http://www.unisdr.org/files/42862_economichumanimpact20052014unisdr.pdf (accessed October 24, 2016).

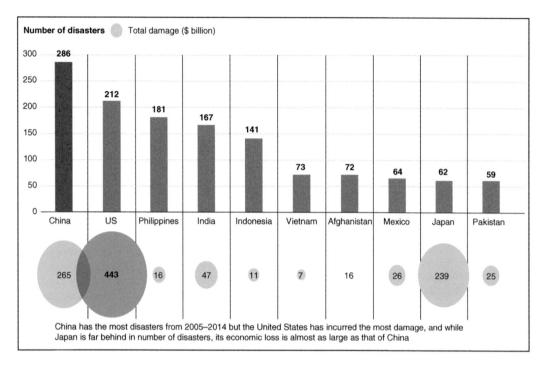

Number of disasters ⬤ Total damage ($ billion)

China has the most disasters from 2005–2014 but the United States has incurred the most damage, and while Japan is far behind in number of disasters, its economic loss is almost as large as that of China

Figure 9.2 The top 10 countries with the most disasters from 2005 to 2014.
Source: UNISDR with data from EM-DAT database, Centre for Research on the Epidemiology of Disasters (CRED), and Munich Re, http://www.unisdr.org/files/42862_economichumanimpact20052014unisdr.pdf, with permission.

under flood waters. The two-year drought in the East Africa region (between 2011 and mid-2012) caused a severe food crisis in six countries (Somalia, Djibouti, Ethiopia, Kenya, Sudan, South Sudan and parts of Uganda), affected the livelihood of 95 million people, and claimed the lives of about 258 000 people in Somalia alone (BBC News, 2011a, b; Woodridge, 2011).

Although developing countries tend to be more prone to natural disasters owing to poorly constructed buildings, rapid population growth, limited resources for disaster response and rebuilding, and the lack of economic safety nets, developed countries have not been spared. In 2012, Hurricane Sandy swept across the US and affected 24 states, costing the government $65 billion in direct damages. That same year, droughts occurred in the American Midwest and cost $35 billion in damages. The 2011 Japan earthquake is the most expensive disaster on record to date. It cost an estimated $210 billion in damages alone.

Complex humanitarian emergencies cause a surge in refugee and displaced persons populations, migration-related mortality, disease outbreaks, injuries, and disability. Socially, they bring about social breakdown that facilitates gender-based violence, the transmis-sion of sexually transmitted diseases, overcrowding in camps, and the separation of families. Psychologically, they cause distress and mental issues such as grief, depression, anxiety, post-traumatic stress disorder, and psychosis, and economically, they cause losses to the means of production and infrastructure, and the redirection of resources from other sectors for recon-struction and rehabilitation efforts in the post-disaster period. Like natural disasters, CHEs also significantly affect food security given the fact that they can damage food-storage facilities, disrupt food production and distribution networks, cause crop and livestock failure, and scarcity of food commodities.

Managing natural disasters and complex humanitarian emergencies

Regardless of how varied disaster response measures are across the globe, they generally tend to focus on a common purpose: disaster management. The ability

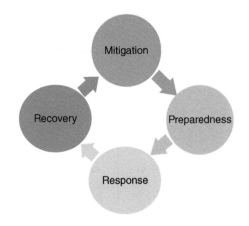

Figure 9.3 Disaster management cycle.

of countries to manage disasters is wide ranging and contingent upon political, economic, cultural, and other factors. Disaster management involves multisectoral mobilization and management of resources and responsibilities to address the humanitarian aspects of an emergency and risk prevention. It also entails preparing for disasters before they occur, responding when they do occur (e.g. emergency evacuation, quarantine, mass decontamination), and rebuilding after they have occured. It further requires continuous effort by affected populations to manage hazards, so as to avoid or minimize the resulting impact. Disaster management does not remove threats. It concentrates on creating plans to decrease the effect of disasters. Failure to create a plan could lead to the calamitous loss of human life, assets, and revenue.

Disaster management consists of four phases: mitigation, preparedness, response, and recovery (see Figure 9.3). Each phase has specific requirements, tools, strategies, resources, and challenges. The duration of each phase is dependent on the type and severity of the disaster.

Mitigation phase

The mitigation phase precedes potential disasters and focuses on measures that can prevent hazards from developing into disasters (World Health Organization, 2011). Unlike the other three phases, this phase concentrates on long-term risk reduction or elimination measures. Mitigation efforts may be structural technological solutions to a hazard, such as the building of levees to prevent floods, or non-structural, such as the creation of policies to avoid unnecessary risks. To be effective, mitigation efforts need to be preceded by risk assessment.

Preparedness phase

The preparedness phase involves predicting disasters where possible and putting in place measures on a continuous basis to prevent or reduce their potential effects on vulnerable populations. Some general preparedness measures include having an easy to understand communication plan ready with a clearly defined chain of command, developing multiagency coordination and incident command centers or emergency operations centers, maintaining and training emergency service providers and emergency volunteers, developing and testing emergency population warning systems, creating emergency shelters and evacuation plans, and stockpiling necessary supplies and equipment.

When done properly, disaster preparedness can facilitate the design of appropriate activities and minimize the duplication of efforts. When rooted in risk reduction, preparedness activities can prevent disaster situations, save lives, and make it possible for affected populations to bounce back quickly after an emergency.

Response phase

This phase occurs immediately after a disaster has occurred and focuses on addressing the immediate threats presented, including rescuing surviving populations from immediate danger, stabilizing their physical and emotional condition, attending to humanitarian needs (food, shelter, clothing, public health, and safety), cleaning up, doing damage assessment, and commencing resource distribution. The response phase is often fraught with some degree of chaos, which may either be short lived (a month) or long lasting, depending on the type of disaster and the extent of damage caused.

With time, response efforts shift from tackling immediate emergency issues to doing repair work, restoring utilities, establishing operations for public services, and completing cleanup activities. Depending on the nature of injuries sustained by victims, climatic conditions, and access to fresh air and water, among others, most people severely affected by a disaster may die within the first 72 hours. Often times, search and rescue teams cease work a week after the occurrence of a major incident. At this point, the event enters a "recovery phase" (Dimersar Academy, 2010).

Recovery phase

Recovery is the fourth phase of disaster management. This phase is primarily concerned with restoring the affected area back to normalcy after needs have been addressed. The recovery effort may be short term, ranging from 6 months to about a year, or long term, lasting for decades. It requires strategic planning and action to address the severe or enduring impacts of a disaster. The International Federation of the Red Cross and Red Crescent Societies (IFC) is active in postdisaster and postconflict relief and rehabilitation efforts worldwide.

Natural disasters and complex humanitarian emergencies management challenges

Globally, there are ongoing challenges around the ability of countries to shift from a response and recovery approach to disaster management to a proactive approach, which focuses more on prevention and mitigation of hazards and the development of community and country capacities to provide timely and effective response and recovery during and after disasters (World Health Organization, 2011). The establishment of common protocols and standards for emergency response within countries and among partners are additional challenges.

In the case of CHEs, feuding factions sometimes hinder response efforts to affected areas. This results in food shortages, outbreak of diseases, and unhealthy living conditions in refugee camps. In recent times, CHEs have created unsafe environments for aid workers. Attacks by road became a frequent practice in the 1990s and 2000s and peaked in 2012, with 167 incidents (Harmer *et al.*, 2013). Between 2001 and 2011, the number of aid workers who died as a result of response-related activities tripled to 100 deaths per year. The kidnapping of aid workers is also on the rise.

Poor coordination, collaboration, undefined roles and responsibilities, and the management and exchange of information among relevant stakeholders affects effective disaster response and decision making. The disjointed nature of the response to the Haiti earthquake in 2010, and the utilization of hierarchical models of information management, among other things, caused the response effort to be less effective than it could have been.

The overcrowding and lack of privacy in camp environments is detrimental to survival and can lead to psychosocial problems, sexual and gender-based violence, and distress. The lack of accountability mechanisms during disaster events do not ensure

that resources donated or deployed are used for the purposes for which they were made available. The poor and marginalized are the population most affected by disasters. Unless intentional, concerted, and conscious efforts are made to protect this population, they will continue to bear the brunt of these events.

Global action and strategies

As several actions need to be taken to respond effectively to disasters, the United Nations (UN) established a priority list of actions including:

- Conducting rapid needs assessment immediately after a disaster to assess the level and impact of damage on affected populations, their needs, potential courses of action, and resources required
- Providing safe water, sanitation, and hygiene (WASH) services to prevent the outbreak of diseases in disaster-affected children and their families
- Ensuring that there is adequate food supply to meet the nutritional needs of all population groups affected by a disaster and where populations are dependent on food assistance, food rations are adequate, meet the minimum energy, protein and fat requirements for survival, and are culturally acceptable for subgroups of the population
- Providing safe and suitable shelters in order to save lives, reduce morbidity, and enable people to live with dignity
- Providing basic physical, mental and preventative care to disaster victims
- Controlling communicable diseases by identifying the main threats, preventing transmission through the maintenance of clean physical environment, establishing a disease surveillance system to ensure early case detection, reporting and monitoring of disease trends, and controlling and managing disease outbreaks by prompt diagnosis and appropriate treatment
- Conducting public health surveillance
- Mobilizing human resources and training health personnel and community-based volunteers to manage the disaster

In 1990, following the adoption of Resolution 44/236, the UN launched the International Decade for Natural Disaster Reduction (IDNDR) from 1990 to 1999. The overall purpose of the decade was to reduce, through international collaboration, the loss of life, property damage, and social and economic disruption caused by natural disasters. Specifically, the goals of the decade were to:

- Improve the capacity of UN Member States to mitigate the effects of natural disasters expeditiously and effectively, pay special attention to assisting developing countries in the assessment of disaster damage potential, and establish early warning systems and disaster-resistant structures when and where needed
- Devise appropriate guidelines and strategies for applying existing scientific and technical knowledge, taking into account the cultural and economic diversity among nations
- Foster scientific and engineering endeavors aimed at closing critical gaps in knowledge in order to reduce loss of life and property
- Develop measures for the assessment, prediction, prevention, and mitigation of natural disasters through programs of technical assistance and technology transfer, demonstration projects, and education and training, tailored to specific disasters and locations, and to evaluate the effectiveness of those programs

In the effort to implement activities towards the achievement of IDNDR goals, UN Member States were to have in place by 2000:

- Comprehensive national assessments of risks from natural hazards that were to be taken into account in the development of disaster management plans
- Mitigation plans at national and or local levels, including long-term prevention and preparedness, and community awareness
- Access to global, regional, national and local warning systems and broad dissemination of warnings

In 2005, the World Conference on Disaster Reduction was held in Hyogo, Japan. The conference facilitated the development of strategic and systematic approaches to reduce disaster-related vulnerabilities (Inter-Agency Task Force on Disaster Reduction, 2004) and risks, and emphasized the need for nations and communities to build resilience to disasters. Following the Hyogo conference, the global community adopted the Hyogo Framework for Action (HFA) on Building the Resilience of Nations and Communities to Disasters. The 10-year (2005–2015) plan endorsed by the UN General Assembly Resolution A/RES/60/195 focused on five priorities for action by countries:

- Ensure that disaster risk reduction is a national and local priority with a strong institutional basis for implementation
- Identify, assess, and monitor disaster risks and enhance early warning
- Use knowledge, innovation, and education to build a culture of safety and resilience at all levels
- Reduce underlying risk factors
- Strengthen disaster preparedness for effective response at all levels

The HFA was conceived to provide further momentum to global efforts under the International Framework for Action for the International Decade for Natural Disaster Reduction of 1989, the Yokohama Strategy for a Safer World adopted in 1994, and the International Strategy for Disaster Reduction of 1999 (United Nations, 2015).

Supported by the UN Office for Disaster Risk Reduction at the request of the UN General Assembly, the Sendai Framework for Disaster Risk Reduction (2015 to 2030) was adopted at the Third UN World Conference in Sendai, Japan in 2015. This framework is the outcome of stakeholder consultations initiated in 2012, and intergovernmental negotiations from 2014 to 2015. It is the successor instrument to the HFA. The Sendai Framework seeks to ensure the continuity of UN Member States and other stakeholders to disaster risk reduction under the HFA. The Sendai Framework calls for:

- Improved understanding of disaster risk in all its dimensions of exposure, vulnerability, and hazard characteristics
- Strengthening of disaster risk governance, including national platforms, accountability for disaster risk management, and preparedness to "Build Back Better"
- Recognition of stakeholders and their roles and the mobilization of risk-sensitive investment to avoid the creation of new risk
- Resilience of health infrastructure, cultural heritage, and workplaces
- Strengthening of international cooperation and global partnership, and risk-informed donor policies and programs, including financial support and loans from international financial institutions

The Vodaphone Foundation Technology Partnership is collaborating with the UN Foundation to provide knowhow and telecommunications resources to help relief workers to quickly establish mobile phone networks for reliable communications, and to allow them to photograph refugees with the goal of reuniting separated families (Center for Disaster Philanthropy, 2015).

The MacArthur Foundation recently financed several initiatives related to CHEs including providing a $225 000 grant to create an international criminal court to try war crimes committed in Uganda. The Foundation further provided an additional $1.5 million to fund programs for children affected by civil war in that country (Center for Disaster Philanthropy, 2015).

The W. K. Kellogg Foundation devoted significant funds to finance the immediate health needs of Haitians during the aftermath of the 2010 earthquake. Specifically, the Foundation provided $65 000 to the Soul Foundation to secure medical care for special-needs orphans. Taking into account long-term efforts, the Kellogg Foundation also provided World Vision with about $600 000 to support programs that help farmers in poor regions increase food supply, and further donated $300 000 to the Nature Conservancy to develop eco-tourism and environmental protection in coastal areas (Center for Disaster Philanthropy, 2015). As part of its mandate, the UNHCR works continually to provide emergency supplies, shelter, and life-saving food, medical care and water to refugees (United Nations High Commission for Refugees, 2016).

Discussion points

1 How different are natural disasters from CHEs?
2 What are some recently occurring natural disasters and CHEs?
3 How do disasters impact global health?
4 How can countries reduce and manage disasters?
5 Discuss the United Nation's priority list for responding to disasters.
6 How significant was the IDNR to disaster reduction?
7 How realistic is the HYOGO Framework for Action?
8 How different is the Sendai Framework from the Hyogo Framework?
9 What activities are private entities engaged in with regards to disaster reduction and management?
10 How would you describe global efforts towards disasters?

REFERENCES

Balkhi, A. (2015) *Twenty-Five Worst Earthquakes in History*, http://list25.com/25-worst-earthquakes-in-history/2/(accessed October 24, 2016).

BBC News (2011a) *Horn of Africa Drought: A Vision of Hell*. Radio news, http://www.bbc.com/news/uk-14078074 (accessed October 24, 2016).

BBC News (2011b) *Horn of Africa Drought: Somalia Aid Supplies Boosted*. Radio news, http://www.bbc.com/news/world-africa-14118507 (accessed October 24, 2016).

Blaikie, P., Cannon, T., Davis, I., and Wisner, B. (2003) *At Risk – Natural Hazards, People's Vulnerability and Disasters*, Routledge, London.

Center for Disaster Philanthropy (2015) *Complex Humanitarian Emergencies*, http://disasterphilanthropy.org/complex-humanitarian-emergencies/#sthash.c81LnALI.dpuf (accessed October 24, 2016).

Dimersar Academy. (2010) *Disaster Management Cycle*, https://sites.google.com/site/dimersarred/disaster-management-cycle (accessed October 24, 2016).

Harmer, A., Stoddard, A., and Toth, K. (2013) *Aid Worker Security Report 2013: The New Normal: Coping with the Kidnapping Threat*, https://aidworkersecurity.org/sites/default/files/AidWorkerSecurityReport_2013_web.pdf (accessed October 24, 2016).

Iceland, C. (2015) *A Global Tour of Seven Different Droughts*, http://www.wri.org/blog/2015/06/global-tour-7-recent-droughts (accessed October 24, 2016).

Inter-Agency Task Force on Disaster Reduction (2004) Extracts Relevant to Disaster Risk Reduction from International Policy Initiatives 1994- 2003, I, ninth meeting 4-5 May, 2004.

MercyCorps (2016) *Quick Facts: What You Need to Know About the Syria Crisis*, https://www.mercycorps.org/articles/iraq-jordan-lebanon-syria-turkey/quick-facts-what-you-need-know-about-syria-crisis (accessed October 24, 2016).

National Geographic (2016) *Tsunami's: Killer Waves*, http://environment.nationalgeographic.com/environment/natural-disasters/tsunami-profile/ (accessed October 24, 2016).

National Weather Service (2008) *Drought*. Public fact sheet, http://www.nws.noaa.gov/os/brochures/climate/DroughtPublic2.pdf (accessed October 24, 2016).

Overseas Development Institute (n.d.) *Doing Cash Differently: How Cash Transfers can Transform Humanitarian Aid*, http://www.odi.org/publications/9876-cash-transfers-humanitarian-vouchers-aid-emergencies (accessed October 24, 2016).

Quarantelli, E. L. (1998) *Where We Have Been and Where We Might Go. In What is a Disaster? A Dozen Perspectives on the Question*, Routledge, London.

Stone, A. (2002) Military's aid and comfort ease 9/11 survivors' burden. *USA Today*, http://usatoday30.

usatoday.com/news/sept11/2002-08-20-pentagon_x.htm (accessed October 24, 2016).

Summers, A. S. and Robbyn, S. S. (2011) *The-Eleventh-Day-The-Ultimate-Account-of-911*, http://www.telegraph.co.uk/culture/books/bookreviews/8722787/(accessed October 24, 2016).

Sydney's desal plant switched on. (2010) *The Sydney Morning Herald* (January 28), http://www.smh.com.au/environment/water-issues/sydneys-desal-plant-switched-on-20100128-n13h (accessed October 24, 2016).

United Nations (2015) *Sendai Framework for Disaster Risk Reduction 2015–2030*, http://www.unisdr.org/files/43291_sendaiframeworkfordrren.pdf (accessed October 24, 2016).

United Nations High Commission for Refugees (2016) *Central African Republic*, http://www.unrefugees.org/where-we-work/car/(accessed October 24, 2016).

United Nations International Strategy for Disaster Reduction (2007) *Hyogo Framework for Action 2005–2015: Building the Resilience of Nations and Communities to Disasters*. Extract from the Final Report of the World Conference on Disaster Reduction (A/CONF.206/6), 2005, http://www.unisdr.org/files/1037_hyogoframeworkforaction english.pdf (accessed October 24, 2016).

United Nations Development Fund Bureau for Crisis Prevention and Recovery (2010) *Disaster Risk Assessment*, http://www.undp.org/content/dam/undp/library/crisis%20prevention/disaster/2Disaster%20Risk%20Reduction%20-%20Risk%20Assessment.pdf (accessed October 24, 2016).

United States Geological Survey (2016) *Historic Earthquakes*, http://earthquake.usgs.gov/earthquakes/states/events/1964_03_28.php (accessed October 24, 2016).

Wachman, R. (2007) Water becomes the new oil as World runs dry. *Guardian*, https://www.theguardian.com/business/2007/dec/09/water.climatechange (accessed October 24, 2016).

Wooldridge, M. (2011) *Horn of Africa Tested by Severe Drought*, http://www.bbc.com/news/world-africa-14023160 (accessed October 24, 2016).

World Health Organization. (2011) *Disaster Risk Management for Health Overview*, http://www.who.int/hac/events/drm_fact_sheet_overview.pdf (accessed October 24, 2016).

World Vision (2015) *Top Humanitarian Crises of 2015*, https://www.worldvision.org/disaster-response-news-stories/top-humanitarian-crises-2015 (accessed October 24, 2016).

FURTHER READING

ABC News. *Timeline: 100 Years of Deadly Tsunamis* [News], http://www.abc.net.au/news/2004-12-29/timeline-100-years-of-deadly-tsunamis/610126 (accessed October 24, 2016).

Altay, N., & Labonte, M. (2004) *Challenges in Humanitarian Information Management and Exchange: Evidence from Haiti Overseas Development Institute*, John Wiley & Sons, Oxford.

CBS News (2003) *9/11 Fund Deadline Passes*. Television news, http://www.cbsnews.com/news/9-11-fund-deadline-passes/(accessed October 24, 2016).

Dechert, S. (2015) *UN All-Nighter Concludes World Disaster Risk Plan*, http://c1cleantechnicacom.wpengine.netdna-cdn.com/files/2015/03/Number-of-people-affected-by-disaster-type.png (accessed October 24, 2016).

Hackman, C. L., Hackman, E. E., and Hackman, M. E. (2001) *Hazardous Waste Operations and Emergency Response Manual and Desk Reference*, McGraw-Hill, New York.

Huber, C., and Reid, K. (2015) *Top Humanitarian crises of 2015*, http://www.worldvision.org/news-stories-videos/top-humanitarian-crises-2015 (accessed October 24, 2016).

Watts, R. J. (1889) *Hazardous Wastes: Sources, Pathways, Receptors*, John Wiley & Sons, New York, NY.

10

Gender and global sexual and reproductive health

Learning objectives

By the end of this chapter, you will be able to:

✔ Discuss the effects of gender and power relations on female reproductive health;

✔ List and explain at least two global sexual and reproductive health challenges;

✔ Describe at least two strategies for improving the sexual and reproductive health of women.

Summary of key points

The social status and role of women in certain societies have implications for their health in general and their sexual and reproductive health in particular. In societies where women have lower social status than men, gender roles, power relations, and gender inequities often determine their access to healthcare, family planning services, and contraceptives. While it has been established that women generally have higher life expectancy than men, it is pertinent to note that it is not because of their ability to seek medical care in time of ill health. Indeed, many women in low- and middle-income countries, especially those who are pregnant, are often unable to access healthcare. This is because of their economic situation and the systematic discrimination and inequities rooted in gender norms prevalent in the societies in which they live. Male dominance in relationships and gender-based violence (GBV) also influence women's access to reproductive healthcare (Whitehead, 1992). This chapter focuses on sexual and reproductive health with an emphasis on how gender, gender roles, and gender power relations affect women's reproductive health globally. It also points out some of the challenges associated with sexual and reproductive health, and global strategies and actions in place for improving the sexual and reproductive health of women.

Gender versus sex

The terms gender and sex are often used interchangeably. While closely linked, the two terms are distinct and do not mean the same thing. Gender refers to the differences between women and men within the same household and within and between cultures, which are socially and culturally constructed, and therefore changeable over time. As a social construct, gender is associated with what society defines as masculine (being aggressive, assertive, competitive, dominant, independent, objective, and rational), or feminine (being intuitive, passive, submissive, subjective, and supportive). Sex on the other hand,

Global Health: Issues, Challenges, and Global Action Lecture Notes, First Edition. Elizabeth A. Armstrong-Mensah.
© 2017 John Wiley & Sons Ltd. Published 2017 by John Wiley & Sons Ltd.

refers to the biological and anatomical differences that define individuals as either male or female. Unlike gender, which is a social construct and therefore changeable, sex is a biological fact, and difficult to change. Although often used to refer to women, the term "gender" embraces both women and men and their interdependent relationships.

Gender roles and gender power relations

Gender roles are the different roles and responsibilities expected of males and females in a given society. They comprise a set of social norms that dictate the attitudes, behaviors, characteristics, and values considered acceptable, appropriate, or desirable in people based on their actual or perceived sex. From childhood to adolescence, males and females are socialized to assume stereotyped roles and are judged by how well they conform to them. The roles they are made to assume influence their personalities, worldviews, and lives, and at times, cause conflict when one sex ceases to feel at ease with their ascribed gender role. Gender roles vary within and across cultures and have implications for decision-making, access to resources, opportunities, gender relations, and gender equality.

Sociological studies indicate that gender roles create a social hierarchy and an unequal division of power between men and women (Connell, 2001, 2005), which manifests in the form of female subordination and male dominance. Raewyn Connell, an Australian sociologist and influential voice in gender relations theorizing, advanced the theory that, masculinities and femininities play out at the societal level and that, although there are varied and multiple forms, they are all molded by social structures and institutions in which men dominate women. Recognizing gender hierarchy, he indicated that hegemonic masculinity is idealized masculinity that subordinates other masculinities and femininities. In his book *Gender and Power,* Connell further indicated that gender hierarchy is the result of labor (domestic and in the market), power (physical and authority), and cathexis (intimate relationships including parenting). He argued that hegemonic masculinity, as evidenced in marriage, paid work, and physical strength, benefit men, and that gender difference is really gender inequality as a result of gender power and hierarchy.

The subordination of women to men, gender division of labor characterized by substantial responsibilities, the limited control and lack of access to resources by women, physical and verbal abuse within intimate relationships; women's insecurity and vulnerability in their relationships with men and their dependence on men negatively affects many areas of their lives including their reproductive health (Avotri and Walters, 2001; Bottorff *et al.*, 2011).

The disempowerment, low status, and restricted decision-making capacity of women in relation to men in certain countries, puts them at risk of high birth and high maternal mortality rates. In Nepal, for example, girls marry as early as 14 years, and after 2 years become pregnant because their husbands want children. The power imbalance in the marriage makes it such that these girls cannot negotiate contraceptive use or delay pregnancy in order to pursue an education. They produce the number of children their husbands request, even if it is at the expense of their health (Regmi *et al.*, 2010). Birth spacing is another gender and power relations issue that affects women's reproductive health. The lack of communication between husband and wife plus culturally ascribed gender roles for women as wives and mothers, robs them of their right to negotiate the frequency of pregnancy.

Concepts of sexual and reproductive health

The concepts of sexual and reproductive health were first articulated at the United Nations International Conference on Development and Population (ICPD) held in Cairo, Egypt, in 1994. These concepts arose as a result of debates between demographers who were concerned with issues related to population growth and its impact on socio-economic development, and advocates of women's health rights, who were concerned about gender imbalances and the health needs of women. Prior to the ICPD, the health needs of women were traditionally addressed within the ambit of maternal and child health.

A noteworthy outcome of the ICPD was the Cairo Program of Action, titled "Gender Equality, Equity and Empowerment of Women," which underscored the empowerment and autonomy of women and the improvement of women's political, social, economic, and health status. Additional outcomes of the ICPD were the focus on the reproductive rights of women, and the development of the definitions of sexual and reproductive health (Finkle, n.d.).

Intent on producing a definition for sexual health and reproductive health, the ICPD Program of Action defined sexual health as:

> A state of physical, emotional, and mental wellbeing related to sexuality: not merely the absence of disease, dysfunction, or infirmity. Sexual health requires a positive and respectful approach to sexuality and sexual relationships, as well as the possibility of having pleasurable and safe sexual experiences, free of coercion, discrimination and violence. For sexual health to be attained and maintained, the sexual rights of all persons must be respected, protected, and fulfilled.

The ICPD Program of Action also defined reproductive health as:

> "A state of physical, mental, and social well-being in all matters relating to the reproductive system at all stages of life. Reproductive health implies that people are able to have a satisfying and safe sex life and that they have the capability to reproduce and the freedom to decide if, when, and how often to do so. Implicit in this are the right of men and women to be informed and to have access to safe, effective, affordable, and acceptable methods of family planning of their choice, and the right to appropriate health-care services that enable women to safely go through pregnancy and childbirth. (United Nations Population Information Network, 1994, paragraph 7.2, p. 43)

In 2002, the World Health Organization (WHO) adopted the ICPD definitions of sexual health and reproductive health as its working definition of the terms. A critique of the definitions is that they are pitched from a wellbeing and health perspectives rather than from a disease and death standpoint, hence making their measurement a challenge.

Reproductive ill health and global disease burden

Reproductive ill health encompasses illnesses, diseases, and disability associated with the reproductive system. Among women, reproductive ill health is caused by childbirth, sexually transmitted diseases, obstetric fistula, and reproductive tract cancers, and among men, by erectile dysfunction and prostate cancer among others. Globally, reproductive ill health is highest among women and infants who inherit health conditions or diseases from their mothers during pregnancy or childbirth. Using a narrow subset of possible reproductive morbidities, the 1990 Global Burden of Disease Study estimated that 21.9% of the disability-adjusted life years (DALYs) lost by women between the ages of 15–44 was due to reproductive ill health (Murray and Lopez, 1996).

Worldwide, pregnancy-related conditions and sexually transmitted diseases account for about 30% of the global burden of disease among women of reproductive age (15–44 years) and an estimated 5–15% of the total global burden of disease. Of the 3.43 million adult deaths that occurred globally in 2000, 98% were related to poor reproductive health. In 2010, about 800 women died from pregnancy and childbirth-related complications including severe bleeding, infections, and obstructed labor globally. Four hundred and forty of those deaths occurred in sub-Saharan Africa and 230 in south Asia.

In sub-Saharan Africa, Asia, the Arab region, Latin America, and the Caribbean, an estimated 2 million women are living with obstetric fistula, with about 50000 to 100000 new cases occurring each year. Obstetric fistula is a debilitating and traumatic childbirth injury that creates an abnormal hole between the vagina and the bladder and/or rectum due to prolonged, obstructed labor without timely medical intervention (Browning, 2004). Fewer than 8000 Ethiopian women (WHO) and between 2500–3000 women in Tanzania develop new fistulas every year. In Kenya, the number of new cases of fistulas stands at an estimated 3000 cases per year with only 7.5% treated cases. The direct consequences of obstetric fistula include constant involuntary leaking of urine, feces, or blood. The leakage causes a foul odor, repeated vaginal or urinary tract infections, and irritation or pain in the vagina or surrounding areas. The indirect consequences of obstetric fistula are social stigma, isolation, marginalization, and economic deprivation, which have implications for affected women, their spouses, children, and extended family.

Cancer of the cervix uteri (cervical cancer), cancers originating in the endometrium, and other cancers, such as ovarian, vulvar, vaginal, fallopian tube, and choriocarcinoma, are reproductive cancers in women that cause morbidity and mortality. Cervical, endometrial, and ovarian cancers are the most common cancers, whereas vulvar, vaginal, fallopian tube cancers, and choriocarcinomas are very rare. Cervical cancer is the third most common cancer in women worldwide with an estimated 530232 new cases in

2008 (Weiderpass and Labrèche, 2012). Over 85% of the global burden of cervical cancer occurs in developing countries. High standardized incidence rates (greater than 20 per 100 000 women) are found in Eastern, Western, and Southern Africa, South-Central Asia, South America, Melanesia, and Central Africa, and low standardized incidence rates are found in Western Asia, North America, and Australia / New Zealand (less than 6 per 100 000 women) (Ferlay et al., 2010). Cervical cancer was responsible for 275 000 deaths in 2008, with about 88% of those deaths occurring in developing countries.

Unsafe abortion

Although global maternal mortality rates have dropped significantly since the 1990s, maternal mortality continues to be a global health issue owing to a number of factors including unsafe abortions. Defined by WHO as "a procedure for terminating an unintended pregnancy performed by persons lacking the necessary skills, in an environment that does not conform to minimal medical standards, or both mostly," unsafe abortion is a health concern of many countries, especially those where abortion is illegal and where there is a lack of skilled medical personnel to perform the procedure.

Globally, 80 million of the 210 million pregnancies that occur are unintended. One in five and one in ten of those pregnancies often culminate in abortions and unsafe abortions, respectively. Performing abortions under unsafe conditions often results in the death of tens of thousands of women and girls around the world annually. It also results in several chronic and often irreversible health conditions. Of the estimated 46 million induced abortions that occur each year globally, about 19 million are performed in unsafe conditions and or by unskilled providers, resulting in the deaths of about 68 000 women and girls. These deaths account for approximately 13% of all pregnancy-related deaths globally.

From 2003 to 2008, unsafe abortions increased from 19.7 million to 21.6 million worldwide. In 2008, the global unsafe abortion rate was 14 unsafe abortions per 1000 women aged 15–44 years. In that same year, the unsafe abortion rate in developing countries was 27 per 1000 women aged 15–44 years, and 16 per 1000 women of the same age group in developed countries. The high unsafe abortion rate in developing countries can be attributed to the

growing unmet contraceptive needs of women and to gender and power relations (World Health Organization, 2012).

Gender-based violence

Gender-based violence is any gender-based act or conduct that results in, or is likely to result in, physical, sexual, or psychological harm or suffering to women or men including threats of such acts, and all forms of coercion or arbitrary deprivations of liberty in both the public and private sphere (Universal Access Project, 2015). It is often directed at women due to their unequal power relations with men and the fact that they are women. Gender-based violence takes various forms such as rape, forced early marriage, female genital mutilation, intimate partner violence (IPV)/domestic violence, sexual violence, sexual exploitation, marital rape, trafficking, and femicide – the violent and deliberate killing of women because of their sex by males. The occurrence and brutality of GBV varies between countries and across continents, but its negative health impacts on individuals and families are universal (United States Agency for International Development, 2010).

Gender-based violence affects women's sexual and reproductive health. It is a prime barrier to pleasurable and safe sexual experience and family planning. Gender-based violence is most prominent in societies where gender roles are strictly defined, observed and enforced, where masculinity is linked with toughness, male honor or supremacy, where the suppression of women and children is accepted, and where violence is the norm for conflict resolution in relationships (Heise et al., 1999; Jewkes, 2002).

Rape

Rape as a weapon of war, acts of sexual violence against women in refugee camps, forced sexual initiation, and the abuse of children are all unacceptable acts. These personal violations not only disrupt communities, but also affect the sexual and reproductive health of those victimized. A cross-sectional study of sexual violence showed that 40% of the first sexual intercourse of women in South Africa, 28% in Tanzania, and 7% in New Zealand were forced and mostly perpetrated by men known to the women (Watts and Zimmerman, 2002).

Early marriage

The early marriage of girls to older men is also a form of GBV. In certain parts of East and West Africa, girls are married off at a very young age (as early as 8 or 14 years) against their will. This predisposes them to childbearing at a very early age and to a wide range of reproductive ill-health issues including obstructed labor, obstetric fistula, and incontinence brought about by prolonged labor and the lack of access to emergency healthcare during childbirth. Girls under the age of 15 are five times more likely to die in childbirth than women in their twenties. This is because the bodies of the latter are more mature and therefore more able to handle pregnancy than those of the former (United Nations Department of International Economics and Social Affairs, 1991).

Female genital mutilation

Female genital mutilation (FGM), also known as "female genital cutting" or "female circumcision," is a culturally supported form of GBV prevalent in more than 29 countries in Africa and the Middle East. In these countries, over 125 million girls between infancy and the age of 15 have been circumcised under the guise that it is crucial for preparing them for adulthood and marriage, and for maintaining cultural norms around femininity and modesty (World Health Organization, 2014).

Female genital mutilation is the intentional alteration, causing of injury to, or the partial or total removal of the external female genitalia for cultural, traditional, or nonmedical reasons. Major reproductive ill-health issues associated with FGM include severe bleeding, chronic pain, complications during childbirth, increased risk of neonatal mortality, cysts, difficulty urinating, infection, infertility, and sexual dysfunction. There are no health benefits associated with FGM. Indeed, it is a selfish health-compromising act perpetrated against women by women in favor of men to ensure premarital virginity and marital fidelity of wives. It violates the human rights of girls and women.

Domestic violence / intimate partner violence

Domestic violence, also known as intimate partner violence, is accepted as "normal" in some societies regardless of its harmful effects on the health of victims. Domestic violence usually manifests in the form of physical, sexual or emotional abusive acts, verbal aggression, or controlling behaviors. Evidence from studies reveal that domestic violence is the leading cause of injury and disability for women in many parts of the world (see Figure 10.1), and is a risk factor for numerous physical, mental, sexual, and reproductive health problems. Domestic violence not only has lasting consequences for the health, development, and wellbeing of the children of female victims. It also has a negative socio-economic impact on society as a whole (Ellsberg et al., 2008).

In 1993, the United Nations (UN) General Assembly, formally recognizing the urgent need for the universal application to women, the rights to equality, security, liberty, integrity and dignity, and a life free of violence, passed the Declaration on the Elimination of Violence Against Women. According to the UN, at least one in three women is beaten, coerced into sex, or abused by an intimate partner in the course of her lifetime. A 2005 WHO study of ten countries and 15 sites, revealed that 15–71% of ever-partnered women had experienced physical or sexual violence, or both, at the hands of an intimate partner. A Demographic and Health Survey (DHS) report on domestic violence in Bolivia, Cameroon, Columbia, Kenya, Peru, and Zambia, also found that over 40% of women had at some point experienced violence from a spouse or partner (Kishor and Johnson, 2004). Domestic violence increases the chances of women contracting sexually transmitted infections and having more children than they would otherwise have liked, as it limits their ability to control the timing of sex and the negotiation of contraceptive use.

Pregnant women have also been found to be at high risk of physical, sexual, and emotional abuse by intimate partners. The violence they experience is often triggered by the presence of an unwanted or unplanned pregnancy. This is the case in Bangladesh, Bolivia, the Dominican Republic, Kenya, Malawi, Moldova, New Zealand, Rwanda, and Zimbabwe. In rural Peru, one out of every four women has experienced violence during pregnancy. Abuse during pregnancy often results in fatal consequences, such as homicide and suicide, or in nonfatal consequences such as hemorrhaging, low birthweight of babies, miscarriage, obstetric complications, poor maternal weight gain, preterm labor or delivery, sexually transmitted infections, unsafe abortions, depression, lack of attachment to children by mothers, and physical impairment (Campbell et al., 2004). Evidence from the United States shows an increased risk of homicide among pregnant women by an intimate partner. Police and medical examiner records in 11 United States cities from 1994 to 2000, attests to this (Campbell et al., 2003).

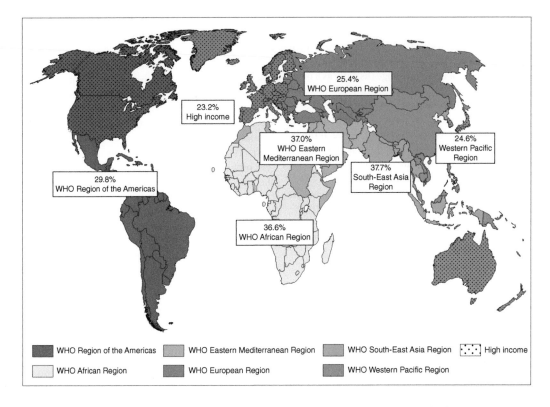

Figure 10.1 Global map showing regional prevalence of rates of intimate partner violence by WHO region, 2010. *Source*: World Health Organization, London School of Hygiene and Tropical Medicine, and South African Medical Research Council (2013), with permission.

Family planning

Having access to family planning and reproductive health services is crucial to the health and survival of women and children. Through family planning, which is controlling of the number of children in a family and the intervals between them, couples are able to regulate whether or not to have children, when to have children, and the number of children to have. Family planning improves upon the health of women and their children because it reduces high-risk pregnancies, stops or delays childbearing, and allows women to give birth at their healthiest time. It also facilitates sufficient spacing between pregnancies, promotes contraceptive use, reduces unsafe abortions or the need for abortion, promotes women's and girls' rights and opportunities for education, employment and full participation in society, and controls fertility and population growth with their concomitant strain on natural resources. Findings from studies

point out that children born 3–5 years apart have a better chance of surviving to the age of 5 than children born less than 2 years apart. According to the United States Agency for International Development, (USAID), the practice of family planning has the tendency to prevent about 30% of the over 287 000 annual global maternal deaths and to save the lives of 1.6 million children under the age of 5 per annum (United States Aigency for International Development, n.d.).

Globally, over 225 million women have unmet contraceptive needs, that is, they want to avoid pregnancy but are not using any form of contraception. This situation is especially true of women in developing countries and is the result of a myriad of factors including culture and GBV. In 2011, an estimated 143 million women worldwide, married or of reproductive age, had an unmet need for family planning. Over 50% of countries in west Africa and the Horn of Africa, as well as in countries in Asia such as Afghanistan, Pakistan, Saudi Arabia, Tajikistan, Timor-Leste, the United Arab Emirates, and Yemen have an estimated contraceptive prevalence rate of below

30%. Bosnia and Herzegovina and Montenegro in Europe have contraceptive prevalence rates of less than 50%. North America has the highest contraceptive prevalence rate in the world (75%) followed by Latin America and the Caribbean (73%), and then Europe (70%) (United Nations, 2013).

Sexually transmitted diseases

Sexual violence, trauma, and forced unprotected sex predispose women to a number of sexually transmitted infections and diseases. Sexually transmitted infections (STIs) are infections that are transferred from one person to another through sexual intercourse (vaginal and anal), kissing, oral-genital contact, or the use of sexual toys. These infections usually have no symptoms. Sexually transmitted diseases (STDs) are also infections that are transmitted during sexual contact. However, these have symptoms and can cause impairment or abnormality. Having an STD means an infection is actually causing one to be sick or is contributing to disease, symptoms are felt by the individual, the infection shows on the body, or is discovered by a doctor through assessment. It must be noted that while all STDs are preceded by STIs, not all STIs become STDs. Sexually transmitted diseases are considered to be dangerous because they can spread easily and cannot be easily detected by just looking at a person (Campbell, 2002).

There are over 25 STDS caused either by bacteria, viruses, or parasites. Chlamydia, gonorrhea, and syphilis are some of the STDs caused by bacteria. The human immunodeficiency virus (HIV), human papilloma virus (HPV), hepatitis B, and herpes are STDS caused by a virus, and trichomoniasis is an STD caused by a parasite. Five of the above-mentioned STDs are discussed in this section.

Human immunodeficiency virus

HIV causes acquired immune deficiency syndrome (AIDS). Among other pathways, it is transmitted through having unprotected sex with an infected person, sharing infected needles, receiving infected blood, and from mother to child during pregnancy, childbirth, or breastfeeding. Symptoms associated with HIV are rapid weight loss, dry cough, recurring fever or profuse night sweats, profound and unexplained fatigue, swollen lymph glands, diarrhea, and white spots or unusual blemishes on the tongue, in the mouth, or throat. Human immunodeficiency virus symptoms do not manifest right away. They usually show about 5–10 years after infection. The virus progressively compromises the body's immune system and reduces its ability to fend off infections and other opportunistic diseases. When an HIV-positive person has a CD4 count of less than 200 cells/mm^3 that person is said to have AIDS. A normal CD4 count ranges from 500 to 1000 cells/mm^3 of blood.

An HIV study conducted in South Africa revealed that power inequality and intimate partner violence increased the risk of HIV infection among young women (Jewkes *et al.*, 2010). A 2008 report on married women in India also showed that HIV prevalence was four times higher among women who had experienced physical and sexual IPV than among nonabused women (Silverman *et al.*, 2008; World Health Organization, 2005). Another study in Tanzania, revealed that young women, aged 18–29, who had been abused by a partner were ten times more likely to be HIV positive than their counterparts who had not been abused (Maman *et al.*, 2001).

Chlamydia

Chlamydia is caused by the bacterium *Chlamydia trachomatis*. It is very common among teens and young adults. Chlamydia is transmitted by having unprotected anal, vaginal, or oral sex with an infected person, through contact with infected body fluids, and from an untreated mother to her baby during childbirth. Chlamydia often has no symptoms, but where there are symptoms, they appear 1–3 weeks after infection. About 80–90% of women who are infected with chlamydia are asymptomatic. Symptoms of chlamydia in women include vaginal discharge caused by an inflamed cervix, lower abdominal pain, low back pain, nausea, fever, pain during intercourse, or unusual bleeding between menstrual periods. In men, there is white, cloudy, and watery discharge from the penis (see Figure 10.2). Chlamydia can cause infertility and ectopic pregnancy in women and infertility in men. It can also cause eye (conjunctivitis) or lung (pneumonia) infections in babies. Women with chlamydia are five times more likely to become infected with HIV.

A cross-sectional analysis of 3521 women in the United States on exposure to various types of interpersonal violence, showed that women who reported that they had experienced four or more types of violence were over five times more likely to report a lifetime of chlamydia diagnosis compared to women

(a) (b)

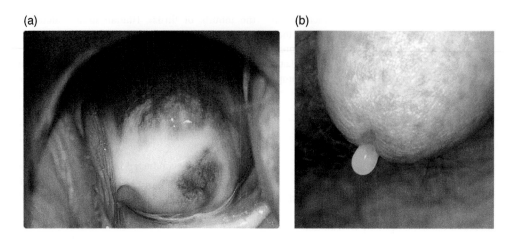

Figure 10.2 Discharge from (a) the cervix and (b) the penis due to chlamydia.
Sources: SOA-AIDS Amsterdam (2014).

(a) (b)

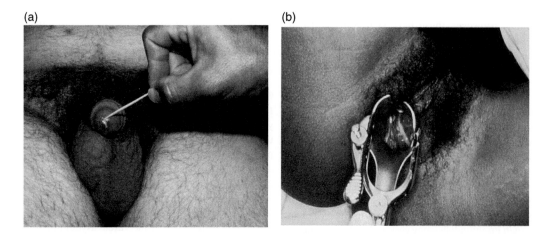

Figure 10.3 Gonorrhea discharge from (a) penis and (b) vagina.
Source: Centers for Disease Control and Prevention, Division of STD Prevention, National Center for HIV/AIDS, Viral Hepatitis, STD, and TB Prevention: Gonorrhea, http://phil.cdc.gov/phil/details.asp (accessed October 24, 2016). Male photo by Renelle Woodall.

who had never experienced interpersonal violence. Women who experience physical and or sexual partner violence are 1.5 times more likely to be infected with syphilis, chlamydia, or gonorrhea.

Gonorrhea

Gonorrhea is caused by the *Neisseria gonorrhoeae* bacterium. It is most common among the reproductive age group and men sleeping with men (MSM). Like chlamydia, gonorrhea is transmitted by having unprotected anal, vaginal, or oral sex with an infected person, through infected body fluids, and from an untreated mother to her baby during childbirth. Gonorrhea is often asymptomatic in women and symptomatic in men. In men, symptoms usually appear 2–5 days after infection. Symptoms include a white, yellow, or green discharge from the penis, burning pain when passing urine, and painful testicles (see Figure 10.3). In women, symptoms appear within 10 days of infection and include cloudy and yellow vaginal discharge, burning when passing

(a)

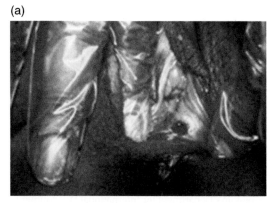

(b)

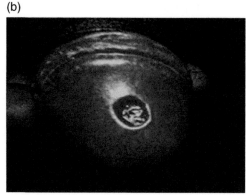

Figure 10.4 Primary stage syphilis on (a) the vagina and (b) the penis.
Source: Centers for Disease Control and Prevention National Center for HIV, STD, & TB. *Syphilis Images*, http://www. cdc.gov/std/syphilis/images.htm (accessed October 25, 2016).

urine, and vaginal bleeding. In the case of an oral infection, there may be a sore throat.

Gonorrhea can infect the eye and rectum, and can cause infertility, brain infections, and eye and skin infections in neonates. Resistance to medication is making the treatment of gonorrhea a major health challenge.

Syphilis

Syphilis is caused by the *Trepenoma pallidum* bacterium. It can be transmitted during vaginal, anal, or oral sex and by direct contact with syphilis sores on the vagina, anus, and lips, and in the rectum and mouth. Pregnant women with the syphilis can pass it on to their unborn babies.

Syphilis is a slowly progressing infection that has several stages. Symptoms of primary-stage syphilis are the appearance of painless ulcers (chancres) at the place where the syphilis bacteria entered the body (see Figure 10.4). Secondary symptoms may include flulike illness, a non-itchy rash, patchy hair loss, and flat, warty-looking growths on the vulva in women and around the anus in both women and men. If not adequately treated, primary stage syphilis can progress to the secondary stage.

Syphilis can cause heart trouble, blindness, deafness, and brain damage if left untreated in neonates. About 4–15% of pregnant women in Africa test positive for syphilis. The Centers for Disease Control and Prevention (CDC) recommends that all pregnant women should be tested for syphilis. Syphilis may predispose one to HIV.

Trichomonas

Trichomonas, also known as "trich," is caused by the protozoan parasite, *Trichomonas vaginalis.* The trich parasite can be transmitted from an infected person to an uninfected person during sex, from a penis to a vagina, from a vagina to a penis, or from a vagina to another vagina. It is not common for the parasite to infect other body parts, like the hands, mouth, or anus. Trich has very few symptoms and is harder to detect in men than in women. Men do not usually have symptoms.Where there are symptoms, they usually appear 5–28 days after exposure. In men, there is itching or irritation inside the penis, burning after urination or ejaculation, or discharge from the penis. In women, there is itching, burning, redness or soreness of the genitals, discomfort with urination, or a thin discharge with an unusual smell, which is usually clear, white, yellow, or green. Trich causes genital inflammation that makes it easy for one to become infected with or transmit HIV to a sex partner.

Sexual and reproductive health challenges

By reason of their sex and marginalized status in society, women and young girls tend to suffer disproportionately from STDs and other sexual and reproductive health-related issues. Their lack of access to contraceptives put them at risk for unintended pregnancies, and unsafe abortions (Barot, 2011).

Harmful cultural norms, male dominance, the lack of women's control over their own bodies and reproductive choices, and the lack of women's access to accurate STI/STD information, contraceptives, appropriate cost-effective interventions, and integrated reproductive health services are some of the sexual and reproductive challenges women face in different parts of the world.

Global strategies and action for improving sexual and reproductive health

In recent years, efforts have been made at the national and global levels to reduce maternal morbidity and mortality. At the national level, countries have created mechanisms to address sexual and reproductive health issues. In Tanzania, for example, the Ministry of Health and Social Welfare (MoHSW) has developed national strategies to decrease maternal deaths and to improve upon reproductive health. These strategies specifically focus on strengthening and improving the provision of antenatal care to pregnant women, expanding emergency obstetric care services, and increasing knowledge and use of contraceptives. The MoHSW has also partnered with multiple nongovernmental organizations including the Bloomberg Philanthropies, which support efforts to improve maternal and neonatal health, by upgrading health facilities to provide quality comprehensive emergency obstetric and neonatal care services in the Kigoma, Pwani, and Morogoro Regions of Tanzania. Bloomberg Philanthropies is currently scaling up activities in the Kigoma Region to incorporate family planning and comprehensive postabortion care into the operations of various health facilities (Centers for Disease Control and Prevention, 2015).

Several policies, programs, and initiatives exist at the global level to tackle the issues of maternal and child morbidity and mortality. In 2010, the UN Secretary-General, Ban Ki-moon, unveiled a global strategy for women's and children's health, which focused on family-planning information and services, antenatal, newborn and postnatal care, emergency obstetric and newborn care, skilled care during childbirth at appropriate facilities, and the prevention of HIV and other STIs. Unlike the Millennium

Development Goals, this strategy was not based on country consensus. Thus, although beneficial to women, it was generally regarded as not carrying as much weight as other UN documents or policies.

At the global level, the G-8 launched Muskoka Initiative also sought to promote comprehensive, high-impact and integrated sexual and reproductive health interventions, including antenatal care, attended childbirth, postpartum care, sexual and reproductive healthcare and services including voluntary family planning (G-8, 2010). The International Alliance for Reproductive, Maternal and Newborn Health, a public-private partnership comprising USAID, the United Kingdom's Department for International Development (DFID), the Australian Agency for International Development (AusAID), and the Bill and Melinda Gates Foundation, seek to reduce unmet family planning needs. They also seek to expand skilled birth attendance and facility-based deliveries, and increase the number of women and newborns receiving quality postnatal care, so as to reduce child mortality and improve maternal health.

The United Nations Populations Fund (UNFPA) supports programs that specifically address the challenges people face at different points in their lives, such as STI prevention services and the treatment of reproductive health illnesses (including breast and cervical cancer). It works with governments, other UN agencies, civil society, and donors to develop comprehensive efforts to ensure universal access to sexual and reproductive healthcare through primary healthcare.

At present, family planning services, screening for lower reproductive tract infections, and other reproductive health services are being integrated in certain countries to ensure that women's reproductive health needs are met during and after pregnancy. Reproductive health service providers in developing countries are becoming sensitive to the social conditions that adversely affect women's reproductive health. Some community leaders and national governments now see the utility and need to sponsor health education programs and interventions on violence against women, FGM, and rape among others, and the need to discourage their perpetration.

Discussion points

1 What is the difference between gender and sex?
2 What is sexual health? How different is it from reproductive health?
3 How do gender roles and gender power relations affect female reproductive health?

4 Explain reproductive ill health. What are some examples and how do these examples affect the reproductive health of women?

5 To what extent is unsafe abortion a reproductive health issue?

6 What two STDS are caused by bacteria? Describe their symptoms and how they are transmitted.

7 What are the causes and effects of the various aspects of gender-based violence on women's reproductive health?

8 What role does culture play on the reproductive health of women?

9 List and explain three sexual and reproductive health challenges.

10 What global strategies and actions are in place to address global sexual and reproductive health issues?

REFERENCES

Avotri, J. Y. and Walters, V. (2001) We women worry a lot about our husbands: Ghanaian women talking about their health and their relationships with men. *Journal of Gender Studies* **10**, 197–211.

Barot, S. (2011). Unsafe abortion: The missing link in global efforts to improve maternal health. *Policy Review*, **14**(2), 24–28.

Bottorff, J. L., Oliffe, J. L., Robinson, C. A., and Carey, J. (2011) Gender relations and health research: a review of current practices. *International Journal for Equity in Health* **10**(60), 1–8.

Browning, A. (2004) Obstetric Fistula in Ilorin, Nigeria. *PLoS Medicine* **1**.1, 022–024.

Campbell, J. (2002) Health consequences of intimate partner violence. *The Lancet* **359**(9314), 1331–1336.

Campbell, J., Garcia-Moreno, C., and Sharps, P. (2004) Abuse during pregnancy in industrialized and developing countries *Violence Against Women* **1**(10), 770–789.

Campbell, J., Webster, D., Koziol-McLain. J., *et al.* (2003) Risk factors for femicide in abusive relationships: Results from a multisite case control study. *American Journal of Public Health* **93**(7), 1089–1097.

Centers for Disease Control and Prevention (2015) *2014 Kigoma Reproductive Health Survey: Kigoma Region, Tanzania*, Centers for Disease Control and Prevention, Atlanta, GA, https://www.cdc.gov/reproductivehealth/global/publications/surveys/africa/kigoma-tanzania/2014-kigoma-reproductive-health-survey_tag508.pdf (accessed October 30, 2016).

Connell, R. (2001) *The Men and the Boys*, University of California Press, Berkeley, CA.

Connell, R. (2005) *Masculinities*, Allen & Unwin, Sydney.

Ellsberg, M., Jansen, H.A., Heise, L., *et al.* (2008) Intimate partner violence and women's physical and mental health in the WHO Multi-country Study on Women's Health and Domestic violence: an observational study. *The Lancet* **371**(9619), 1165–1172.

Ferlay, J., Shin, H. R., Bray, F., *et al.* (2010) Estimates of worldwide burden of cancer in 2008: GLOBOCAN (2008). *International Journal of Cancer* **127**(12), 2893–2917.

Finkle, J. L. (n.d.) *Impact of the 1994 International Conference on Population and Development*, http://www.un.org/esa/population/publications/completingfertility/RevisedFINKLEpaper.PDF (accessed October 24, 2016).

G-8 (2010) *Muskoka Declaration: Recovery and New Beginnings*, https://www.whitehouse.gov/sites/default/files/g8_muskoka_declaration.pdf (accessed October 28, 2016).

Heise, L., Ellsberg, M., and Gottemoeller, M. (1999) Ending violence against women. *Population Reports, L*(**11**).

Jewkes, R. (2002) Intimate partner violence: causes and prevention *The Lancet*, **359**(9315), 1423–1429.

Jewkes, R., Dunkle, K., Nduna, M., and Shai, N. (2010) Intimate partner violence, relationship power inequity, and incidence of HIV infection in young women in South Africa: A cohort study. *The Lancet* **376**(9734), 41–48.

Kishor, S., and Johnson, K. (2004) *Profiling Domestic Violence – A Multi-Country Study*, ORC Macro, Calverton, MD.

Maman, S., Mbwambo, J., Hogan, M., *et al.* (2001) *HIV and Partner Violence: Implications for HIV Voluntary Counseling and Testing Programs in Dar es Salaam, Tanzania*, http://pdf.usaid.gov/pdf_docs/PNACL410.pdf (accessed October 25, 2016).

Murray, C. J. L., and Lopez, A. D. (eds.) (1996) *The Global Burden of Disease: A Comprehensive Assessment of Mortality and Disability from Diseases, Injuries, and Risk Factors in 1990 and Projected into 2020*, Harvard School of Public Health, Cambridge, MA.

Regmi, K., Smart, R., and Kottler, J. (2010) Understanding gender and power dynamics within the family: A qualitative study of Nepali women's experience. *The Australian and New Zealand Journal of Family Therapy* **31**(2), 191–201.

Silverman, G., Decker, M., Saggurti, N., *et al.* (2008) Intimate partner violence and HIV infection among married Indian women. *Journal of the American Medical Association* **300**(6), 703–710.

SOA-AIDS Amsterdam (2014) *Chlamydia-Trachomatis-Female*, https://commons.wikimedia.org/wiki/File:SOA-Chlamydia-trachomatis-female.jpg (accessed October 28, 2016).

STD (2005) *Chlamydia Symptom Photo – Male*, http://www.std-gov.org/std_picture/chlamydia.htm (accessed October 25, 2016).

United Nations (2013) *World Contraceptive Patterns*, http://www.un.org/en/development/desa/population/publications/pdf/family/worldContraceptivePatternsWallChart2013.pdf (accessed October 25, 2016).

United Nations Department of International Economics and Social Affairs (1991) *The World's Women: Trends and Statistics 1970–1990*, United Nations, New York, NY.

United Nations Population Information Network (1994) *Report of the International Conference on Population and Development*, http://www.un.org/popin/icpd/conference/offeng/poa.html (accessed October 25, 2016).

United States Agency for International Development (2010) *Gender-Based Violence: Impediment to Reproductive Health*, http://www.prb.org/igwg_media/gbv-impediment-to-RH.pdf (accessed October 25, 2016).

United States Agency for International Development. (n.d.) *Family Planning and Reproductive Health*, https://www.usaid.gov/what-we-do/global-health/family-planning (accessed October 25, 2016).

Universal Access Project (2015) *Briefing Cards: Sexual and Reproductive Health: Sexual and Reproductive Health and Rights (SRHR) and Sustainable Development*, http://www.universalaccessproject.org/wp/wp-content/uploads/2015/06/BriefCards_RH_6.30.2015.pdf (accessed October 25, 2016).

Watts, C., and Zimmerman, C. (2002) Violence against women: global scope and magnitude. *The Lancet*, **359**(9313), 1232–1237.

Weiderpass, E. and Labrèche, F. (2012) Malignant tumors of the female reproductive system. *Safety and Health at Work* **3**(3), 166–180.

Whitehead, M. (1992) The concepts and principles of equity and health. *International Journal of Health Services* **22**(3), 429–445.

World Health Organization (2005) *Multi-Country Study on Women's Health and Domestic Violence*, http://www.who.int/gender/violence/who_multicountry_study/Introduction-Chapter1-Chapter2.pdf (accessed October 25, 2016).

World Health Organization (2012) *Unsafe Abortion Incidence and Mortality: Global and Regional levels in 2008 and Trends during 1990–2008*, http://apps.who.int/iris/bitstream/10665/75173/1/WHO_RHR_12.01_eng.pdf (accessed October 25, 2016).

World Health Organization (2014) *Female Genital Mutilation*. Fact sheet no. 241, http://collections.infocollections.org/ukedu/en/d/Js0519e/ (accessed October 25, 2016).

World Health Organization, London School of Hygiene and Tropical Medicine, and South African Medical Research Council. (2013) *Global and Regional Estimates of Violence Against Women*, http://apps.who.int/iris/bitstream/10665/85239/1/9789241564625_eng.pdf (accessed October 25, 2016).

FURTHER READING

Gender, Hierarchy, Power and Inequality: What Sociological Theory Adds to our Understanding of Sex-Discrimination, http://www.westminsterlawreview.org/downloads/Gender%20Hierarchy%20Power%20and%20Inequality%20UoWSLR%20Article%20Feb%202012.pdf (accessed October 25, 2016).

World Health Organization (2002) *World Report on Violence and Health*, http://apps.who.int/iris/bitstream/10665/42495/1/9241545615_eng.pdf (accessed October 25, 2016).

World Health Organization (2005) *World Health Report 2005: Make Every Mother Count*, http://www.who.int/whr/2005/whr2005_en.pdf (accessed October 25, 2016).

11

Health systems and global health

Learning objectives

By the end of this chapter, you will be able to:

- ✔ Define health system and health system strengthening;
- ✔ List and explain at least two health system goals;
- ✔ Identify and discuss at least two health system building blocks;
- ✔ Discuss at least two challenges associated with health systems;
- ✔ Discuss global action and strategies for addressing health system challenges.

Summary of key points

While there is no perfect health system, an effective and well-functioning health system is essential for the improvement and maintenance of a population's health. Unlike high-income countries, health systems in most low- and middle-income countries (LMICs) are often unable to provide the needed medicines, vaccines, care, or treatment in an affordable, effective, or timely manner for the populations they serve. Thus, people in this part of the world often tend to suffer or die from diseases that could have been prevented. While countries around the world use diverse health system models to meet the healthcare needs of their populations, they all generally strive to improve health, treat the sick, and where possible, protect patients from financial ruin that could arise from the payment of huge medical bills (World Health Organization, 2015). To be effective, health systems need to improve the health status of populations,

individuals and communities, and provide access to population-centered care as and when needed. This chapter focuses on the models, goals, and building blocks of health systems. It discusses health system resources and their management, and then goes on to describe health systems in LMICs. This chapter goes on to provide a brief overview of health system strengthening, unveils some of the challenges associated with health systems, and finally, describes global actions and strategies employed to address those challenges.

The concept of a health system

Also referred to as healthcare system, a health system is the mobilization of people, institutions, and resources that provide healthcare services to meet the health needs of target populations. It is also:

Global Health: Issues, Challenges, and Global Action Lecture Notes, First Edition. Elizabeth A. Armstrong-Mensah.
© 2017 John Wiley & Sons Ltd. Published 2017 by John Wiley & Sons Ltd.

The people, institutions and resources, arranged together in accordance with established policies, to improve the health of the population they serve, while responding to people's legitimate expectations and protecting them against the cost of ill-health through a variety of activities whose primary intent is to improve health. (World Health Organization, 2007)

From the definitions, it is clear that health systems not only comprise of healthcare providers, health facilities, and health insurance organizations working together to provide health services, but also parents taking care of their sick children at home, behavior change interventions, health and safety legislation, and intersectoral actions geared towards improving a population's health.

Health system models, goals, and building blocks

Health systems are modeled differently from country to country, but generally take one of four forms:

- The Beveridge model, named after William Beveridge, the social reformer who designed Britain's National Health Service. This model focuses on healthcare provision through government taxation. It is used in Great Britain, Spain, and most of Scandinavia and New Zealand.
- The Bismarck model, named after the Prussian Chancellor, Otto von Bismarck, who is credited with inventing the welfare state as part of the unification of Germany in the nineteenth century. This model emphasizes healthcare provision through health insurance schemes financed jointly by employers and employees through the payroll deduction system. It is used in Belgium, Germany, France, Japan, the Netherlands, Switzerland, and to some degree in Latin America.
- The National Health Insurance Model, which comprises elements of both the Beveridge and Bismarck models. This model focuses on private-sector healthcare provision and government-run citizen contribution to health insurance programs. It is used in Canada and in some newly industrialized countries including Taiwan and South Korea.
- The Out-of-Pocket Model, which requires patients to pay healthcare providers directly for services

they receive. This model is prevalent in various forms in Australia and many countries in sub-Saharan Africa (Physicians for a National Health Program, 2010).

Health system goals and functions

Irrespective of how health systems are modeled, their primary goal, according to WHO, should be to improve upon the health of the populations they serve, respond to the population's legitimate healthcare expectations through the provision of quality services, provide fair financial protection against the cost of ill health, and to use available resources efficiently. However, the extent to which health systems actually achieve these goals varies from country to country.

To achieve WHO-identified healthsystems goals, health systems need to establish certain mechanisms and perform certain functions. Among other things, health systems need to have a well trained, well paid, responsive, and productive workforce that can efficiently provide health services. They need to set up real-time surveillance systems to collect reliable health information that can be used to inform decision making and policies. They also need to ensure that all patients, irrespective of their socioeconomic status, have equal access to, and receive quality, safe, and cost-effective medical products, vaccines, and technologies. In addition, health systems need to mobilize adequate funds to cover the health expenditure of patients, so as to protect them from becoming bankrupt or impoverished after seeking care. Finally, health systems need to have able leadership that can provide effective oversight and ensure proper governance and accountability (World Health Organization, 2007).

Ideally, the above mentioned functions should be set in motion and assured by national governments, but in reality this is not the case in some countries. This is because of a number of factors in addition to the lack of managerial capacity, and the poorly organized nature of many health systems. Effective health system oversight and management have the propensity to improve health system performance and to identify potential areas for reform.

Figure 11.1 shows WHO's health systems framework. It highlights the ideal goals and functions of health systems.

System building blocks   Overall goals/outcomes

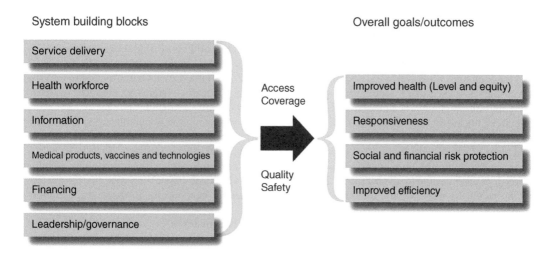

Figure 11.1 The World Health Organization health system framework.
Source: World Health Organization (2007), with permission.

Health system resources and management

Health-system resources are the means available to a healthcare system to deliver services to a population. There are three main categories of health-system resources: physical capital, consumables, and human capital. Physical capital comprises nonhuman healthcare infrastructure such as ambulances, clinics, equipment, hospitals, and hospital furnishings including beds and operating tables. Consumables are disposable resources such as adhesive bandages, gauze, medical gloves, paper, pharmaceuticals, and syringes that are used on a day-to-day basis in healthcare delivery. Worldwide, the cost associated with consumables in the delivery of healthcare account for an enormous portion of daily health system expenditure. In 2011 alone for example, England's 165 hospital trusts spent an estimated £4.6 billion on consumables (Matheison, 2011). Human capital, often regarded as the most important health system resource, comprises trained clinical and nonclinical health personnel who are responsible for the provision of public and individual health interventions (Kabene *et al.*, 2006). These health personnel include allied healthcare professionals, dentists, doctors, nurses, midwives, and pharmacists. In certain parts of the world, they also include trained community health workers. A well educated, skilled, and motivated workforce is the key to successful health system performance.

Globally, human capital costs account for over 66% of a country's health system recurrent costs.

Access to health system resources in LMICs is a challenge and its management is an even greater challenge. The efficient and effective management of health system resources prevents a mismatch and imbalance of resources, ensures that the right number and mix of trained healthcare professionals are fairly distributed geographically throughout a country and not concentrated in the urban areas, facilitates the delivery of necessary quality health services to populations, and aids with the accurate projection of future physical capital, consumables, and human capital needs.

Health systems in low-middle- and high-income countries

After gaining independence from their colonial masters, the governments of some LMICs sought to provide their populations with quality healthcare services. Thus, they established teaching hospitals and clinics. These institutions were located in urban areas and created access issues for populations living in rural areas. These populations thus had to depend on missionary hospitals and clinics for their healthcare needs. By the 1970s, the health status of rural communities in LMICs was on the decline, as morbidity and mortality rates were on the rise (Bennett, 1979).

This state of affairs, coupled with other factors, caused WHO and the United Nations Children Fund (Unicef) to advocate for fundamental changes in the delivery of healthcare services. They emphasized the need for equitable access to healthcare at an affordable cost and for disease prevention, while still providing appropriate curative health services. Hence, in 1978, WHO organized the International Conference on Primary Health Care (PHC) at Alma-Ata in Kazakhstan. This conference culminated in the adoption of the Declaration of Alma-Ata, which expressed the need for urgent action by all governments, health and development workers, and the international community, to protect and promote the health of all people by the year 2000, regardless of their gender, income, or education. Countries were to achieve this goal by using the primary healthcare (PHC) approach, which involves universal community-based preventive and curative services, with substantial community involvement (Hall and Taylor, 2003). The Declaration of Alma-Ata affirmed access to basic health services as a fundamental human right.

In the bid to implement the Declaration of Alma-Ata, LMICs embarked on health system reforms, part of which focused on the strengthening of health systems. Despite their efforts, they were unsuccessful in achieving health for all by 2000. One of the reasons offered to explain this failure was the fact that not all aspects of the reforms were implemented, especially those associated with cross-sectoral initiatives to address socio-economic factors that affect healthcare, and those that focused on securing sufficient human and other resources to provide health services akin to those in high-income countries. Another reason was the unwillingness of experts and politicians in LMICs to allow communities to plan and provide their own healthcare services. A further reason was the economic recession of the 1970s, which tempered the enthusiasm of the international community to financially support a comprehensive approach to PHC in LMICs. Thirty-seven years after the adoption of the Declaration of Alma-Ata, many people, especially those in LMICs still lack equitable access to basic health services and the gap is greater in certain parts of the world than others.

Health systems in low- and middle-income countries

The health systems of many LMICs can at best be described as far from satisfactory. They are poorly structured and lack adequate funding. Whereas high-income countries spend an average of 7% of their gross domestic product on the health of their populations, middle-income countries expend less than 4%, and low-income countries, less than 3%. With low national expenditures on health and the inability of health systems to mobilize funds to finance healthcare, health systems in LMICs are unable to provide the populations they serve with comprehensive, high-quality, affordable, and universally accessible healthcare. Therefore, health inequity, manifested in the form of inequitable access to critical diagnostics, treatment, care, and medications, becomes the norm, with the affluent having more access to quality healthcare. In LMICs healthcare is primarily achieved through government-run schemes based on the collection of taxes.

Health systems in LMICs often tend to lack an adequate, efficient, and well trained health workforce. This is because most of the well trained health personnel frequently migrate to high-income countries in search of better paying jobs. Recent WHO estimates show that there is a shortage of over 4 million health workers globally and that, 57 of the poorest countries in the world have fewer than 2.5 doctors, nurses, and midwives per 1000 people. Sub-Saharan Africa, which accounts for about 24% of the global disease burden, has only 3% of the health workforce it needs. As stated by the International Organization for Migration, there were more Ethiopian physicians practicing medicine in Chicago in 2006, than there were in Ethiopia itself (Evans and Rasanathan, 2015).

Health facilities in LMICs are inadequately equipped and ill prepared to respond to and provide care and treatment to their populations in times of emergencies and disease outbreaks. This was evidenced during the Ebola outbreak in Guinea, Liberia, and Sierra Leone in 2014. Due to the water and power situations in LMICs, some health facilities lack access to clean water and experience interrupted power supply during service delivery.

Well established and functioning realtime health surveillance systems that monitor, collect, and provide accurate and timely information, enable policymakers, managers, and individual service providers to make informed decisions about patient care, budgets, and treatment. Unfortunately, such systems are either nonexistent or not functioning the way they should in LMICs. It is therefore not strange that the health focus of health systems in these parts of the world is primarily curative (MEASURE, n.d.).

High-income countries

Health systems in high-income countries are highly structured and efficient. They have strong regulatory frameworks and relatively sufficient numbers of skilled personnel to run them (Zakus and Bhattacharyya, 2007). In high-income countries and most recently, the United States, health systems seek to provide some form of comprehensive universal health coverage to their citizens. In these countries, the goal is to ensure that all people receive quality, essential health services without experiencing financial hardship. In high-income countries, universal healthcare is achieved through various mechanisms: government-run schemes based on the collection of government taxes, such as Britain's National Health Service (NHS), a combination of government and privately run schemes where the government pays the larger share, as is the case in France and Canada, and private health insurance schemes where insurance companies receive government subsidies to pay for healthcare for citizens and where insurance companies are regulated to ensure universal coverage so as to avoid discrimination due to pre-existing conditions. This is the case in Switzerland, which has one of the best health systems in the world (World Health Organization and World Bank, 2015). In Switzerland, the government subsidizes healthcare for the poor on a graduated basis. The aim is to prevent individuals from spending more than 10% of their income on health insurance.

High-income countries do not experience the same level of health workforce shortages as LMICs. Indeed, these countries absorb the well trained health workers who migrate from their home countries. In high-income countries like France where healthcare is almost completely funded, people have easy and equal access to primary care physicians and specialists. The approach to medicine in these countries unlike low-income countries, is preventative care. As health systems in high-income countries are mostly technology driven, healthcare costs can be high, and since almost everyone has access to healthcare through a national health insurance scheme, the burden on the healthcare workforce is great, and can affect the quality of services provided.

Health system strengthening

Defined as "Any array of initiatives and strategies that improves one or more of the functions of the health system and that leads to better health through improvements in access, coverage, quality, or efficiency" (Islam, 2007), health systems strengthening is vital to global health security. The suddenness, swiftness, and extent to which infectious diseases, both emerging and re-emerging, plague the world, make it necessary for health systems to be strengthened, so as to be better equipped and prepared to respond to global health threats.

Rationale for health systems strengthening

Until the twentieth century, health systems in LMICs were set up to treat infectious diseases and health issues related to women and children, poor water and sanitation, and nutrition. With the epidemiological transition, these countries now find themselves in a situation where they not only have to deal with the socio-behavioral illnesses and communicable diseases that they are familiar with, but also with noncommunicable diseases they are unfamiliar with and lack the skills to effectively handle. The treatment and care of people with noncommunicable diseases requires a different set of knowledge, health personnel, medications, research, technology, vaccines, and shifts from traditional care to institutional care, all of which are foreign to many LMICs.

As a result of globalization, health systems need to be on the alert and ready to handle global health threats when they arise within or outside their territories. Thus, they need to build the capacity of their health workforce, establish or improve laboratory and health surveillance capacity to collect quality data for decision making, improve upon processes, logistics, and supply systems to ensure that essential drugs, equipment, and personnel can be transported to where they are needed, increase health financing, reduce financial risk protection, and ensure accountability, oversight, and the development of appropriate health-policy frameworks. Strengthened health systems save lives, protect and enhance human capital, help to achieve global health security, improve life expectancy and productivity, and promote economic growth and development.

In the attempt to support the strengthening of health systems in LMICs, the Global Alliance for Vaccines and Immunizations (GAVI) works with poor countries to identify and address immunization coverage weaknesses and needs. In the area of workforce development, GAVI has trained healthcare workers in 13 of the poorest provinces in Afghanistan and has created a network of new health centers and mobile health teams across five provinces (Global Alliance for Vaccines and Immunizations, 2015).

Between 2013 and 2014, Britain's Department for International Development (DFID) spent an estimated £360 million on strengthening health systems as part of its technical assistance to governments and health providers in LMICs (House of Commons International Development Committee, 2014). The United States President's Emergency Plan for AIDS Relief (PEPFAR) also supports health systems strengthening initiatives in LMICs. Specifically, PEPFAR has helped to improve the quality and access to laboratory services for human immunodeficiency virus (HIV) and other health needs. Through injection safety programs, PEPFAR has assisted with the reduction of the medical transmission of HIV and other blood-borne pathogens. PEPFAR has also promoted the use of mobile phones as a means for health information reporting and communication (PEPFAR, n.d.). In 2010, the World Bank financed a $130 million five-year health systems strengthening project in Uganda to improve upon the health workforce, physical health infrastructure, management, leadership, and accountability for health service delivery (World Bank, 2016).

Health system challenges

There are several challenges that plague health systems globally. In 2015 for example, the government of Malawi faced challenges related to the sustainable financing and efficient management and delivery of quality healthcare to its citizens. The government was also saddled with an acute shortage of adequately trained health personnel across all professional fields, as well as with health supply chain management, infrastructure, and equipment issues (United States Agency for International Development, 2015).

In 2014, the Norwegian Agency for Development Cooperation (Norad) found that weak health systems negatively impacted the performance of immunization programs in LMICs. Reasons proffered for this outcome included the presence of few and under-trained staff, the lack of transportation or funds for immunization activities at the district level, insufficient tracking of district immunization coverage and vaccine stock levels, and inadequate health infrastructure in postconflict situations.

Recent surveys on essential medicines in 39 LMICs found a wide variation when it came to availability. The average availability of essential medicines in the public sector was 20% and 56% in the private sector. As mentioned earlier, there are major shortages in the health workforce in LMICs because of "brain drain."

Globally, 57 countries are experiencing extreme shortages of healthcare workers and 36 of these countries are in Africa. High-income countries also face some challenges when it comes to securing an adequate health workforce. These countries usually rely on migrant health workers from developing countries to meet and fill in the gap of their health workforce needs.

People, especially the poor, elderly, and those with chronic conditions continue to suffer great financial consequences after seeking healthcare (Shah, 2011). Indeed, the lack of financial protection from the high cost of health care, causes about 100 million people to be pushed below the poverty line each year, thus, making it even more difficult for people to seek care in times of ill health (Mills, 2014).

Health surveillance and data collection remains a challenge in LMICs. Less than 25% of deaths in over 60 countries are recorded by vital registration systems. This makes it difficult for the world to know what people are dying from. Inappropriate technology is another health system challenge experienced globally. An estimated 50% of medical equipment either donated or purchased by LMICs cannot be used due to the lack of know-how, and the unavailability of spare parts on the local market to maintain them. In some cases, ambulances purchased have become unusable as the make and/or models ordered were not compatible with the local terrain. In certain high-income countries, poor health system design causes poor hygiene and safety standards, which in turn leads to high rates of hospital-acquired infections, which sometimes cause illness or death.

Additional health system challenges are the continued focus on curative medicine by LMICs rather than on preventative medicine and the location of health centers in places only accessible to urban dwellers. The external funding of vertical or disease-specific programs and the relative underfunding of the broader health care infrastructure in LMICs, are further challenges to health systems.

Global action and strategies

To address the issue of health workforce shortages, a draft global strategy on human resources for health has been developed by the international community. The final version of the strategy was considered by WHO Member States at the 69th World Health Assembly in May 2016. The goal of the strategy is to ensure the availability, accessibility, acceptability, and quality of the health workforce through adequate investments, and the implementation of effective policies at the national, regional, and global levels, to ensure healthy lives for all in all age groups, and for promoting equitable socio-economic development through decent employment opportunities (World Health Organization and Global Health Workforce Alliance, n.d.).

In order to track health systems' response to increased inputs, impact on health outcomes, accountability, the strengthening of health system gaps, and to inform accurate decision making by governments at the country and global levels, a global monitoring and evaluation framework was put in place in 2010, spearheaded by WHO. This framework is the result of a collaborative process with inputs from country health systems experts from around the world as well as WHO, the World Bank, the Global Fund to Fight AIDS, Tuberculosis and Malaria, GAVI; MEASURE, Health Metrics Network, and Unicef among others. The evaluation framework guides the collection of data around a set of indicators on the six WHO health systems building blocks (World Health Organization, 2010).

Over one billion people do not have access to the health services they need because those services are inaccessible, unavailable, unaffordable, or are of poor quality. To address these issues, WHO assists Member States to create resilient health systems and to move towards universal health coverage by supporting them to develop, implement, and monitor solid national health policies, strategies and plans, encouraging Member States to assure the availability of equitable integrated people-centered health services at an affordable price, facilitating access to affordable, safe and effective medicines and health technologies and by helping Member States to strengthen their health information systems and evidence based policy-making.

Discussion points

1 What is the difference between health system and health system strengthening?
2 What is the relevance of health systems to global health?
3 How should health system resources be managed to realize maximum benefits?
4 Describe WHO health system building blocks and show how they link to the functions of health systems.
5 How are health systems in LMICs different from those in high-income countries?

6 Identify and describe three health-system challenges globally.
7 How are multilateral organizations helping to strengthen health systems in LMICs?
8 What global strategies are in place to address health system strengthening challenges?
9 Should the international community assist LMICs to improve upon their health systems? Why?
10 What should LMICs do to make their health systems more effective and efficient?

REFERENCES

Bennett, F. (1979) Primary health care and developing countries. *Social Science and Medicine* **13A**, 505–514.

Evans, T. and Rasanathan, K. (2015) *Primary Care in Low- and Middle-Income Countries*, http://www.mhprofessionalresources.com//mediacenter/hpim18/assets/pdf/Harr18_e01.pdf (accessed October 25, 2016).

Global Alliance for Vaccines and Immunizations (2015) *Health System Strengthening Support*, http://www.gavi.org/support/hss/ (accessed October 25, 2016).

Hall, J. J. and Taylor. R. (2003) Health for all beyond 2000: The demise of the Alma-Ata Declaration and primary health care in developing countries. *Medical Journal of Australia* **178**(1), 17–20.

House of Commons International Development Committee (2014) *Strengthening Health Systems in Developing Countries Fifth Report of Session 2014–15 Report*, http://www.publications.parliament.uk/pa/cm201415/cmselect/cmintdev/246/246.pdf (accessed October 25, 2016).

Islam, M. (ed.) (2007) *Health Systems Assessment Approach: A How-To Manual*, http://www.urc-chs.com/sites/default/files/Health_Systems_Assessment.pdf (accessed October 25, 2016).

Kabene, S. M., Orchard, C., Howard, J. M. *et al.* (2006) The importance of human resources management in health care: a global context. *Human Resources for Health* **4**, 20.

Matheison, S. A. (2011) Hospitals could save £500m on consumables, says NAO. *Guardian*, http://www.theguardian.com/healthcare-network/2011/feb/02/hospitals-save-500m-consumables-nao-nhs (accessed October 25, 2016).

MEASURE (n.d.) *Health Information Systems*, http://www.cpc.unc.edu/measure/our-work/health-information-systems (accessed October 25, 2016).

Mills, A. (2014) Health care systems in low- and middle-income countries. *New England Journal of Medicine* **370**, 552–557.

PEPFAR (n.d.) *Health Systems Strengthening*, http://www.pepfar.gov/about/strategy/ghi/134854.htm (accessed October 25, 2016).

Physicians for a National Health Program (2010) *Health Care Systems, Four Basic Models*, http://www.pnhp.org/single_payer_resources/health_care_systems_four_basic_models.php (accessed October 25, 2016).

Shah, A. (2011) *Health Care around the World*, http://www.globalissues.org/article/774/health-care-around-the-world (accessed October 25, 2016).

United States Agency for International Development (2015) *Malawi's Health Systems Strengthening*. Fact sheet, http://www.usaid.gov/malawi/global-health/health-systems-strengthening (accessed October 25, 2016).

World Bank (2016) *Uganda Health Systems Strengthening Project* http://www.worldbank.org/projects/P115563/uganda-health-systems-strengthening-project?lang=en (accessed October 25, 2016).

World Health Organization (2015) *Health Systems*, http://www.who.int/topics/health_systems/en (accessed October 25, 2016).

World Health Organization (2007) *Everybody's Business: Strengthening Health Systems to Improve Health Outcomes: WHO's Framework for Action*, http://www.who.int/healthsystems/strategy/everybodys_business.pdf (accessed October 25, 2016).

World Health Organization (2010) *Monitoring the Building Blocks of Health Systems: A Handbook of Indicators and their Measurement Strategies*, http://www.who.int/healthinfo/systems/WHO_MBHSS_2010_full_web.pdf?ua=1 Accessed (accessed October 25, 2016).

World Health Organization and Global Health Workforce Alliance (n.d.) *Health Workforce 2030. A Global Strategy on Human Resources for Health*, http://www.who.int/workforcealliance/knowledge/resources/strategy_brochure9-20-14.pdf?ua=1 (accessed October 25, 2016).

World Health Organization and World Bank (2015) *Tracking Universal Health Coverage: First Global Monitoring Report*, http://apps.who.int/iris/bitstream/10665/174536/1/9789241564977_eng.pdf?ua=1 (accessed October 25, 2016).

Zakus, D. and Bhattacharyya, O. (2007) *Health Systems, Management, and Organization in Low- and Middle-Income Countries*, https://cdn1.sph.harvard.edu/wp-content/uploads/sites/114/2012/10/RP248.pdf (accessed October 25, 2016).

FURTHER READING

Lewis, T., Synoweic, C., Lagomarsino, G. and Schweitzer, J. (2012) E-health in low- and middle-income countries: Findings from the Center for Health Market Innovations. *Bulletin of the World Health Organization* **90**, 332–340.

Gillam, S. (2008) Is the declaration of Alma Ata still relevant to primary health care? *British Medical Journal*, **336**(7643), 536–538.

12

Financing global health

Learning objectives

By the end of this chapter, you will be able to:

- ✔ Describe at least two functions of health financing;
- ✔ List and explain at least two sources of global health financing;
- ✔ List and explain at least two determinants of global health expenditure;
- ✔ Discuss at least two global health financing challenges;
- ✔ Discuss global action and strategies for addressing global health financing challenges.

Summary of key points

Adequate financing is crucial for the existence and effective functioning of health systems. Among other things, it determines the extent to which a country can provide quality healthcare services to meet the expectations of the population it serves. Many developing countries, due to their modest economic performance and limited financial resources, are unable to meet the health needs of their citizens and therefore rely heavily on external financial flows in the form of development assistance for health (DAH) to finance health. While DAH continues to be available to developing countries, its volatility and inadequacy, coupled with the burden it places on developed countries, has prompted a global search for innovative financial mechanisms to fill the financial gap for healthcare provision in developing countries. This chapter focuses on the concept, functions, methods, and sources of global health financing. It discusses health expenditures in developing and developed countries, the challenges associated with financing global health, and select innovative mechanisms for global health financing.

The concept of health financing

Health financing re-emerged as a vital component of the global health debate, as developing countries struggled to meet the health-related Millennium Development Goals (MDGs) by the end of 2015, and as DAH from the donor community was becoming volatile and inadequate. Per the World Health Organization (WHO), health financing is the:

> Function of a health system concerned with the mobilization, accumulation and allocation of money to cover the health needs of the people, individually and collectively, in the health system...the purpose of health financing is to make funding available, as well as to

Global Health: Issues, Challenges, and Global Action Lecture Notes, First Edition. Elizabeth A. Armstrong-Mensah.
© 2017 John Wiley & Sons Ltd. Published 2017 by John Wiley & Sons Ltd.

set the right financial incentives to providers, to ensure that all individuals have access to effective public health and personal healthcare. (World Health Organization, 2010, p. 72)

Health financing is also the collection of funds from various sources, pooling of funds, spreading of risks across larger population groups, and the allocation or use of funds to purchase services from public and private providers for healthcare. Through adequate health financing, countries are able to provide their citizens with essential health services, reduce health inequalities, provide financial protection against impoverishment owing to huge unforeseen healthcare costs, and ensure that healthcare providers are remunerated adequately for their services.

Mechanisms for financing healthcare differ across countries and are largely determined by political, economic, and social factors. The amount of funds governments allocate for healthcare affects health outcomes, and the equitableness and efficiency of health systems (Schieber *et al.*, 2006).

Functions of health financing

Health systems perform three main functions: revenue collection, pooling of resources, and purchasing of services. Combined, these functions enhance health system performance and effectiveness.

Revenue collection is the method used by health systems to mobilize funds from businesses, the government, households, individuals, or external sources to finance healthcare. Methods of revenue collection are varied and include taxation, national health insurance, private or voluntary health insurance, and out-of-pocket payments (Murray and Fenk, 2000).

Pooling of resources is the accumulation and management of funds collected by health systems to ensure that members of a pool pay an average expected cost for healthcare in advance, so as to protect themselves from huge unforeseen health expenditures in time of ill health. Through the pooling of resources, health spending between high- and low-risk individuals (risk subsidies) and high- and low-income individuals (equity subsidies) are redistributed to cover all in the pool.

Health purchasing is the means through which public and private agencies pay for and provide health services to beneficiaries. Health-service purchasing may be passive (purchasing based on predetermined budgets or the payment of bills when presented), or strategic (purchasing based on seeking out better quality services at low prices). Health services may be purchased directly by governments through the payment of healthcare providers with general government revenues or insurance contributions for their services, or indirectly by purchasing agencies such as health insurance companies. Purchasers of health services usually include Ministries of Health (MoH), social security agencies, insurance organizations, individuals, or households.

Methods of health financing

The methods employed by countries to finance healthcare is very much contingent upon their level of development, mobilization infrastructure, and the mechanism they deem most appropriate. Methods of financing healthcare may be internal or external to countries.

Internal/local methods

Internal methods of health financing comprise means used by national governments to mobilize funds from within their own economies to finance health. In certain parts of the world, both developed and developing, governments rely exclusively on one type of internal method to finance health while others rely on a combination of internal methods. Internal methods for health financing discussed in this section include general taxes, national health insurance, private health insurance, community-based health insurance, and out-of-pocket- payments.

General taxation

General taxation is a relatively new, but widely utilized mechanism for financing healthcare expenditures worldwide. Revenue from general taxation is derived directly from income tax, property tax, or taxes levied on households and enterprises, or indirectly from value added taxes, or sin taxes on alcohol and tobacco. Countries like Australia, Canada, Denmark, Finland, Ghana, Greece, Ireland, Italy, Portugal, Spain, Sweden, and the United Kingdom have health systems that are exclusively financed by taxes. Tax-based health financing has the ability to pool funds on a continuous basis from a large number of people and to distribute risks across health status, income levels, and entire populations (Guy, 2003).

National health insurance

National health insurance (NHI) is a compulsory insurance scheme that, by law, requires eligible groups of people in a country to enroll and purchase a set of health benefits. Social security, Medicare, the Railroad Retirement program, state-sponsored unemployment insurance programs in the United States, and the Canada Pension Plan (CPP) are all examples of NHI programs.

Administered by the public or private sector, or a combination of both, NHI is either totally or partly funded with tax money and varies by revenue collection mechanism, programs, and service provision. In Australia and the United Kingdom, NHI contributions to the Medicare system and the National Health Service system, respectively, are made exclusively through government taxation. These countries have single-payer healthcare systems where funding for healthcare is made by a single public body; from a single fund. Unlike Australia and the United Kingdom, Ghana's NHI scheme is funded from four different sources: (i) Value-added tax, which is a 2.5% tax levied on goods and services and accounts for 70% of tax revenue; (ii) An earmarked portion of social security taxes from formal sector workers, which accounts for 23% of tax revenue; (iii) Individual premiums, which account for about 5% of tax revenue; and (iv) Miscellaneous funds from investment returns, or Parliament, which account for 2% of tax revenue (Blanchet *et al.*, 2012).

National health insurance schemes provide standard minimum coverage for everyone enrolled without discrimination on grounds of age, occupation, or existing health conditions. Protection for members and insurance companies under this scheme is provided by an equalization pool, which allows risks to be spread between the various funds. Governments sometimes contribute to the equalization pool through healthcare subsidies. This model is used in the Netherlands.

In Germany and Belgium, NHI schemes are implemented through sickness funds, which are primarily funded through huge contributions from employers and a minimum portion from employees. Health services under the NHI scheme are provided by publicly owned or privately owned healthcare providers. Like tax-based systems, most NHI schemes have the benefit of pooling large numbers of people and transferring risk to the government. Through prepayment, NHI schemes make it possible for persons enrolled to seek care from healthcare facilities and to obtain prescriptions in times of ill health.

Private health insurance

Private health insurance (PHI) involves the voluntary purchase of an insurance package. Through PHI, employers, private businesses, individuals, or households enter into private contracts with insurance companies and prepay specified premiums in exchange for insurance packages that meet their health needs. Private health insurance also involves pooling resources and risks. For individuals, PHI premiums are calculated based on individual pre-existing risk conditions and for groups, on risk factors across age, gender, and health status. Unlike NHI programs, which are compulsory, PHI is voluntary.

Community-based health financing

Community-based health financing is an insurance scheme organized at the community level to provide financial resources to promote better health, protect individuals and households against direct financial cost of illness, and to release the poor from the trap of social exclusion. Community-based health financing is organized on the principles of community cooperation, local self-reliance, and prepayment. It is especially prevalent in low- and middle-income countries and targets people who are self-employed, work in the informal sector, and who are socially marginalized and cannot be reached by government or market-based health financing schemes (Jakab and Krishnan, 2001). Contributions to community-based health financing schemes are not risk related. They involve high levels of community participation in the pooling, allocation and management of resources, and are typically financed by individual collections, government grants, and donor support. Funds raised through this scheme for healthcare are often inadequate.

Out-of- pocket payment

Out-of-pocket payments, also known as direct payments or user fees, are payments made by patients to healthcare providers at the time of service delivery. They often take the form of co-insurance, co-payments, deductibles, or the raw cost of healthcare. Out-of-pocket payments as a means of health financing are prevalent in both developing and developed countries. The amount of money a person pays out of pocket for healthcare is primarily dependent on the type of insurance they have or the lack of it, their age, and the health issues they suffer from. In most cases, out-of-pocket payments can be high and unexpected, and can lead to financial impoverishment and hardship. A study conducted in Australia found that patients who were financially challenged and in poor health, were the ones who suffered the heaviest out-of-pocket cost for medication and medical services. The same study also found that senior citizens and persons suffering from chronic conditions like cancer, high blood pressure, diabetes, or depression also had higher out-of-pocket expenditures (Islam *et al.*, 2014).

External methods

External methods of health financing are financial flows for healthcare that formally originate from outside a country. These external sources are generally referred to as development assistance for health (DAH). Development assistance for health is a primary source of global health funding in many developing countries.

Sources of development assistance for health

Development assistance for health is made available to beneficiary countries from various sources including: (i) bilateral development assistance agencies represented by governments of donor countries such as the Danish International Development Agency (DANIDA); (ii) multilateral development assistance entities such as the World Bank and regional development banks; (iii) United Nations (UN) agencies through public-private partnerships such as the Global Fund to Fight AIDS, Tuberculosis, and Malaria (GFTAM) and the Global Alliance for Vaccines Initiative (GAVI); (iv) nongovernmental organizations (NGOs); and (v) private foundations like the Bill and Melinda Gates Foundation (World Vision International, 2013).

Funding channels and modalities for development assistance for health

Multilateral organizations, which are organizations whose funding sources include multiple governments, disburse all DAH funding directly to national governments through credits and grants. International financing institutions (IFIs) such as the World Bank and the three regional development banks (the African Development Bank, the Asian Development Bank, and the Inter-American Development Bank) disburse DAH loans and grants directly to national governments based on country plans. United Nations agencies, both implementing organizations and channels of donor funding, expend a huge portion of their health budget on their own programs, agency research, and technical assistance, and disburse a small portion of their health budget on national government programs, research, and health systems.

The GFTAM, a new UN public-private multilateral organization for financing rapid prevention, care, and treatment of HIV, malaria, and tuberculosis (TB), disburses grants directly to civil society organizations, national governments, and the private sector (World Vision International, 2013). The GAVI, another new UN public-private multilateral organization, also disburses the majority of its grants to national governments in developing countries for the strengthening of vaccine delivery systems and for piloting new or underused vaccines.

Bilateral organizations, which are government agencies responsible for providing aid, use various mechanisms to disburse DAH to recipient countries. The majority of them disburse funds through NGOs. The United States and Canada, two of the largest bilateral donors, disburse 52% and 48% of DAH, respectively through NGOs. Australia and Ireland also disburse over 33% of their DAH through NGOs, while South Korea channels 80.6% of its DAH through government entities. Most European countries channel DAH through the European Commission (EC) or multilateral organizations. Finland and Austria for instance, allocate a high percentage of their DAH to the United Nations Populations Fund (UNFPA), whereas France supports the GFTAM with 35% of its DAH. Germany, Japan, and Italy disburse a greater part of their DAH through bilateral and multilateral organizations, and only 10% through NGOs. Although bilateral organizations employ different modalities to fund NGOs, almost all of them do so through competitive calls for proposals and tenders. In 2010, about 38% of funding for health by bilateral organizations was channeled through NGOs, 25% through governmental entities, and the remaining 36% was split among UN agencies and other multilaterals (World Vision International, 2013).

Development assistance for health trends

Development assistance for health grew significantly after 2000 due to a number of factors including the adoption of the MDGs, increased bilateral and multilateral funding, and the establishment of new global health partnerships and private foundations. In 2010, total DAH from all sources increased from $5.6 billion in 1990 to \$28.2 billion. Bilateral disbursements were the most significant, accounting for 45% of all DAH, with the United States government being the largest single bilateral donor, disbursing \$7 billion annually, representing 25% of the total global DAH portfolio in 2010 (Schieber *et al.*, 2006).

Among multilateral organizations, the UN provided 17% of total DAH in 2010. This was a decrease of 24% compared to 2001 levels. From 2011 to 2012, the percentage of DAH from all UN agencies increased modestly due to increased health expenditures by the United Nations Children's Fund (Unicef). In 2010, the GFTAM disbursed over \$3.3 billion, accounting for 11% of the total DAH portfolio. Although relatively smaller, GAVI rapidly increased its disbursements in 2012 to \$1.8 billion. Also a UN agency, the World Bank accounted for 5% of all DAH in 2010, down from 17% in 2001. Nevertheless, between 2011 and 2012, the World Bank's disbursements increased by 22%. The three regional development banks provided about 2% of all health funding in 2008, and less than 1% in 2010, with no change in the previous two years (World Vision International, 2013).

DAH areas of priority

With regards to priority areas (see Figure 12.1), HIV/AIDS received the most funding of \$7.7 billion in 2011, accounting for 25.1% of all DAH (Institute of Health Metrics and Evaluation, 2013). The size of the disbursement can be attributed to the burden of disease it causes, the quest to achieve MDG6 which focuses on HIV/AID and other diseases, the establishment of the United States President's Emergency Fund for AIDS Relief (PEPFAR), the establishment of GFTAM in 2002, and the successful implementation of mother-to-child HIV/AIDS prevention programs.

Maternal, newborn, and child health (MNCH) received the second largest DAH disbursement of \$6.1 billion in 2011. Although not as much as that allocated to HIV/AIDS, DAH allocation to this area increased by 17.7% and accounted for 23.3% of all DAH in 2011. The increment in funding was influenced by global efforts, including the Group of 8 (G8) Muskoka Initiative to accelerate progress towards the attainment of MDGs 4 and 5 (Institute of Health Metrics and Evaluation, 2013; Shukla, 2015).

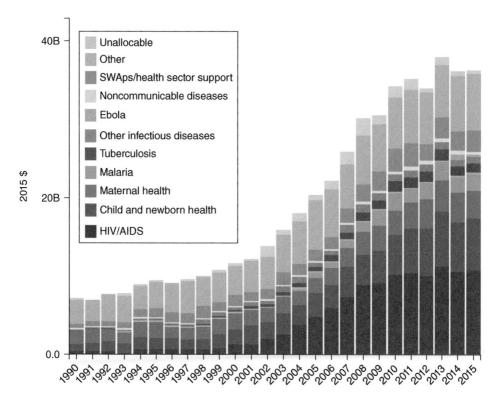

Figure 12.1 Health focus areas for development assistance for health, 1990–2015.
Source: Institute for Health Metrics and Evaluation (2015), with permission.

Development assistance for health expenditure on MNCH was specifically in the areas of childhood vaccinations, antenatal care, postnatal care, and the maintenance of maternal and child health.

Noncommunicable diseases (NCDs) did not receive that much donor funding in 2011. Although what it received ($377 million) was an increase from previous years, it was only 1.23% of total DAH for that year. To date, NCDs continue to receive the least DAH funding compared to other health areas, irrespective of the fact that diseases such as cancer, diabetes, and ischemic heart disease among others, now account for about 50% of the burden of disease in low- and middle-income countries. In 2011, DAH for HIV/AIDS was 20 times higher than that allocated to NCDs.

Development assistance for health system strengthening and the improvement of population health increased by 6% to $1.3 billion from 2010 to 2011, accounting for 4.3% of total DAH in 2011 (Institute of Health Metrics and Evaluation, 2013a). Development assistance for malaria was $1.8 billion in 2011, accounting for 5.8% of DAH in that year. This was a reduction of 13.9% compared to 2010 levels. Development assistance for health for TB from 2000 to 2011 was $1.3 billion, a little less than that allocated to malaria. Disbursements for TB represented 4.1% of total DAH in 2011. The size of TB disbursements can be attributed to decreases in TB incidence, prevalence, and death rates during that period. It must be noted that although HIV received the highest DAH from 2010 to 2011, MNCH and NCDs received the most increases per health area.

DAH recipients by region and country

Low- and middle-income countries are the primary recipients of DAH (see Figure 12.2). By region, sub-Saharan Africa, South Asia, East Asia, and the

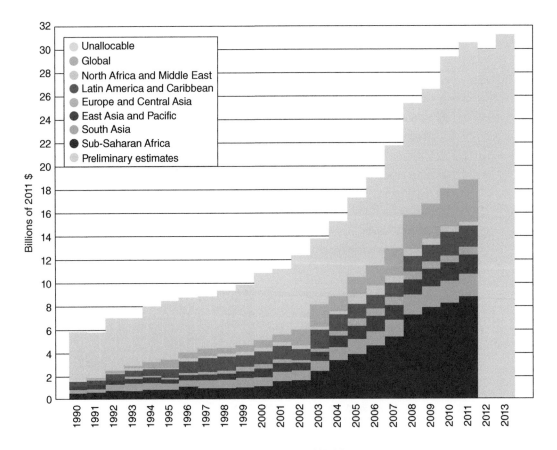

Figure 12.2 Development assistance for health by focus region, 1990–2011.
Source: Institute for Health Metrics and Evaluation (2014), with permission.

Pacific regions received the highest levels of DAH compared to the Latin America and Caribbean, Europe and Central Asia, and the North Africa and Middle East regions in 2011. Development assistance for health to sub-Saharan Africa alone was 46.5% of total DAH in 2011. The level of disbursement to sub-Saharan Africa was driven by country income level, disease burden, and epidemiological trends related to infectious diseases such as HIV/AIDS, malaria, and TB. South Asia received the second highest DAH of $2 billion, accounting for 10.7% of DAH due to its large population and the prevalence of infectious diseases (Institute for Health Metrics and Evaluation, 2013b).

Development assistance for health disbursed to Europe and Central Asia from 2010 to 2011 was $656 million, accounting for 3.5% of total DAH, while that for North Africa and the Middle East for that period was $429 million.

Figure 12.3 shows the top ten recipients of cumulative DAH by country from 2009–2011. India, one of the most populous middle-income countries, received the largest DAH of $2.54 billion, followed by eight sub-Saharan countries:

Nigeria, Ethiopia, Tanzania, Kenya, South Africa, Uganda, Mozambique, and the Democratic Republic of Congo. In 2010, Mexico, another populous middle-income country (in Latin America) received $1.05 billion in DAH from the World Bank Group's International Bank for Reconstruction and Development (IBRD) to strengthen health insurance coverage and health system performance. The number of sub-Saharan African country recipients on the top ten list underscores the role of income level and infectious disease burden in the determination of DAH disbursements.

The bulk of DAH received by the top ten DAH recipient countries from 2009–2011 were from US bilateral agencies. Bilateral DAH from the United States accounted for over 40% of DAH disbursed to six of the top ten recipient countries. The United Kingdom was responsible for the largest share of DAH to India. Second to the United States, the GFTAM also made significant DAH disbursements to the top ten countries from 2009–2011. Due to civil strife and political unrests, the Democratic Republic of Congo received DAH from several sources (Institute for Health Metrics and Evaluation, 2013b).

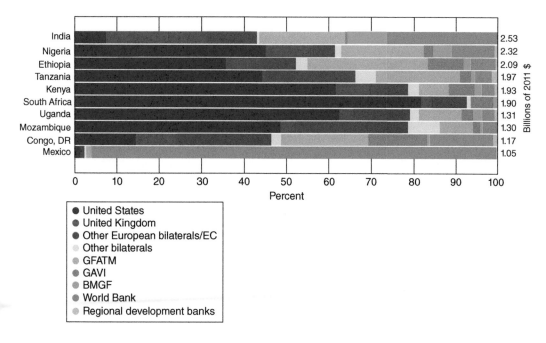

Figure 12.3 Top ten country recipients of DAH by channel of assistance, 2009–2011.
Source: Institute for Health Metrics and Evaluation (2014), with permission.

Health expenditure in low-, middle-, and high-income countries

Health expenditure is the sum of money expended on health-related goods and services, such as equipment, medication, medical education and training, and research and development with the aim of to promoting, restoring, or maintaining the health of a population. Health expenditure is calculated as a percentage of a country's gross domestic product (GDP). It varies significantly across countries and is typically determined by the status of a countries epidemiological transition, level of economic development, and wealth. The assumption is that, the wealthier a country is, the greater the likelihood that it will spend a higher percentage of its GDP on the health of its population, hence the disparities in health spending between high-income and low-income countries.

Generally, low- and middle-income countries spend much less on healthcare than high-income countries. In 2012, the United States, the Netherlands, and France spent 18% and 12%, respectively of their GDP on health. That same year, Liberia and Sierra Leone, both low-income countries, spent 16% and 15%, respectively of their GDP on health. While the GDP percentage of Liberia and Sierra Leone exceeded that of some developed countries in 2012, it must be noted that in terms of raw dollar amounts, the amounts allocated by Liberia and Sierra Leone did not compare to that which was allocated by developed countries with higher GDPs.

In 2000, the average health expenditure per person in low-income countries was $10 and that for high-income countries was $2253. Total global expenditure for health per person per year in 2012 was $948. In terms of countries, the United States spent the most ($8362) on health per person per year in 2012, and Eritrea spent the least ($12) per person per year that same year. When it came to government spending on health per person per year in 2012, Luxembourg was in the lead, spending $6906, while the government of Myanmar brought up the rear, spending $2 per person per year. WHO's estimate of minimum spending per person per year in order to provide basic, life-saving health service is $44. In 2012, the health spending of 34 WHO Member States, including spending by governments, households, the private sector, and funds provided by external donor amounted to less than $50 per person per year (World Health Organization, Geneva, 2012).

Determinants of health expenditure

A host of factors determine the amount of funds that are expended on healthcare. How long people live, rising healthcare costs related to a number of domains, epidemiological transition, life style choices, medical liability, administrative costs, and wasteful healthcare spending are some of these determinants. While these determinants prevail in most countries, they impact health expenditures in different ways.

Ageing population

Although high-income countries have the highest number of ageing people due to the advanced stage of the epidemiologic transition they are currently experiencing, the number of this population is also growing rapidly in low- and middle-income countries. The proportion of the world's population aged 60 and over, grew from 8% in 1950 to 12% in 2013. This was a 2% increase in 1950 and a 23% increase in 2013. In 2013, there were 841 million old people (aged 60 and over) in the world. This was four times higher than the 202 million in 1950. In 1900, life expectancy did not exceed 50 years. Now it exceeds 83 years in countries like Japan and is at least 81 years in many other high-income countries.

Increased life expectancy and decreased mortality rates can increase healthcare expenditure. As people live longer, they tend to end up with conditions or chronic diseases such as Alzheimer's disease, arthritis, asthma, cardiovascular disease, cancer, cataract, dementia, diabetes, hypertension, and osteoporosis, all of which are expensive to treat and manage. An analysis of global cancer trends conducted by the Economist Intelligence Unit (EIU) found that there were about 13 million new cancer cases in 2009, with an associated cost of at least $286 billion. Owing to global aging, the incidence of cancer is projected to rise to 17 million by 2020, and 27 million by 2030 (National Institute of Aging, 2011). Access to acute care, institutional long-term care services, and medical care services by the elderly in developed countries, puts upward pressure on overall healthcare spending.

Rising healthcare costs

The use of medical health information technologies, such as electronic health records and computerized provider order entry (COPE) systems, drives healthcare spending, especially in high-income countries. While these technologies make patient health information readily accessible and help to reduce errors associated with poor handwriting of medication orders, the cost associated with their installation and implementation can be in the millions of dollars, with annual maintenance costs in the hundreds of thousands of dollars. These costs are transferred to patients in due course, driving up the cost of healthcare.

The development of new and advanced medical technologies such as robotic surgery, magnetic resonance imaging (MRIs), and therapies that expand treatment options for diseases, are now on the rise, especially in high-income countries. Inasmuch as these technologies and therapies improve the overall quality of healthcare, they are high-cost procedures that create increased medical costs for patients. According to the United States Congressional Budget Office, about 50% of increased healthcare expenditure in the United States is associated with medical technological advances. Rising hospital fees, high provider charges, high patient deductibles and out-of-pocket payments for healthcare, as well as the cost of goods and services utilized in patient care and treatment, also drive global health expenditure.

Medical liability

Medical liability is another driver of healthcare costs globally. In order to avert potential lawsuits arising from medical malpractice, physicians, especially those in high-income countries, practice defensive medicine. They purchase medical malpractice insurance to protect themselves from potential medical claims that could lead either to financial harm or bankruptcy. In the United States, the most common malpractice insurance policies sold by insurers to physicians provide $1 million of coverage per incident and $3 million of total coverage per year. Premiums for medical liability vary by specialty, with physicians practicing high-risk specialties such as obstetrics, paying higher premiums than those practicing internal medicine. The consequence of physicians paying huge amounts in medical malpractice premiums often results in increases in health insurance premiums for patients (US General Accounting Office, 2003).

Administrative expenses

Healthcare administrative tasks including the coding and translation of medical records for billing, the maintenance of physical infrastructure like buildings and equipment, the purchase of software and hardware for information technology systems, and the costs associated with salaries and benefits for staff, telephone bills, postage used for the business, and office supplies such as paper and ink, increase health expenditure. A study of healthcare systems conducted in eight countries including Canada, England, France, Germany, the Netherlands, and the United States, found that the United States has the highest hospital administrative costs, spending about $361 billion annually on healthcare administration, which is more than twice its total spending on heart disease and more than thrice its total spending on cancer (Cutler, Wikler, & Basch, 2012).

Wasteful healthcare spending

Defined as spending that can be eliminated without harming patients or reducing the quality of care patients receive, wasteful spending in health systems also affects health expenditure. Patient overtreatment, including unnecessary tests and diagnostic procedures caused by defensive medicine, affects healthcare expenditure. With regards to unnecessary admissions and the length of hospital stays, studies conducted in Canada found that over 24% to 90% of admissions and over 27% to 66% of inpatient days were inappropriate (DeCoster *et al.*, 1997). According to the United States Institute of Medicine (IOM), unnecessary health spending in the United States amounted to $750 billion in 2009, with the most wastes arising from the practice of defensive medicine and redundant, inappropriate, or unnecessary medical tests and procedures.

Global health financing challenges

Financing global health through internal or external means is fraught with many challenges. Regardless of the challenges these mechanisms pose, they provide the much-needed funds required by governments to meet the basic health needs of their citizens. In this section, health financing challenges associated with taxation, National Health Service systems, and DAH are discussed.

Taxation

Using general taxation as a means of financing health in low-income countries often presents challenges. Poor tax collection infrastructure, a weak tax base, a large informal sector, low tax collection capacity, poor accountability, and tax evasion hamper the realization of adequate revenue. While low-income countries like Benin, Ghana, and Zimbabwe have shown that it is possible to rely on general taxation to support health sector expenditures, they have also shown that a total reliance on this mechanism is insufficient and that other mechanisms like DAH are needed to supplement healthcare expenditure.

National health service system

The majority of low-income country governments use a national health service system run by the Ministry of Health to provide their citizens with basic health services. This mode of health financing includes significant and often high out-of- pocket payments, which limit access to healthcare, especially by the poor and marginalized. Added challenges of the utilization of national health service systems as a means of health financing are inadequate government financing, the heavy reliance on traditional and inefficient financing mechanisms, mismanagement of funds, the lack of accountability, corruption, underfunding, and misallocation of expenditures.

Development assistance for health

Development assistance for health supplements the finances of developing countries and thus, provides them with some of the funds they need to finance health. This notwithstanding, developing country governments cannot rely entirely on DAH to finance health, as its disbursement is volatile, irregular, insufficient, and uncertain. The volatility and insufficiency of DAH flows have implications for the provision of basic health services, the supporting of long-term health system efforts, and the meeting of recurring costs, such as the purchasing of drugs and the payment of healthcare personnel salaries. Factors contributing to DAH volatility include short-term donor commitments, variable gaps between disbursements and commitments, backloading of disbursements, and making aid conditional on the mobilization of additional financing (Lane and Glassman, 2008).

Development assistance for health is to be used by developing countries to supplement their health budgets. Unfortunately, this is not what actually happens in some countries. At times, DAH, once received, ends us up becoming the sole source of health financing and is not added to pre-existing domestic health budgets. On other occasions, the infusion of DAH is repurposed to cope with aid volatility. Thus, it is not surprising that after DAH infusion, some developing countries still appear to fall short of the finances they need to provide basic and effective health services. Although it is believed that some displacement of funds occurs, there is however, no evidence that this is really the case.

Donor focus on particular diseases, as manifested in the diseases they tie their DAH to, raises concerns about donor countries using aid as an instrument of foreign policy to advance their interests in developing countries. According to Kickbusch (2002), global health priorities are often a reflection of the economic and political interests of donor countries. To him, greater United States engagement in global health since the mid-1990s, has increasingly been due to national interests or enlightened self-interest (Kickbusch, 2002).The result is, the nonalignment of the health priorities of donor countries with those of recipient countries.

Global action and strategies

As the cost of improving health status globally is enormous, and as existing financing mechanisms such as taxation and DAH have been unable to provide adequate funds to close the health financing gap in low-income countries, various innovative mechanisms to finance health have been established. In addition to complementing existing global health financing efforts, the objective of the new financing mechanisms among others is to ensure that funding for global health is adequate, consistent, and sustainable. Innovative mechanisms developed to finance health globally and currently in use include the international financing facility for immunization (IFFIm), the advance market commitment for vaccines (AMC), taxes on airline tickets, and debt swaps. To date these innovative mechanisms have raised over $2 billion dollars per annum. Other innovative financing mechanisms under exploration and yet to be implemented globally include levies on foreign currency exchange transactions, business value-added tax (VAT) waivers, and the auctioning of permits to emit greenhouse gases.

International financing facility for immunization

Regarding innovative mechanisms currently being implemented to complement health financing globally, the IFFIm, managed by GAVI, uses long-term pledges made by the governments of rich developed countries as collateral to issue vaccine bonds on capital markets, so as to provide "frontloaded" access to funds to pay for immediately needed important health products, such as childhood vaccines needed in poor countries, while delaying donor payments for 20 years. Income from vaccine bonds provides a more predictable source of funding for childhood vaccines and healthcare. To date, through the IFFIm facility, GAVI has been able to raise $5 billion from donors. Further pledges from IFFIm donors including the United Kingdom, France, Italy, Norway, Australia, Spain, the Netherlands, Sweden, and South Africa, will make available over $6.5 billion to the IFFIm over a 23-year period. These funds will be used to reimburse IFFIm bondholders.

Advance market commitment

The advance market commitment (AMC) for vaccines is a legally binding contract typically offered by donor governments and organizations to prepay for the purchase of new life-saving vaccines yet to be manufactured by pharmaceutical companies, so as to protect against specific preventable diseases causing high morbidity and mortality in developing countries. The aim of this mechanism is to encourage accelerated pharmaceutical industry investments in research, development, and the manufacture of urgently needed vaccines for diseases that would under normal circumstances be neglected, and to reward vaccine manufacturers who successfully develop and make available new generations of life-saving vaccines and medicine for developing countries, with a ready attractive market for their products. Through the AMC mechanism, manufacturers produce and sell a fixed number of vaccines at affordable prices to developing countries for a certain period of time, or license their technology to other manufacturers. Under the AMC, vaccines are purchased only when they meet predetermined standards of efficacy and safety, and only when they are demanded for by developing countries. The first AMC pilot was launched in 2009 by Canada, Italy, Norway, Russia, the United Kingdom, and the Bill and Melinda Gates Foundation with a combined pledge of $1.5 billion for the development of a new vaccine to combat childhood pneumonia and meningitis, which kill hundreds of thousands of children each year in developing countries. The pilot was a public-private partnership led by the GAVI Alliance and the World Bank and implemented with Unicef and WHO (Cernuschi *et al.*, 2011). Since 2010, pneumo vaccines have been made available to 28 countries under the AMC facility and over 100 million doses of the vaccines were purchased in 2012 (United Nations Children's Fund, 2013).

UNITAID / solidarity levy on airline tickets

UNITAID is a pioneer global health organization based in Geneva that utilizes innovative mechanisms to complement the financing of health globally. Established in 2006 by the governments of Brazil, Chile, France, Norway, and the United Kingdom as an international drug-purchasing facility, UNITAID obtains about 50% of its revenue by imposing small levies on the purchase of airline tickets in a number of countries worldwide. In 2014, UNITAID collected $1.48 billion through airline ticket levies. Revenue realized was used to support the efforts of global health agencies by promoting the production of affordable health products, creating improved access to nutritional supplements for children, and improving the diagnosis and treatment of HIV/AIDS, malaria, and TB in developing countries. Through its enormous purchasing power, UNITAID not only ensures that drug prices are reduced and affordable, but also ensures that needed drugs by developing countries are available. It does this by assuring the purchase of a minimum volume of drugs and health products. Currently, UNITAID finances projects in 94 countries. Between 2006 and 2014, Nigeria, Uganda, and Kenya received health products in the form of cumulative United States dollars from UNITAID, with Nigeria receiving the most ($243 357 136). At present, UNITAID membership includes countries like Cameroon, Congo, Guinea, Luxembourg, Madagascar, Mali, Mauritius, Niger, and Spain, and organizations like the Bill and Melinda Gates Foundation (Hecht *et al.*, 2010; UNITAID, 2016).

Debt swaps

Debt swap is the process by which rich developed creditor countries or organizations cancel the external debts of developing countries with the assurance that the debtor countries will use the debt amount forgiven for socio-economic development projects.

A variation of debt swap, the debt-to-health (Debt2Health) Conversion Scheme of the GFTAM is a global health financing initiative developed in 2007, that allows bilateral and multilateral creditors to write off debts owed them by developing nations, with the guarantee that a portion of the face value of the amount owed will be converted to local currency and transferred to the GFTAM to enable it support additional health sector activities, (such as basic disease control) in those countries. The first Debt2Health agreement was signed in 2007, between the governments of Indonesia and Germany, with Germany cancelling €50 million of Indonesia's bilateral debt. Under that agreement, Indonesia was to transfer the local currency equivalent of €25 million (€5 million annually from 2008 to 2012) to the GFTAM to enable it finance additional health activities in Indonesia. While some perceive Debt2Health as an effective mechanism for reducing developing country indebtedness and for increasing their access to funds for basic health needs, this mechanism in reality is not sustainable and does not generate sufficient funds to improve health, as there is no guarantee that bilateral donors will always be willing to write off debts (Cassimon *et al.*, 2008).

Proposed innovative mechanisms under exploration

There are additional innovative mechanisms proposed for global health financing, which are yet to be implemented. The development of these mechanisms was driven by the 2008 high-level Task Force on Innovative Financing for Health Systems, chaired by Gordon Brown, (former Prime Minister of the United Kingdom) and by Robert Zoellick (former President of the World Bank) with the aim of identifying additional innovative mechanisms for strengthening health systems in the 49 countries with the lowest-incomes in the world. These mechanisms include VAT, green house gas emission permits, and the currency transactions levy. The currency transactions levy is to operate as a voluntary national levy of 0.005% imposed on all foreign exchange transactions anywhere they occur in the world on the four major currencies (the United States dollar, the Japanese yen, the euro, and the British pound sterling) as a means of generating funds to finance clean water and basic sanitation, global pandemics and disease, and humanitarian emergencies (Cassimon *et al.*, 2008; Hillman *et al.*, 2007).

Arguments in support of the currency transactions levy state that, the foreign exchange market trades about $4 trillion a day, thus, a small tax levied on the four major currencies could yield about $33 billion in revenue annually. The levies are to be collected by large-scale foreign-exchange settlement systems, such as the Continuous Linked Settlement (CLS) Bank and SWIFT (Society for Worldwide Interbank Financial Telecommunication).

Regardless of their benefits, the innovative mechanisms for financing global health have been criticized as lacking ambition, having a voluntary charitable approach, being consumption based, and as a smoke screen by donor countries to renege on their commitments to provide systematic and reliable DAH flows to developing countries. For global health to be financed effectively, it is important that all countries, especially those in the developing world, prioritize revenue mobilization and come up with efficient and sustainable mechanisms to generate funds to meet their short- and long-term healthcare needs. To avoid frustration with DAH volatility, local revenues and funding sources should be relied upon for the bulk of health financing, which means, developing countries will have to take drastic steps to significantly improve upon their income and earning levels. If national and per capita income increase and if payroll tax collection and the tax collection infrastructure are improved to reach people within the taxable bracket, taxes could generate more income to finance health.

Discussion points

1 What is health financing?
2 Describe the mechanisms for health financing.
3 Why do developing countries rely on DAH to finance healthcare?
4 How different is ODA from DAH?
5 What are some of the sources and channels of DAH?
6 Why are the traditional mechanisms for global health financing problematic?
7 List and explain three global health financing challenges.
8 What innovative mechanisms are in place and which ones are yet to be implemented to finance global health?
9 Should the developed world provide funding to finance health in developing countries? Why?
10 In your opinion, how should global health be financed?

REFERENCES

Blanchet, N. J., Fink, G., and Osei-Akoto, I. (2012) The effect of Ghana's National Health Insurance Scheme on health care utilisation. *Ghana Medical Journal* **46**(2), 76–84.

Cassimon, D., Renard, R., and Verbeke, K. (2008) Assessing debt-to-health swaps: a case study on the

Global Fund Debt2Health Conversion Scheme. *Tropical Medicine and International Health* **13**(9), 1188–1195, doi: 10.1111/j.1365-3156.2008.02125.x

Cernuschi, T., Furrwe, E., Schwalbe, N., *et al.* (2011) Advance market commitment for pneumococcal vaccines: putting theory into practice. *Bulletin of the World Health Organization* **89**, 913–918.

Cutler, D., Wikler, E., and Basch, P. (2012) Reducing administrative costs and improving the health care system. *New England Journal of Medicine* **367**(20), 1875–1878.

DeCoster, C., Roos. N. P., Carriere, K. C., and Peterson, S. (1997) Inappropriate hospital use by patients receiving care for medical conditions: targeting utilisation review. *Canadian Medical Association Journal* **157**, 889–896.

Guy, C. (2003) *Community based Health Insurance Schemes in Developing Countries: Facts, Problems and Perspectives*, http://apps.who.int/iris/bitstream/ 10665/69023/1/EIP_FER_DP.E_03.1.pdf?ua=1 (accessed October 26, 2016).

Hecht, R., Palriwala, A., and Rao, A. (2010) *Innovative Financing for Global Health A Moment for Expanded US Engagement? A Report of the CSIS Global Health Policy Center*, https://csis-prod.s3. amazonaws.com/s3fs-public/legacy_files/files/ publication/100316_Hecht_InnovativeFinancing_ Web.pdf (accessed October 26, 2016).

Hillman, D., Kapoor, S., and Spratt, S. (2007) *Taking the Next Step: Implementing a Currency Transaction Development Levy*, https://mpra.ub.uni-muenchen. de/4054/1/MPRA_paper_4054.pdf (accessed October 26, 2016).

Institute of Health Metrics and Evaluation (2013a) *Development Assistance for Health to Specific Health Focus Areas*, Chapter 3, http://www.healthdata.org/ sites/default/files/files/policy_report/2014/ FGH2013/IHME_FGH2013_Chapter3.pdf (accessed October 26, 2016).

Institute for Health Metrics and Evaluation (2013b) *Recipients of DAH in Financing Global Health*. Chapter 2, http://www.healthdata.org/sites/default/files/files/ policy_report/2014/FGH2013/IHME_FGH2013_ Chapter2.pdf (accessed October 26, 2016).

Institute for Health Metrics and Evaluation (2014) *Financing Global Health 2013: Transition in an Age of Austerity*, IHME, Seattle, WA, http://www.healthdata. org/sites/default/files/files/policy_report/2014/ FGH2013/IHME_FGH2013_Full_Report.pdf (accessed October 26, 2016).

Institute for Health Metrics and Evaluation (2015) *Financing Global Health*, IHME, University of

Washington. Seattle, WA, http://vizhub.healthdata. org/fgh/ (accessed October 26, 2016).

Islam, M., Yen, L.,Valderas, J. M., and McRae, I. (2014) Out-of-pocket expenditure by Australian seniors with chronic disease: the effect of specific diseases and morbidity clusters. *BMC Public Health* **14**, 1008.

Jakab, M. and Krishnan, C. (2001) *Community Involvement in Health Care Financing: A Survey of the Literature on the Impact, Strengths, and Weaknesses. HNP Discussion Paper Series,* World Bank, Washington, DC, https://openknowledge. worldbank.org/handle/10986/13706 (accessed October 26, 2016).

Kickbusch, I. (2002) Influence and opportunity: reflections on the US role in global public health. *Health Affairs (Millwood)* **21**(6), 131–141.

Lane, C. and Glassman, A. (2008) *Smooth and Predictable Aid for Health: A Role for Innovative Financing?* http://www.brookings.edu/research/ papers/2008/08/global-health-glassman (accessed October 26, 2016).

Murray, J. L. and Fenk, J. A. (2000) *A WHO Framework for Health System Performance Assessment,* http:// www.who.int/healthinfo/paper06.pdf (accessed October 30, 2016).

National Institute of Aging (2011) *Assessing the Costs of Aging and Health Care,* https://www.nia.nih. gov/research/publication/global-health-and- aging/assessing-costs-aging-and-health-care

Schieber, G., Baeza, C., Kress, D., and Maier, M. (2006) Financing health systems in the twenty-first century. In *Disease Control Priorities in Developing Countries* (eds. Dean T. Jamison, J. G. Breman, A. R. Measham, *et al.*), 2nd edn. World Bank, New York, NY.

Shukla, S. (2015) *Rise in Global Health Financing but Funding Priorities Shifts,* http://www.weeklyblitz. net/2014/04/rise-in-global-health-financing-but- funding-priorities-shift/ (accessed October 26, 2016).

UNITAID (2016) *About UNITAID,* http://www.unitaid. eu/en/who/about-unitaid (accessed October 26, 2016).

United Nations Children's Fund (2013) *The Advance Market Commitment for Pneumococcal Vaccine,* http://www.unicef.org/supply/index_60990.html (accessed October 26, 2016).

US General Accounting Office. (2003) *Excerpts from Medical Malpractice and Access to Healthcare* (GAO-03-836), http://www.policyalmanac.org/ health/archive/medical_malpractice.shtml (accessed October 26, 2016).

World Health Organization, Geneva. (2012) *Spending on Health: A Global Overview*. Fact sheet, http://

www.who.int/mediacentre/factsheets/fs319/en/ (accessed October 26, 2016).

World Health Organization. (2010) *Health Systems Finanacing,* http://www.who.int/healthinfo/systems/WHO_MBHSS_2010_section5_web.pdf(accessed October 26, 2016).

World Vision. (2013) *Development Assistance for Health; Donor Landscape for Health Financing,* http://www.wvi.org/health/publication/development-assistance-health (accessed October 26, 2016).

FURTHER READING

Ekman, B. (2004) Community-based health insurance in low-income countries: a systematic review of the evidence. *Health Policy Plan* **19**(5):249–70.

Hopkins., S. (2010) Health expenditure comparisons: Low, middle and high income countries. *Open Health Services and Policy Journal* **3**, 111–117.

Lanthaume, P. (2012) *Tax-Financed Health Systems: National Health Services,* http://www.social-protection.org/gimi/gess/ShowTheme.do?tid=3125 (accessed October 26, 2016).

Leach-Kemon, K., Chou, D. P., Schneider, M. T., and Tardif, A. (2012) The global financial crisis has led to a slowdown in growth of funding to improve health in many developing countries. *Health Affairs* **31**(1), 228–235.

Murray, C. J., Ortblad, K. F., Guinovart, C., *et al.* (2014) Global, regional, and national incidence and mortality for HIV, tuberculosis, and malaria during 1990–2013: a systematic analysis for the Global Burden of Disease Study 2013. *The Lancet* **384**(9947), 1005–1070, doi: 10.1016/S0140-6736(14)60844-8

Poullier, J. P., Hernandez, P., Kawabata, K., and Savedoff, W. D. (2002) *Patterns of Global Health Expenditures: Results for 191 Countries,* http://www.who.int/healthinfo/paper51.pdf (accessed October 26, 2016).

Savedoff, W. (2004) *Tax-Based Financing for Health Systems: Options and Experiences,* http://www.who.int/health_financing/taxed_based_financing_dp_04_4.pdf (accessed October 30, 2016).

Shah, A. (2014) *Foreign Aid for Development Assistance,* http://www.globalissues.org/article/35/foreign-aid-development-assistance (accessed October 26, 2016).

United Nations Education and Social Commisssion Courier. *Pearson Report: A Strategy for Global Development,* http://unesdoc.unesco.org/images/0005/000567/056743eo.pdf (accessed October 26, 2016).

13

Ethics in global health research, design, and practice

Learning objectives

By the end of this chapter, you will be able to:

✔ Discuss the significance of ethics in global health research;

✔ Describe at least two ethical issues associated with the conduct of global health research in resource-poor settings;

✔ Describe at least two challenges of global health research;

✔ List and explain at least two global strategies in place to address the issue of ethics in global health research.

Summary of key points

Conducting global health research is crucial to addressing health issues and reducing disparities. Although frequently undertaken in the developed world, the converse is true in the developing world, even though it accounts for a great portion of the world's disease burden. This contradiction begs for an explanation. The dearth of global health research in the developing world is not due to researcher apathy, but to a number of factors that stand in the way of both the researcher and the researched. Conducting global health research in developing countries is fraught with a number of ethical challenges, including the fact that expatriate researchers sometimes fail to take cognizance of the cultural, economic, political, and social context of the host countries and communities in which they carry out their activities, and the fact that some researchers fail to obtain consent, safeguard human subject privacy, and protect human subjects from harm. For global health research to be considered ethical, researchers must adhere to international and national guidelines for the ethical conduct of health research.

This chapter opens with a brief overview of the concept of ethics, traces the evolution of ethics in health research, describes the rationale for ethics in global health research, and discusses ethical issues to be considered in global health research in resource-poor settings. It goes on to discuss challenges associated with global health research and global action to address them.

The concept of research ethics

Research ethics focuses on ethical issues related to the involvement of humans in health research. Its first objective is to protect human subjects, its

Global Health: Issues, Challenges, and Global Action Lecture Notes, First Edition. Elizabeth A. Armstrong-Mensah.

second is to ensure that research serves the interests of individuals, groups and/or society as a whole, and its third is to examine the ethical soundness of research activities and projects with a focus on risk management, protection of confidentiality, and the obtainment of informed consent (Family Health International, 2004).

Historical background of ethics in health research

Prior to the 1940s, researchers were not held to any standards for research involving human subjects. It was assumed that they would exercise good judgment and treat research subjects ethically. The atrocities committed by Nazi German scientists, the thalidomide tragedy, and the Tuskegee Syphilis Study proved this assumption wrong.

The Nuremberg War Crimes Trials

In August 1947, two years after World War II, 23 doctors in Nazi Germany concentration camps were tried in Nuremberg and found guilty of breaching the code of medical ethics because they performed horrifying medical experiments on prisoners without their consent. The verdict of the trial led to the creation of the Nuremberg Code, which among other things, advocated for obtaining voluntary informed consent in research involving human subjects, the proper formulation of scientific research, and the practice of beneficence towards humans in scientific clinical experiments. Although the Code lacked the force of law, it represented the genesis of discussions around the ethical treatment and rights of humans in medical research. The Nuremberg War Crimes Trials heightened international concerns about ethical issues surrounding research experiments involving humans. Today, the Code continues to serve as a blue print for safeguarding human subjects in health research.

The thalidomide tragedy

In the 1940s and early 1950s, pregnant women in certain parts of the world who experienced morning sickness and anxieties during the first trimester of pregnancy, were given barbiturate sedatives for relief. The barbiturate sedatives were highly toxic and could be lethal if ingested in large quantities. Therefore, as a safer alternative, the Chemise Grünenthal group

released a new drug, thalidomide, in 1957. While thalidomide was effective in treating morning sickness in women in Brazil, Canada, Europe, Japan, and South America, it caused severe defects in newborn babies. Thus, about 12 000 babies were born with missing and malformed limbs, serious facial deformities, and defective organs. While approved as a sedative in Europe in 1950, thalidomide was not approved by the United States Food and Drug Administration (FDA). The FDA inspector at the time, Frances Kelsey, doubted the safety of the drug. Lessons from the thalidomide tragedy underscored the need for testing new drugs on animals and the need for tightly regulated human clinical trials to determine drug safety prior to their use by humans.

The Tuskegee Syphilis Study

An additional landmark event in history, which underscored the need for the regulation of scientific research involving human subjects, was the Tuskegee Syphilis Study. In 1932, the United States Public Health Service in collaboration with the Tuskegee Institute began a study to record the natural progression of untreated syphilis in 400 African American men without their consent. During the study, treatment was withheld from these men, even though penicillin, a safe and effective treatment for syphilis, had been discovered. The men were made to believe that the spinal taps they received was treatment. Following public outcry over a story published by the Associated Press in 1972 on the Tuskegee Study, an ad hoc advisory panel was appointed to review the study. The panel found that the study was medically unjustified and ordered its immediate termination. The panel also found that although the men had agreed to be examined and treated as part of the study, they were not provided with all the information they needed to make an informed decision about their participation. They were misinformed about the need for some of the procedures they underwent. Following the advisory panel's discoveries, the 93rd United States Congress passed the National Research Act and created the National Commission for the Protection of Human Subjects of Biomedical and Behavioral Research to regulate the utilization of human subjects in research.

The Nuremberg War Crimes Trials, the thalidomide tragedy, the Tuskegee Syphilis Study, the Belmont Report, and the Acts of the United States Congress drew attention to the fact that research involving human subjects has the potential to cause harm if there are no regulations or standards in place to guide research. They also underscored the need to hold researchers accountable for their actions.

Global health research

Global health research is the study of problems that have a disproportionate health burden on low and middle-income countries. Its goal is to understand the complexities of health determinants and their contribution to the development of effective, equitable, sustainable, and ethically sound solutions to health problems, and to create health equity between and among populations. Global health research recognizes that knowledge is a key driver of health and seeks to address the 10/90 gap; the statistical finding of the Global Forum for Health Research that only 10% of worldwide expenditure on health research and development is devoted to health problems that affect the poorest 90% of the world's population.

Global health research facilitates the investigation of health issues that are important to a population, informs policy, and provides evidence for the development of appropriate and effective global health programs. It ensures that "measures proposed to break out of the vicious cycle of ill health and poverty are based, as much as possible, on evidence, so that resources available to finance these measures are used in the most efficient and effective way possible" (Delisle *et al.*, 2005). Global health research broadens the base for scientific endeavor by investing in excellent scientists in low- and middle-income countries who have the greatest potential to advance knowledge, and ensures that they have the resources they need to carry out their work. It further supports public engagement programs by raising the profile of research in low- and middle-income countries, and by promoting informed discussions about their implications for those societies and how ideas can be shared.

Ethical issues in global health research in resource-poor settings

The main ethical issues with global health research in resource-poor settings have to do with obtaining informed consent from potential research subjects, maintaining their privacy and confidentiality, protecting vulnerable populations, respecting cultural and traditional practices, ensuring equity and fairness in research subject selection, the sharing of research benefits, the determination of the standard of care to provide, assessment of risk, and scientific integrity. Some of these ethical issues are described below.

Informed consent

When conducting research of any kind (clinical, biomedical, or behavioral), informed consent must be obtained from all potential research subjects, regardless of which part of the world they live. Informed consent gives researchers permission to involve research subjects in a study. Through the informed consent process, researchers explain a number of things to research subjects: the purpose, duration and procedures to be followed, products to be experimented (drugs, biologics, or technology), foreseeable risks or discomforts (such as physical, psychological, social), benefits to be gained, how subject confidentiality will be maintained, and what compensation and or medical treatments will be available should subjects sustain any injury during the study. Through the consent process, research subjects are also given the opportunity to decide whether or not to participate in a study. They also receive information on who to contact for any additional questions they may have subsequent to the session.

The informed consent form is not merely a legal requirement or a document to be signed between the researcher and his subjects. It is a communication tool between the two that starts even before the research is initiated and continues throughout the life of the study (see Figure 13.1). Unfortunately, some researchers, due to language barriers, time constraints, personal agendas, ignorance, and a number of other reasons, have failed to obtain informed consent from their research subjects, especially those in developing countries. This has culminated in several problems including those related to the infringement on the rights of human research subjects. F. Van den Borne's article, "Using mystery clients to assess condom negotiation in Malawi" (Van den Borne, 2007) is an example of an informed consent process that was not transparent.

Privacy and confidentiality

Respect for the confidentiality and privacy of research subjects is central to informed consent. Information obtained during research is to be kept confidential and not divulged without permission. It should be protected, not used outside the scope for which it was collected, and not handled in a manner that makes it easy to trace the research subject. Personal identifiers

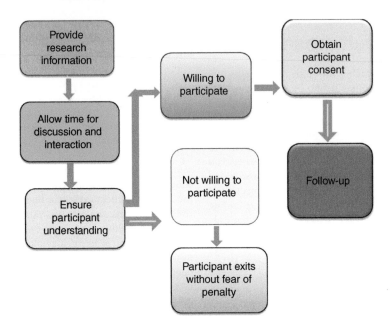

Figure 13.1 Process for obtaining informed consent.

such as names, birthdates, postal addresses, social security and telephone numbers must be kept confidential. The intentional or unintentional disclosure of research subject information can embarrass, harm, stigmatize, or cause them economic loss. The utilization of computers and other social devices for health research make issues of confidentiality and privacy around data protection and access a great challenge.

Protection of vulnerable populations

During research, it is very common for vulnerable populations such as prisoners, children, and pregnant women to be exploited. This should not be the case. The research design should safeguard their rights and provide them with extra protection. They should not be asked to waive their rights, or absolve an investigator, research sponsor, institution, or its agents in the event of negligence or misconduct.

Equity and fairness

At times, researchers exclude certain populations from research studies based on their age, culture, ethnicity, sex, language, health status, disability, or race. While nonparticipation spares some populations from the burden of research, it also causes them to end up not benefiting from the findings of research. Historically,

women have been left out of some research studies. This has resulted in their exposure to unforeseen health consequences, especially in situations where research findings from male-only clinical drug research trials were generalized and applied to them.

Sharing of benefits

Ahead of embarking on research, some researchers have failed to discuss their expectations and to explain to research subjects how benefits (both direct and indirect) derived from the research will be shared. Prior to the commencement of research, it is of prime importance that researchers discuss their expectations with research subjects, and outline the scope and nature of potential benefits to be gained during and after the research. Where the research deliverable is a product (a drug), there should be prior agreement on how it will be made available and shared. All exceptions should be justified and agreed upon by all parties beforehand.

Assessing risk

Information on the extent of risk of harm to human research subjects during research is not always well articulated. Researchers, sponsors of research, host countries, and research ethics committees need to protect human subjects by ensuring that discussions on risks associated with research are not overlooked. Questions about risks that are acceptable in light of anticipated research benefits, who will be asked to accept those risks and why, and who will determine the level of risk that is acceptable should all be addressed prior to conducting research. It is important to note that risk of harm may occur during the research process, or after research results have been disseminated.

Controversies and challenges in global health research

There is global debate on why 90% of the $70 billion devoted to global health research and development (R&D) per year is spent on conditions prevalent in developed countries, and only 10% of that amount is spent on diseases that affect 85% of people living in developing countries (Commission on Health Research for Development, 1990). The argument put forward by some development experts is that, to be fair, the distribution of global research funds should be more balanced.

Although most research guidelines emphasize the importance of obtaining informed consent from potential research subjects, there are no guidelines to help them understand the research project. This is evidenced by the fact that none of the procedures involved in administering and recording the consent process, assesses whether participants understand the nature and implications of the research they are about to participate in.

In the developed world, potential research subjects have autonomy and can therefore make their own decisions about whether or not to participate in a research. The contrary is true in the developing world, where participation in research is for the most part seen as a communal affair for which the decision to participate is often left to village chiefs or male household heads. Individual research subjects in such societies are often the last on the list to give their consent. On occasion, this communal mode of consenting has led to tension, especially in situations where community leaders consented on behalf of the community, but community members were unwilling to participate in the research, and when community leaders declined to consent, but community members wanted to participate in the research. Obtaining informed consent from the community is vital when conducting health research, but this activity can be time consuming, labor intensive, and can delay the conduct of research.

Informed consent forms usually contain complex language and scientific terminologies which often do not have local equivalents. This negatively impacts the informed consent process, as people are unable to totally follow what is being discussed. In situations where participants can neither read nor write, consent forms have to be translated. The general notion is that, in such situations, much of the vital information necessary to understand the research, either gets lost or is misinterpreted. For the most part, informed consent is considered valid when signed by research participants. However, many research subjects in developing countries are illiterate and cannot give informed consent through the signing of forms.

Researchers in developed countries conducting research in developing countries are sometimes faced with the dilemma of not knowing what research guidance to adhere to. In practice, some have gone ahead and done their research as they deemed fit without compliance to any national research code of ethics. The lack of ethics committees in developing countries gives researchers free reign to implement research protocols that may be scientifically unsound, naïve, or inappropriate.

There are also challenges when it comes to the sharing of research benefits. The issues often center on what the ratio of the distribution should be, what point in the life of the research benefits should be shared, and who the beneficiary target should be – individuals, the community, or the host country? Power struggles between collaborating researchers, differences in research focus, inequalities in the publication of knowledge and access to information, noncollective agenda setting, marginalization, and the lack of research capacity are additional challenges associated with global health research.

Global action and strategies

At the first International Conference on Health Research for Development convened in Bangkok in 2000, important recommendations were made to correct the 10/90 misallocation of resources gap in the field of health research at the global, regional, and national levels.

First adopted in 1964, The World Medical Association's Declaration of Helsinki, provides guidance to physicians and other participants engaged in medical research involving human subjects. It expressly states that the wellbeing of the human subject should take precedence over the interests of science and society, and that, medical research should be guided by ethical standards that encourage respect for all human beings and protects their health and rights; especially those of vulnerable populations, the economically and medically disadvantaged, and those who are unable to provide or refuse consent for themselves. The Declaration states that experiments involving human subjects should have a protocol that should be vetted and approved by an ethics review committee that is independent of the investigator, sponsor, or any kind of undue influence. It emphasizes that the risks of research should not outweigh the potential benefits to subjects, that the rights of research subjects must always be respected, and that every precaution should be taken to protect the privacy of subjects, and the confidentiality of the subjects' information. The Declaration also underscores the need to minimize the impact of the study on subjects' physical and mental integrity and on the personality of subjects. The Declaration further states that human subjects must be adequately informed about the aims, methods, sources of funding, possible conflicts of interest, institutional affiliations of the researcher, the anticipated benefits and potential risks of the research, and the discomfort it may cause. In addition, subjects should be informed of their right to decline or withdraw from the research at anytime without any consequence and should be informed about the aspects of care they can receive by participating in the research (World Health Association, 2008). While not a legally binding instrument under international law, the Declaration of Helsinki is widely referenced when it comes to ethics in human research.

Jointly established by the World Health Organization (WHO) and the United Nations Educational, Scientific and Cultural Organization (UNESCO) in 1949, the Council for International Organizations of Medical Sciences (CIOMS), an international nongovernmental organization, oversees the scientific interests of the international biomedical community. Through its 1993 *International Ethical Guidelines for Biomedical Research Involving Human Subjects*, it addresses issues including informed consent, standards for external review, and the recruitment of research subjects among others. The Guidelines provide instructions and principles for ethical biomedical research.

While ethics in health research is new in the developing world, the government of Ethiopia has established national, regional, and institutional level research ethics committees to review and provide guidelines for ethics in research. The Ethiopian Science and Technology Commission (ESTC), now the Ministry of Science and Technology (MoST) created in 1994, is responsible for guiding, coordinating, and facilitating all science and technology activities in the country, including health.

Discussion points

1 What are the contributions of the Nuremberg War Crimes Trials, the thalidomide tragedy, and the Tuskegee Syphilis Study to the inclusion of ethics in human subjects research?
2 What is informed consent? Why is it relevant to global health research?
3 Discuss the informed consent process.
4 What should be done in situations where people are not literate enough to sign an informed consent form?
5 What is the difference between confidentiality and privacy? Why and how should they be maintained?
6 How does community consent get in the way of research in resource-poor settings?
7 What international documents provide guidance for medical research involving humans as subjects? Describe their principles.
8 What is the significance of equity and fairness in global health research?
9 In your opinion, should expatriate researchers follow the same ethical procedures they observe when preparing for research in their home countries in resource-poor settings? Explain your response.
10 What should the governments of developing countries do to prevent the exploitation of their citizens during research?

REFERENCES

Commission on Health Research for Development (1990) *Health Research: Essential Link to Equity in Development*, http://www.cohred.org/downloads/open_archive/ComReports_0.pdf (accessed October 27, 2016).

Delisle, H., Hatcher Roberts, J., Munro, M., *et al.* (2005) The Role of NGOs in global health research for development. *Health Research Policy and Systems* **3**(3). doi: 10.1186/1478-4505-3-3

Family Health International (2004) *Research Ethics Training Curriculum for Community Representatives Informed Consent as a Process*, http://www.fhi360.org/sites/default/files/webpages/RETC-CR/en/RH/Training/trainmat/ethicscurr/RETCCREn/ss/Contents/SectionV/b5sl45.htm (accessed October 30, 2016).

Van den Borne, F. (2007) Using mystery clients to assess condom negotiation in Malawi. *Studies in Family Planning* **38**, 322–330.

World Health Association (2008) *World Medical Association Declaration of Helsinki Ethical Principles for Medical Research Involving Human Subjects*, http://www.wma.net/en/30publications/10policies/b3/17c.pdf (accessed October 27, 2016).

FURTHER READING

Beauchamp, T. L. and Childress, J. F. (1994) *Principles of Biomedical Ethics* (4th edn.). Oxford University Press, New York, NY.

Bhutta1, Z. A. (2002) Ethics in international health research: a perspective from the developing world *Bulletin of the World Health Organization*, **80**, 114–120.

Bloom, B. R., Michaud, C. M., La Montagne, J. R., and Simonsen, L. (2006) Priorities for Global Research and Development of Interventions, in *Disease Control Priorities in Developing Countries* (2nd ed.) (eds. D. T. Jamison, J. G. Breman, A. R. Measham, *et al.*). Oxford University Press and World Bank, Washington DC.

Boga, M., Davies, A., Kamuya, D., *et al.* (2011) Strengthening the informed consent process in international health research through community engagement: The KEMRI-Wellcome Trust Research Programme experience. *PLoS Medicine* **8**(9), 1–4.

Claremont Graduate University. (2016) *History of Ethics*, http://www.cgu.edu/pages/1722.asp (accessed October 27, 2016).

Council for International Organizations of Medical Sciences and the World Helath Organization (2002) *International Ethical Guidelines for Biomedical Reasearch Involving Human Subjects*, http://cioms.ch/publications/layout_guide2002.pdf (accessed October 27, 2016).

General Assembly of the World Medical Association (2014) World Medical Association Declaration of Helsinki: ethical principles for medical research involving human subjects. *Journal of the American College of Dentists* **81**(3), 4–8.

Government of Canada, Panel on Research Ethics (2012) *Tri-Council Policy Statement: Ethical Conduct for Research Involving Humans*, Fairness and equity in research participation: Best practices for health research involving children and adolescents, http://www.pre.ethics.gc.ca/eng/policy-politique/initiatives/tcps2-eptc2/chapter4-chapitre4/ (accessed October 27, 2016).

Kim, J. H. and Scialli, J. R. (2011) Thalidomide: the tragedy of birth defects and the effective treatment of disease. *Toxicological Sciences* **122**(1), 1–6.

Koplan, J. P., Bond, T. C., Merson, M. H., *et al.* (2009) Towards a common definition of global health. *The Lancet* **373**(9679), 1993–1995.

Krogstad, D. J., Diop, S., Diallo, A., *et al.* (2010) Informed consent in international research: the rationale for different approaches. *American Journal of Tropical Medicine and Hygiene* **83**(4), 743–747.

Lloyd. G. E. R. L. (1983) *Hippocritic Writings (Introduction)*, Penguin Classics, Harmondsworth.

Marshall, P. (2010) Module 3: Public Health Research and Practice in International Settings: Special Ethical Concerns, http://www.slideshare.net/Medresearch/module-3-public-health-research-and-practice-in-international (accessed October 27, 2016).

National Human Genome Research Institute (1993) *Protecting Human Research Subjects: Office for Protection from Research Risks, 1993 Institutional Review Board Guidebook*, https://www.genome.gov/10001752/ (accessed October 27, 2016).

Parker, M. and Bull, S. (2009) Ethics in collaborative global health research networks. *Clinical Ethics* **4**(4), 165–168.

Pedroni, J. A. and Pimple, K. D. (2001) *A Brief Introduction to Informed Consent in Research With Human Subjects*, https://ccts.osu.edu/sites/default/files/Subject%20Management%20and%20Site%20Activities_Informed%20Consent%20in%20Research%20(Attachment).pdf (accessed October 30, 2016).

Stephen, C. and Daibes, I. (2010) Defining features of the practice of global health research: an examination of 14 global health research teams. *Global Health Action* **3**. doi: 10.3402/gha.v3i0.5188

14

Health-related millennium development goals and global health

Summary of key points

At the Millennium Summit held in September 2000, 189 United Nations (UN) Member States signed the UN Millennium Declaration and agreed to work towards achieving a set of eight time-bound Millennium Development Goals (MDGs) by the year 2015. The MDGs committed world leaders to address a range of global issues ranging from the elimination of poverty to the establishment of global partnerships for health. They represented a partnership between developed and developing countries, and created an environment that was conducive to human development. Each of the eight MDGs had specific targets and indicators that were used to monitor progress from 1990 levels. Three of the eight MDGs (MDGs 4, 5, and 6) expressly focused on health-related issues. These three goals are the focus of this chapter.

Health-related Millennium Development Goals targets and indicators

All told, the MDGs comprised eight goals, 21 targets, and 61 indicators. The eight MDGs were:

1 Eradicate extreme poverty and hunger
2 Achieve universal primary education
3 Promote gender equality
4 Reduce child mortality
5 Improve maternal mortality

Global Health: Issues, Challenges, and Global Action Lecture Notes, First Edition. Elizabeth A. Armstrong-Mensah.
© 2017 John Wiley & Sons Ltd. Published 2017 by John Wiley & Sons Ltd.

6 Combat HIV/AIDS, malaria and other diseases

7 Ensure environmental sustainability

8 Develop a global partnership for development

While several of the MDGs had health-related indicators, three of them were expressly related to health. They are MDG 4-Reduce Child Mortality, MDG 5-Improve Maternal Mortality, and MDG 6-Combat HIV/AIDS, Malaria and Other Diseases.

MDG4 – reduce child mortality

Also known as under-five mortality rate, child mortality rate is the probability of a newborn child dying by age five expressed in terms of the number of such deaths per 1000 live births. This statistic often includes neonatal and infant deaths measured by the number of deaths of infants under age 1 per 1000 live births in a given year, and the number of deaths of infants under 28 days of age per 1000 live births in a given year, respectively. Globally, an estimated 9.2 million children die annually, with about 27 000 of those deaths occurring on a daily basis from diarrhea, malaria, pneumonia, complications related to childbirth, malnutrition, and the lack of access to safe water and improved sanitation (see Figure 14.1).

Regarding neonatal deaths, an estimated 4 million newborns die in the first 4 weeks of life, accounting for about 40% of child mortality (Joint United Nations Programme on HIV/AIDS, 2016). In 2015 alone, about 2.7 million neonatal deaths occurred (about 45% of all child mortality), with about 1 million of those deaths occurring on the day of delivery, and close to 2 million during the first week of life. Also in that same year, 4.5 million infants (about 75% of all under-five deaths) died within the first day of their life. Since 1990, the proportion of neonatal deaths as a share of child mortality has been on the rise in all six WHO regions (World Health Organization, 2015b).

The risk of a child dying prior to its fifth birthday is greatest in 42 developing countries, with the most deaths occurring in sub-Saharan Africa and South-East Asia. Nigeria, the Democratic Republic of Congo, China, India, and Pakistan account for approximately 50% of under-five deaths in the aforementioned regions. Combined, these countries account for over a third of all global child mortalities. The child mortality rate (81 per 1000 live births) in the WHO African Region is about

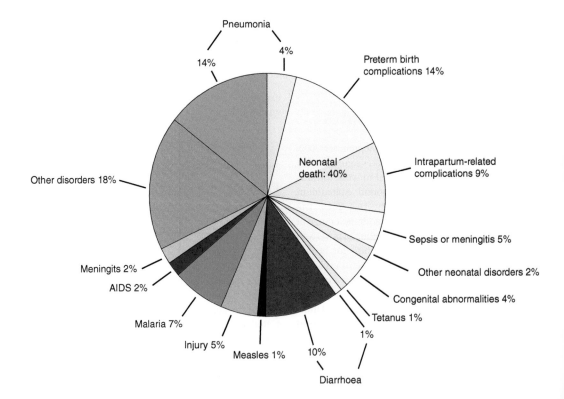

Figure 14.1 Global causes of childhood deaths in 2010.
Source: Liu *et al.* (2012), with permission.

seven times higher than that in the WHO Europe Region (11 per 1000 live births).

It must be noted that while child mortality rates are high in developing countries, they vary between wealthy and poor households. An article authored by Save the Children, an international nongovernmental organization (NGO), found that children from the poorest households in India were three times more likely to die before reaching their fifth birthday than their counterparts in the richest households in that same country (Save the Children, 2015).

Immunization

Through immunization, children all over the world are kept healthy and protected from the six childhood killer diseases: whooping cough, diphtheria, measles, polio, tetanus, and tuberculosis. It was to reduce health disparities and to save the lives of children across the world that world leaders committed to adopting MDG4. The targets and indicators they strive to achieve and monitor through various projects and interventions are presented in Table 14.1.

MDG5 – Improve maternal health

Defined as the health of women during pregnancy, childbirth, and the postpartum period of life, maternal health is measured in terms of maternal mortality ratio (MMR), which is the number of women who die

as a result of pregnancy and childbirth complications per 100 000 live births in a given year. Maternal health involves family planning, preconception, prenatal and postnatal care, and efforts that seek to reduce maternal morbidity and mortality (World Health Organization, 2016a).

Maternal morbidity and mortality

Motherhood is supposed to be a time of joy and fulfillment for women, but in certain parts of the world, this experience comes with suffering, illness, disability, or even the loss of life. The causes of maternal morbidity and mortality (see Figure 14.2) may be direct or indirect. Direct causes include severe bleeding after childbirth, blood clots, eclampsia, infection usually after childbirth, unsafe abortion, and obstructed labor. Indirect causes include the lack of access to healthcare services and pre-existing conditions prior to pregnancy such as anemia, diabetes, HIV, malaria, and pregnancy-induced high blood pressure (pre-eclampsia and eclampsia) (World Health Organization, 2015c).

On a daily basis, approximately 830 women die from preventable causes related to pregnancy and childbirth. Almost 99% of maternal deaths occur in developing countries (World Health Organization, 2015c) with over 50% of those deaths occurring in sub-Saharan Africa, and about 30% occurring in South Asia. Globally, there were an estimated 287 000 maternal deaths in 2010; developing countries accounted for 99% (284 000) of those deaths. In 2013, sub-Saharan Africa and South Asia accounted for 85% of global maternal deaths.

Of the 40 countries identified with very high MMRs, Sierra Leone ranked the highest with a MMR of 1100 deaths per 100 000 live births in a given year. Sub-Saharan African countries with very high MMRs in 2013 were Chad (980), Central African Republic (880), Somalia (850), Burundi (740), Democratic Republic of the Congo (730), South Sudan (730), and Cote d'Ivoire (720). Cabo Verde and Mauritius were the

Table 14.1 Reduce child mortality (MDG4) targets and indicators.

Target	Indicators to measure progress
Target 4A: Reduce by two thirds, between 1990 and 2015, the under-five mortality rate	4.1 Under-five mortality rate
	4.2 Infant mortality rate
	4.3 Proportion of 1-year-old children immunized against measles

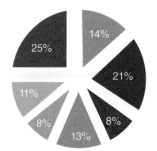

	Unsafe abortion
	Severe bleeding
	Infection
	Eclampsia
	Obstructed labor
	Other direct causes
	Indirect causes*

*Indirect causes include: anemia, malaria, heart disease

Figure 14.2 Causes of maternal deaths worldwide.
Source: UNFPA Turkmenistan. (2014), with permission.

only two sub-Saharan African countries with low MMR in 2013; 53 and 73 maternal deaths per 100 000 live births, respectively. Afghanistan (400) and Haiti (380) were the two non-sub-Saharan countries with high MMRs in 2013 (World Health Organization, United Nations Children's Fund, United Nations Population Fund, The World Bank, and the United Nations Population Division, 2014), In 2015, MMR was 239 per 100 000 live births in developing countries and 12 per 100 000 live births in developed countries.

Maternal mortality is higher among women with low incomes and women who live in rural areas than among women with high incomes and women who live in urban areas. It is also higher among young female adolescents than in women, owing to the complications the former experience during pregnancy and childbirth. Indeed, complications related to pregnancy and childbirth are the second cause of death among girls aged 15–19-worldwide. The likelihood that a 15-year-old adolescent female will die from a maternal-related cause is 1 in 4900 in developed countries compared to 1 in 180 in developing countries (World Health Organization, 2015c). In general, women in developing countries have more children and hence more pregnancies than women in developed countries, causing their lifetime risk of death due to pregnancy to be higher (World Health Organization 2015d).

Skilled attendant at birth

Being attended to by a skilled health professional during delivery is likely to increase the chances of survival for mother and child. A skilled attendant is an accredited health professional with the requisite knowledge and skills to provide safe and effective healthcare during childbirth to women and their infants in the home, health center, and in hospital settings (MEASURE Evaluation, n.d.). Globally, over 25% of babies and their mothers do not have access to crucial medical care during childbirth. This number varies by region, with coverage ranging from universal and nearly universal (96%) in Eastern Asia and the Caucasus and Central Asia, to a low of about 52% in sub-Saharan Africa and Southern Asia. Sub-Saharan Africa and South Asia are the regions with the highest rates of maternal and newborn mortality in the world. Access to skilled attendants at birth varies by income level and by the rural urban divide.

Per WHO recommendations, women need to have a minimum of four antenatal care visits during pregnancy to safeguard their life and that of their unborn babies. During these visits, they are to receive basic care including nutritional advice and information on

warning signs that warrant the need to seek help during delivery (United Nations, 2015b).

Contraceptive use

Contraceptive use prevents sexually transmitted diseases as well as unwanted pregnancies and its concomitant complications. It also delays childbearing, thus, allowing women and girls to give birth at their healthiest time. Globally, almost 230 million women of reproductive age lack information and access to a variety of contraceptive methods. This dearth is driven by increasing population size and a scarcity of family planning services. In the regions of Africa, Asia, and Latin America and the Caribbean, the levels of womens' unmet contraceptive need are 23.3, 10.9 and 10.4%, respectively (United Nations Department of Economic and Social Affairs, 2013).

Adolescent birth rate

Approximately 16 million adolescent girls give birth to 11% of all the children born in the world per annum (World Health Organization, 2016b). Over 80% of these births occur in low- and middle-income countries. Adolescent fertility rate, which is the number of births per 1000 women aged 15–19, is about 2% in China, 18% in Latin America and the Caribbean, and over 50% in sub-Saharan Africa. Fifty percent of all adolescent births occur in Bangladesh, Brazil, the Democratic Republic of the Congo, Ethiopia, India, Nigeria, and the United States (World Health Organization, 2016b). Global MDG targets and indicators set for measuring maternal health are presented in Table 14.2.

Table 14.2 Improve maternal health (MDG5) targets and indicators.

Target	Indicators to measure progress
Target 5A: Reduce by three quarters, between 1990 and 2015, the maternal mortality ratio	5.1 Maternal mortality ratio 5.2 Proportion of births attended by skilled health personnel
Target 5B: Achieve, by 2015, universal access to reproductive health	5.3 Contraceptive prevalence rate 5.4 Adolescent birth rate 5.5 Antenatal care coverage (at least one visit and at most four visits) 5.6 Unmet need for family planning

MDG6 – HIV/AIDS, malaria, and other diseases

The goal of MDG6 is to stop and reverse HIV/AIDS, malaria, and other diseases globally. The human immunodeficiency virus is a retrovirus that infects and destroys the human immune system. Its advanced stage is AIDS. Globally, there were 36.9 million people living with HIV in 2014. This was slightly lower than in 2013. This decline may be attributed to increased access to antiretroviral therapy and the fact that people with HIV are living longer. In 2013, over 75% of new HIV infections occurred in 15 sub-Saharan African countries with an estimated 50% of these cases occurring in Nigeria, South Africa, and Uganda.

Around 2.7 million people aged 15 to 24 are living with HIV in eastern and southern Africa. This is over 50% of the global total. In Botswana, Lesotho, and Swaziland where HIV prevalence is highest, more than 1 in 10 young people are living with HIV. More young women are infected with HIV than men. This is the case in Swaziland where 15.6% of young women aged 15 to 24 are HIV positive, compared to 6.5% of their male counterparts (United Nations Children's Fund, n.d.).

The youth in many countries still do not have adequate knowledge of HIV and thus, engage in risky sexual behavior. In 2014, only 30% of young women and 37% and young men aged 15–24 had comprehensive, correct HIV knowledge, and only three of the 11 sub-Saharan African countries with the highest incidence of HIV, had condom use rates of 45% or greater among females. There are disparities when it comes to income level, geographic location, and HIV knowledge among the youth; it is 17% for young women living in poor households and 35% for young women living in rich households. For young men, it is 25% for men living in poor households and 36% for men living in rich households (United Nations Children's Fund, 2011). Young women in urban areas (36%) have more comprehensive HIV knowledge than their rural counterparts (23%) and the same can be said for young men living in urban (46%) and rural (32%) areas (United Nations, 2015b).

In 2013, nearly 17.7 million children below the age 18 worldwide had lost a parent or both to AIDS, raising concerns about their economic support, protection, and education.

Malaria

Malaria is an infectious mosquito-borne disease caused by the *Plasmodium* parasite. It is transmitted from person to person through the bite of an infected female Anopheles mosquito. The symptoms of malaria include fever, fatigue, vomiting, headaches, and in severe cases, yellow skin, seizures, coma, or death. Globally, 97 countries and territories are malaria endemic and about 3.2 billion people are at risk for malaria (World Health Organization, 2015a). In 2015, there was an estimated 214 million cases of malaria and 438 000 malaria-related deaths (United Nations, 2015b). Sub-Saharan Africa accounted for 89% of those cases and 91% of the deaths.

The incidence of malaria is highest and most deadly among children under the age of five. In 2015, about 305 000 children in sub-Saharan Africa died from malaria before their fifth birthday (World Health Organization, 2015a). Pregnant women are also at high risk for malaria. Thus, to protect them and their fetuses from malaria and malaria-related complications (such as spontaneous abortion, premature delivery, stillbirth, severe maternal anemia, and low-birth-weight babies), WHO recommended that pregnant women living in moderate to high malaria transmission areas in Africa, be given malaria intermittent preventive treatment in pregnancy (IPTp) with sulfadoxine-pyrimethamine (IPTp-SP) after the first trimester of pregnancy, during scheduled antenatal visits (World Health Organization, 2016d).

Tuberculosis

Tuberculosis (TB) is an airborne respiratory disease that affects the lungs and other parts of the human body. It is caused by the *Mycobacterium tuberculosis* bacterium and is transmitted when people with active TB cough or sneeze. There are two types of TB infections: latent TB and TB disease. People with latent TB are asymptomatic and thus, not contagious. However, when TB bacteria become active in the body and multiply, a person with latent TB may become sick with TB disease, which can be fatal if left untreated. About 30% of the world's population has TB disease. In 2013, 1.1 million HIV-negative people and about 360 000 HIV positive people died from TB disease, respectively (United Nations, 2015b). In 2014, global TB disease incidence was 9.6 million with about 58% of new TB cases occurring in the WHO regions of South-East Asia and the Western Pacific (World Health Organization, n.d.). Compared to the global average of 133, sub-Saharan Africa had the highest TB disease burden of 281 cases per 100 000 population in 2014 (World Health Organization, n.d.). Some TB bacteria are resistant to two of the most powerful first-line anti-TB drugs: isoniazid and rifampicin. Multi-drug resistant TB exists in many countries and, as such, poses a challenge to TB prevention and control (World Health

Table 14.3 HIV/AIDS, malaria, and other diseases (MDG6) targets and indicators.

Target	Indicators to measure progress
Target 6A: Have halted by 2015 and begun to reverse the spread of HIV/AIDS	6.1 HIV prevalence among population aged 15–24 years
	6.2 Condom use at last high-risk sex
	6.3 Proportion of population aged 15–24 years with comprehensive correct knowledge of HIV/AIDS
	6.4 Ratio of school attendance of orphans to school attendance of non-orphans aged 10–14 years
Target 6B: Achieve, by 2010, universal access to treatment for HIV/AIDS for all those who need it	6.5 Proportion of population with advanced HIV infection with access to antiretroviral drugs
Target 6C: Halt and begun to reverse the incidence of malaria and other major diseases	6.6 Incidence and death rates associated with malaria
	6.7 Proportion of children under 5 sleeping under insecticide-treated bed nets
	6.8 Proportion of children under 5 with fever who are treated with appropriate antimalarial drugs
	6.9 Incidence, prevalence and death rates associated with TB
	6.10 Proportion of TB cases detected and cured under directly observed treatment short course

Organization, Geneva, 2015f). Global efforts towards HIV, malaria, and TB are measured by the targets and indicators presented in Table 14.3.

Health-related MDG progress

Efforts towards achieving the health-related MDGs were tackled with earnest in certain parts of the world. With 1990 as the baseline, some MDGs chalked significant gains, while others did not. Gains in the health-related MDGs were not even across the regions of the world or between countries. Majority of countries in the developing world were lagging behind as their progress was hindered by a host of factors including conflict, economic hardship, high levels of HIV/AIDS, and the lack of adequate commitment, and capacity. The report card for the health-related MDGs presented data on how countries were closing in on the set targets. Akin to the other five MDGs, some countries were on track to achieving targets while other countries were not.

MDG4 Target 4A: Reduce by two-thirds, between 1990 and 2015, the under-five mortality rate

Under-five mortality rates have dropped significantly in all regions of the world. Globally, between 1990 and 2015, global, under-five mortality rates dropped by 53% from an estimated 91 deaths per 1000 live births, to 43 deaths per 1000 live births, respectively. The annual rate of reduction from 2000 to 2015 was 3.9%, compared to 1.8% from 1990 to 2000. Despite population growth in certain developing countries, child mortality rates declined from 12.7 million in 1990 to almost 6 million in 2015 globally (United Nations, 2015b).

Regarding infant mortality, the world experienced a decreased rate of 32 deaths per 1000 live births in 2015 compared to 63 deaths per 1000 live births in 1990. The annual infant mortality rate dropped from 8.9 million in 1990 to 4.5 million in 2015 (World Health Organization, 2016c). In 2011, sub-Saharan Africa and Southern Asia achieved child mortality rate reductions of 39% and 47%, respectively and sub-Saharan Africa reduced its average child mortality rate from 3.1% per annum between 1990 and 2000, to 1.5% per annum between 2000 and 2011. Ethiopia, Madagascar, Malawi, Niger, and Rwanda in sub-Saharan Africa, and Bhutan and Nepal in Southern Asia, saw reductions in child mortality rates of at least 60% since 1990.

Vaccination of children in the appropriate age group against measles prevented nearly 15.6 million deaths between 2000 and 2013. During this period, an estimated 84% of children aged 12–23 months received at least one dose of measles-containing vaccine (MCV1) (World Health Organization, 2015c). The most notable progress was in sub-Saharan Africa, where coverage increased to 74% in 2013. Between 2000 and 2013, 66% of UN Member States achieved immunization coverage rates of 90%, thus, dropping child measles deaths by 74% (from 481,000 to 124,000) (World Health Organization, 2015c). With World Bank International Development Association (IDA) support, approximately 600 million children in the poorest countries of the world were immunized. Through IDA funding, immunization coverage for children in Afghanistan almost tripled from 11% in 2003 to 30% in 2011, and that for Ghana rose from 69% in 2003 to 79% in 2008.

Gains in global immunization coverage can be attributed to improvements in routine coverage among children in the appropriate age group who received MCV1, and to the success of supplementary immunization activities (SIAs). Despite these gains, about 21.6 million children, especially the poorest and those living in hard- to reach areas, did not receive MCV1 in 2013. Notwithstanding the significant decreases in global under-five mortality rates between 1990 and 2015, the MDG target of a two thirds reduction, from 1990 levels was not achieved by 2015. Global progress was insufficient.

MDG5 Target 5A: Reduce the maternal mortality ratio by three-quarters, between 1990 and 2015

Between 1990 and 2013, all regions of the world decreased MMR by 37%. Regions that made significant progress during that period were Eastern Asia (65%) followed by Southern Asia (64%), Northern Africa (57%), South-eastern Asia (57%), Oceania (51%), Sub-Saharan Africa (49%), the Caucasus and Central Asia (44%), Western Asia (43%), and Latin America and the Caribbean (40%). The highest decline per annum (5.2%) occurred in Eastern Asia. During this period, 19 countries including Belarus (96% reduction in MMR), Maldives (93%), Bhutan (87%), Cambodia (86%), Israel (84%), Equatorial Guinea (81%), Poland (81%), and Rwanda (76%) had already achieved the three quarters (75%) reduction in MMR far ahead of the 2015 deadline. Countries like Botswana and South Africa initially registered increases in MMR between 1990 and 2000, primarily due to the onslaught of the HIV epidemic, but began to experience a decline in mortality as antiretroviral therapy became more available (World Health Organization, United Nations Children's Fund, United Nations Population Fund, The World Bank, and the United Nations Population Division, 2014).

From 1990 to 2014, over 71% of pregnant women were delivered by a skilled attendant during childbirth, accounting for a 59% increase from 1990 levels. Impressive as this number was, the gains were uneven across the world. Globally, access to skilled care was the least in low-income countries, where coverage of skilled attendant at delivery was 46% compared to 64% in lower middle-income countries, and 95% in upper middle-income countries. In developing countries, skilled attendants at childbirth was 56% in rural areas compared with 87% in urban areas. Declines in maternal mortality rates between 1990 and 2013 can be attributed to individual country efforts and interventions towards the achievement of MDG5 (World Health Organization, 2016e).

MDG5 Target 5B: Achieve, by 2015, universal access to reproductive health

Global contraceptive use among women aged 15–49, married or in a union, increased from 55% in 1990 to 64% in 2015. The proportion of contraceptive use in sub-Saharan Africa increased from 13% to 28% and from 39% to 59% in Southern Asia between 1990 and 2015 (United Nations, 2015b).

All regions of the world saw a drop in adolescent birth rates between 1990 and 2015. Global rates among girls aged 15–19 declined from 59 births per 1000 girls in 1990 to 51 births in 2015, with the most progress observed in Eastern Asia, Oceania, and Southern Asia. The least progress was in sub-Saharan Africa where adolescent birth rate was 116 births per 1000 adolescent girls in 2015 (United Nations, 2015b).

From 2007 to 2014, 84% of women received antenatal care at least once during pregnancy. Unfortunately, the numbers were not as high (64%) when it came to the recommended WHO minimum of four or more antenatal visits during pregnancy (United Nations, 2015b). Though there were significant reductions in maternal mortality by 2015, and although certain countries achieved their MMR targets before the 2015 deadline, the rate of decline was insufficient to achieve the three quarters target established globally.

MDG6 Target 6A: Halt the spread of HIV/AIDS by 2015 and begun to reverse it

Since 2000, HIV incidence has dropped by 35%. In 2014, there were 2 million new global cases of HIV, down from 3.1 million in 2000. Between 2000 and 2013, there was a 40% drop in HIV incidence from 3.5 million to 2.1 million. During this period, 10 countries recorded drops of over 75% and 27 countries experienced drops of 50%. Sub-Saharan Africa remains severely affected by the HIV epidemic, with 1.5 million new infections in 2013. Nevertheless, South Africa, the country with the highest number of people living with HIV, recorded the largest decline in new infections, with 98 000 fewer new infections occurring in 2013 than in 2010. Additionally, the number of new HIV infections among young people aged 15–24 in that region declined by 45% between 2000 and 2013 (Joint United Nations Programme on HIV/AIDS, 2016).

Comprehensive HIV knowledge among people aged 15–24 worldwide increased by a small margin. In sub-Saharan Africa, 30% of young women and 37% of young men had correct comprehensive HIV knowledge, representing a 10% increase from 2000. In 2000 and 2014, condom use among this population revealed higher use by young men than young women, thus revealing the inadequacy of prevention efforts in tackling the unique vulnerability of young women. Differences in comprehensive, correct HIV knowledge persisted by income level and location among young women and men aged 15–24. It was 17% for women living in the poorest households and 35% for their counterparts who lived in the richest households (Joint United Nations Programme on HIV/AIDS, 2016).

Trends in the number of orphaned versus nonorphaned children aged 10–14 attending school were also encouraging. The school attendance ratio between orphaned and nonorphaned children showed an increase of 0.80 in 2000 to 0.96 in 2014 (United Nations, 2015b).

MDG6 Target 6B: Achieve, by 2010, universal access to treatment for HIV/AIDS for all those who need it

In June 2014, 13.6 million people living with HIV globally had access to antiretroviral therapy (ART). This was a significant increase from the 2003 level of 800 000. All told, ART prevented the loss of 7.6 million lives to AIDS between 1995 and 2013. To date, Botswana, Cambodia, Cuba, Dominican Republic, Guyana, Mexico, Namibia, Rwanda, Swaziland, and Zambia have attained universal access to antiretroviral therapy, defined as coverage of at least 80% of the population in need. Laudable as this may be, only 36% of the 31.5 million people living with HIV in the developing world had access to ART in 2013. While sub-Saharan Africa has the highest number of

people living with HIV, 78% of people living with HIV in that region, do not have access to ART (United Nations, 2015b).

MDG6 Target 6C: Halt and begun to reverse the incidence of malaria and other major diseases by 2015

Global malaria morbidity and mortality rates decreased by 60% in all age groups and by 65% among children under the age of five since 2000 (World Health Organization, 2015e). This was due to the implementation of malaria control measures such as, the distribution of insecticide-treated bed nets, indoor residual spraying, and the promotion of intermittent preventive treatment for pregnant women. Worldwide, the proportion of children who slept under an insecticide-treated bed net in sub-Saharan Africa increased from less than 2% in 2000 to approximately 68% by 2015. Globally, the MDG target of halting by 2015 and beginning to reverse the incidence of malaria was met (World Health Organization, 2015e).

The Millennium Development Goal target to reverse TB incidence by 2015 was also met. Global TB incidence rates peaked at 141 per 100 000 people in 2002, but begun to fall slowly since then. From 1995 to 2011, 51 million TB patients were successfully treated under the Directly Observed Treatment Short Course (DOTS) strategy and its successor, the Stop TB Strategy launched in 2006. About 20 million lives were saved. Between 2010 and 2011, the annual global incidence of TB fell by 2.2%. Between 1990 and 2015, TB mortality rates dropped by 47% throughout the world (United Nations, 2015b) and during that same year, the 11 countries with the highest TB cases experienced a decline of about 55% (World Health Organization, 2015e). Tuberculosis-related deaths among people living with HIV dropped by 32% since 2004 and 77% of HIV-positive people with TB were on antiretroviral treatment in 2014 (World Health Organization, n.d.).

In addition to reversing HIV, malaria, and TB, MDG6 sought to halt neglected tropical diseases, thus, human African trypanosomiasis, guinea worm, leprosy, visceral leishmaniasis, and lymphatic filariasis were targeted to be eliminated by 2020 (World Health Organization, Geneva, 2015e). Despite the progress made in reducing malaria-related deaths and halting and reversing the incidence of TB, MDG 6 was not achieved by 2015. Global progress was insufficient.

Critique of the health-related MDGs

Like the other five MDGs, the health-related MDGs were also criticized. To the high modernists the MDGs including those related to health were a blueprint for human development. To other critics, they were poorly thought through and lacked analytical power, justification (Deneulin & Shahani, 2009; Kabeer, 2010), and legitimacy, in that, the voices they were supposed to serve (local people in developing countries and women) were not sufficiently involved in their development. For Samir Amin, (an economist), the MDGs, including those related to health were a litany of pious hopes that committed no one and therefore were not be taken seriously, as their promoters (the United States, Western Europe, and Japan) only implemented them as and when it was convenient. Additional criticisms leveled against the health-related MDGs include the fact that they were too expensive and ambitious, needed more than 15 years to achieve, and lacked reliable data to measure progress.

John McArthur and Jeffrey Sachs, both MDG proponents, counter argued that the MDGs were valid, regardless of how difficult they were to measure. To them, all the MDGs, including those related to health, provided a political and operational framework for global development that had hitherto not been in existence. They pointed out that by prioritizing interventions for MDG achievement, developing countries were able to make decisions about how much of their funds (internal and external) to allocate towards their MDG efforts (McArthur, Sachs, & Schmidt-Traub, 2005). According to McArthur, the MDGs "have helped to provide an objective framework for establishing priorities in collaboration with international partners" and "are an important reminder of humanity's common purpose."

Health-related MDG challenges

Working towards achieving the health-related MDGs have been fraught with challenges, especially for developing countries. In these countries, inadequate internal and external financing for health interventions, low priority accorded to health in national development policies, weak vital registration systems (unavailable or poor-quality data on live births, deaths, fetal deaths, etc.), conflict, and instability among others, stood in the way of progress.

Although child and infant mortality rates dropped from 1990 levels globally by 2015, they still remained high and far from the set target. Similarly, while maternal mortality decreased from 1990 levels, it was far from the 2015 target of 162 per 100 000 live births. The lack of access to skilled attendants at birth and poor health infrastructure, roads, and transport networks especially in rural areas, continue to negatively impact the life and health of women and girls during pregnancy and childbirth.

Prevention of mother-to-child transmission (PMTCT) of HIV remains a challenge in rural areas, as over 75% of antenatal care facilities that provide PMTCT services are located in urban areas, inadequately covering the health needs of women in rural areas. While TB treatment has been successful since 2007, the emergence of multi-drug-resistant tuberculosis (MDR-TB) is threatening to reverse achievements.

Global action and strategies

Child and maternal health are major concerns of WHO. As such, WHO works with the governments of developing countries to strengthen their local health systems and to promote interventions that focus on policies and strategies that are effective, pro-poor, and cost-effective. The WHO builds effective partnerships to mobilize resources and to minimize the duplication of efforts that improve maternal and newborn health. Advocating for investments in maternal and child health, WHO also highlights the inherent social and economic benefits, and emphasizes maternal mortality as a human rights and equity issue.

During the 2015 UN General Assembly meeting in New York, former UN Secretary-General, Ban Ki-moon launched the Global Strategy for Women's, Children's and Adolescents' Health to be implemented from 2016 to 2030. The Global Strategy is a framework for the newly adopted Sustainable Development Goals (SDGs) and seeks to bring to an end all preventable maternal, child, and adolescent deaths by creating an environment that not only promotes the survival of this population, but also transforms their health and well-being. Among other things, the Global Strategy's goal of ending preventable maternal mortality, requires WHO to work with Member States to:

- Address inequalities in access to and quality of reproductive, maternal, and newborn healthcare services
- Ensure universal health coverage for comprehensive reproductive, maternal, and newborn healthcare

- Address all causes of maternal mortality, reproductive and maternal morbidities, and related disabilities
- Strengthen health systems to respond to the needs and priorities of women and girls, ensuring accountability in order to improve quality of care and equity (United Nations, 2015a)

Post MDGs

After 15 years of implementation, the era of the MDGs came to an end in December 2015, and was replaced with the era of the SDGs. Also known as the global goals, the SDGs focus on sustainable development for the entire world based on a triple bottom-line approach to human wellbeing; economic development, environmental sustainability and social inclusion. Unlike the MDGs that mainly targeted poor countries and sought rich country participation through financial and technological assistance among others, the SDGs focus on challenges that are applicable to all countries and require global collaboration to be achieved.

Approved by the 70th Session of the UN General Assembly, the SDGs were adopted by UN Member States on September 25, 2015. They cover a wide range of issues and comprise 17 goals and 169 targets to be achieved over 15 years (December 2030). The SDGs seek to end poverty, protect the planet, and ensure prosperity for all.

The third SDG relates to MDGs 4, 5, and 6. Sustainable Development Goal 3 specifically seeks to reduce the global maternal mortality ratio to less than 70 per 100 000 live births and to end preventable deaths of newborns and children under five years of age. Under this SDG, all countries will in addition, aim to reduce neonatal mortality to at least as low as 12 per 1000 live births and under-five mortality to at least as low as 25 per 1000 live births. Sustainable Development Goal 3 also seeks to end the epidemics of AIDS, TB, malaria, and neglected tropical diseases and to combat hepatitis, water-borne diseases, and other communicable diseases (see Figure 14.3).

The SDG development process was state led with broad participation from major groups and other civil-society stakeholders. Inputs for the SDGs were provided by an open working group of the UN General Assembly, the report of an intergovernmental committee of experts on sustainable development financing, and UN General Assembly dialogues on technology facilitation, among many others. These inputs were synthesized into a report by the UN Secretary General, at the behest of the UN General Assembly in 2014. The UN facilitated global conversations that led up to the adoption of the SDGs (United Nations, 2015c).

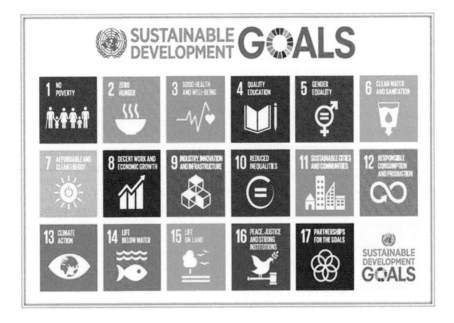

Figure 14.3 The sustainable development goals.
Source: https://sustainabledevelopment.un.org/topics/sustainabledevelopmentgoals (accessed October 28, 2016).

Discussion points

1 What are the MDGs
2 Which of the MDGs are health related? List them all.
3 What are some of the causes of global child mortality?
4 Describe progress made towards MDGs 4, 5, and 6.
5 Which health-related MDG targets were achieved by December 2015?
6 What are some of the critiques levelled against the health-related MDGs?
7 What are some of the challenges with the achievement of the health-related MDGs in developing countries? Explain your response.
8 What was the WHO's role in accelerating progress towards the attainment of the health-related MDGs?
9 What are the SDG?
10 How are the SDGs associated with MDGs 4, 5, and 6?

REFERENCES

Deneulin, S. and Shahani, L. (2009) *An Introduction to the Human Development and Capability Approach: Freedom and Agency*, Earthscan International Development Research Centre, Sterling, Virginia Ottawa, Ontario.

Joint United Nations Programme on HIV/AIDS (2016) *Fact Sheet 2016*, http://www.unaids.org/en/resources/fact-sheet (accessed October 28, 2016).

Kabeer, N. (2010) *Can the MDGs Provide a Pathway to Social Justice? The Challenge of Intersecting Inequalities*, http://www.cbm.org/article/downloads/82788/Can_the_MDGs_provide_a_pathway_to_social_justice_ISD_and_MDG_Achievement_Fund.pdf (accessed October 28, 2016).

Liu, L. Johnson, H.L., Cousens, S., *et al.* (2012) Global, regional, and national causes of child mortality: An updated systematic analysis for 2010 with time trends since 2000. *The Lancet* **379**(9832), 2151–2161.

McArthur, J. W., Sachs, J. D., and Schmidt-Traub, G. (2005) Response to Amir Attara. *PLoS Medicine* **2**(11), 379.

MEASURE Evaluation. (n.d.) *Family Planning and Reproductive Health Indicators Database*, https://www.measureevaluation.org/prh/rh_indicators (accessed October 30, 2016).

Save the Children. (2015) *Inequalities in Child Survival: Looking at Wealth and other Socio-Economic Disparities in Developing Countries*, http://resourcecentre.savethechildren.se/library/inequalities-child-survival-looking-wealth-and-other-socio-economic-disparities-developing (accessed October 28, 2016).

UNFPA Turkmenistan (2014) Harnessing Data to Improve Maternal Health, http://www.unfpa.org.tm/en/pressroom/news/local-news/harnessing-data-to-improve-maternal-health/ (accessed October 28, 2016).

United Nations. (2015a) *Global Strategy for Women's, Children's and Adolescents' Health, 2016–2030*, United Nations, New York.

United Nations. (2015b) *Millennium Development Goals Report 2015*, http://www.un.org/millenniumgoals/2015_MDG_Report/pdf/MDG%202015%20rev%20%28July%201%29.pdf (accessed October 28, 2016).

United Nations. (2015c) *Sustainable Development Knowledge Platform*, https://sustainabledevelopment.un.org/post2015 (accessed October 28, 2016).

United Nations Children's Fund (2011) *Fact of the Week*, http://www.unicef.org/factoftheweek/index_59254.html (accessed October 28, 2016).

United Nations Children's Fund (n.d.) *Preventing HIV Infection among Adolescents and Young People*, http://www.unicef.org/esaro/5482_HIV_prevention.html (accessed October 28, 2016).

United Nations Department of Economic and Social Affairs (2013) *World Contraceptive Patterns 2013*, http://www.un.org/en/development/desa/population/publications/family/contraceptive-wallchart-2013.shtml (accessed October 28, 2016).

World Health Organization (2015a) *10 Facts on Malaria*, http://www.who.int/features/factfiles/malaria/en/ (accessed October 28, 2016).

World Health Organization (2015b) *Global Health Observatory Data Child Mortality and Causes of Death*, http://www.who.int/gho/child_health/mortality/causes/en/ (accessed October 28, 2016).

World Health Organization (2015c) *Maternal Mortality. Fact sheet*, http://www.who.int/mediacentre/factsheets/fs348/en/ (accessed October 28, 2016).

World Health Organization (2015d) *MDG5: Improve Maternal Health*, http://www.who.int/topics/millennium_development_goals/maternal_health/en/ (accessed October 28, 2016).

World Health Organization(2015e) *Millennium Development Goals. Fact sheet*, http://www.who.int/mediacentre/factsheets/fs290/en (accessed October 28, 2016).

World Health Organization (2015f) *Multi-drug Resistance TB. Fact sheet*, http://www.who.int/tb/challenges/mdr/mdr_tb_factsheet.pdf (accessed October 28, 2016).

World Health Organization (2016a) *Maternal Health*, http://www.who.int/topics/maternal_health/en/ (accessed October 28, 2016).

World Health Organization (2016b) *Adolescent Pregnancy*, http://www.who.int/maternal_child_adolescent/topics/maternal/adolescent_pregnancy/en/ (accessed October 28, 2016).

World Health Organization (2016c) *Infant Mortality*, http://www.who.int/gho/child_health/mortality/neonatal_infant_text/en/ (accessed October 28, 2016).

World Health Organization. (2016d) *Intermittent Preventive Treatment in Pregnancy (IPTp)*, http://www.who.int/malaria/areas/preventive_therapies/pregnancy/en/ (accessed October 28, 2016).

World Health Organization (2016e) *Skilled Attendant at Birth*, http://www.who.int/gho/maternal_health/skilled_care/skilled_birth_attendance_text/en/ (accessed October 28, 2016).

World Health Organization (n.d.) *Ten Facts about Tuberculosis*, http://www.who.int/features/factfiles/tb_facts/en/index9.html (accessed October 28, 2016).

World Health Organization, United Nations Children's Fund, United Nations Population Fund, The World Bank, and the United Nations Population Division (2014) *Trends in Maternal Mortality 1990 to 2013*, http://apps.who.int/iris/bitstream/10665/112682/2/9789241507226_eng.pdf?ua= (accessed October 30, 2016).

FURTHER READING

Conde-Agudelo, A., Belizan, J. M., and Lammers, C. (2005) Maternal-perinatal morbidity and mortality associated with adolescent pregnancy in Latin America: Cross-sectional study. *American Journal of Obstetrics and Gynecology* **192**(2), 342–349.

Cousens, S., Blencowe, H., Stanton, C. *et al.* (2011) National, regional, and worldwide estimates of stillbirth rates in 2009 with trends since 1995: a systematic analysis. *The Lancet* **377**(9774), 1319–1330.

Patton, G. C., Coffey, C., Sawyer, S. M. *et al.* (2009) Global patterns of mortality in young people: A systematic analysis of population health data. *The Lancet* **374**(9693), 881–892. doi:10.1016/S0140-6736(09)60741-8

Say, L., Chou, D., Gemmill, A., *et al.* (2014) Global causes of maternal death: A WHO systematic analysis. *The Lancet Glob Health* **2**(6), e323–333. doi:10.1016/S2214-109X(14)70227-X

Sikazwe, E. J. (2014) *Achieving The MDGs: Progress and Challenges. Social Watch Report 2014*, http://www.socialwatch.org/node/15959 (accessed October 28, 2016).

United Nations Children's Fund. *Preventing HIV Infection Among Adolescents and Young People*, http://www.unicef.org/esaro/5482_HIV_prevention.html (accessed October 28, 2016).

United Nations Children's Fund, World Health Organization, The World Bank, and United Nations Population Division (2015) *The Inter-agency Group for Child Mortality Estimation (UN IGME). Levels and Trends in Child Mortality Report*, http://www.childmortality.org/files_v20/download/IGME%20Report%202015_9_3%20LR%20Web.pdf (accessed October 28, 2016).

15

Global health partnerships and governance

Learning objectives

By the end of this chapter you will be able to:

✔ Discuss the purpose of global health partnerships and governance;

✔ List at least two examples of global health partnerships;

✔ Discuss the benefits of global health partnerships;

✔ Discuss at least two global health partnership successes;

✔ List and explain at least two challenges of global health partnerships and governance.

Summary of key points

Recognizing the scope and complexity of global health issues and the impossibility of acting alone to address the challenges they pose, countries, organizations, individuals, and other entities, have found it necessary to form global health partnerships (GHPs). To date, there are over 100 global partnerships for health working on a variety of issues across a variety of sectors. For GHPs to be effective and efficient, they need to be governed, so the plethora of actors and their activities are properly coordinated and managed. In this chapter, the purpose, characteristics, focus, actors, funders, and successes of GHPs are discussed. This is followed by deliberations on the purpose of global health governance (GHG), the challenges associated with GHPs and GHG, and actions and strategies suggested for addressing GHP and GHG challenges.

The concept of global health partnerships

Global health partnerships are alliances among public and private entities to implement worldwide agreed goals on the health of the public. They are also "relatively institutionalized initiatives established to address global health problems, in which public and private-for-profit sector organizations have a voice in collective decision-making." While GHPs are formed at the global level, their implementation takes place at the national level within individual countries. Some examples of GHPs are presented in Box 15.1.

Global Health: Issues, Challenges, and Global Action Lecture Notes, First Edition. Elizabeth A. Armstrong-Mensah.
© 2017 John Wiley & Sons Ltd. Published 2017 by John Wiley & Sons Ltd.

Purpose and benefits of global health partnerships

In an interconnected world where diseases are no respecter of persons or boundaries, GHPs have become the norm. These partnerships:

> Bring groups – including governments, donors, NGOs, and a variety of private-sector representatives – into a formal, collaborative relationship dedicated to the pursuit of a shared health goal. Typically, the partnerships work directly with the governments of affected countries to develop and implement plans for aid.
> (Conway *et al.*, 2006)

Global health partnerships encourage the public and private sectors to work together in areas where the former lacks expertise and experience (e.g., product development, manufacturing, management, marketing and distribution) so as to save lives. As a relatively new approach to health, GHPs draw attention to critical global health issues and diseases and encourage countries to craft better policies and plans for the future health of their citizens, as was the case in Angola. After decades of civil war, GHP funds enabled the government of Angola to increase its national budgetary allocation to health to more than what it was (5%) prior to the war. As Angola transitioned from a war environment to a post-war environment, donor and GHP funding from the Global Fund to Fight AIDS, TB and Malaria (GFTAM), and the World Bank also helped the government to embark on strategies to control the spread of the human immunodeficiency syndrome and acquired immune deficiency syndrome (HIV/AIDS), as people who were once isolated by the war could now move about freely and potentially spread the disease (Bill and Melinda Gates Foundation and McKinsey Company, 2005).

Global health partnerships increase stakeholder participation in the health sector. In Bangladesh and Zambia for example, where more than 50% of healthcare is provided by the private sector, non-governmental organizations (NGOs) have been able to bid for and receive GFTAM grants to finance their HIV/AIDS activities. Global health partnerships allow donors and governments to undertake large scale global health initiatives they could otherwise not have undertaken on their own. Thus, the GFTAM, the Global Alliance for Vaccines and Immunization (GAVI), and UNITAID for example, are able to embark on large-scale global health activities because of the considerable sums of money they are able to raise (over $4 billion per year). When managed properly, GHPs further help to reduce duplication of investments and efforts. They create awareness of health problems at national, regional, and international levels, promote health research and education, facilitate new product development such as drugs for malaria, tuberculosis (TB), and neglected diseases, introduce new ways of working, play a key role in meeting the critical health needs of low- and middle-income countries, and help to build health-system capacity. With limited resources and funding capacity, developing countries depend to a great extent on GHPs to meet the health needs of their populations.

Characteristics of good global health partnerships

For GHPs to function effectively, collaborating parties must have a shared and clearly defined set of realistic goals. Roles and responsibilities have to be delineated and agreed upon from the onset, and the benefits to be gained from the collaboration spelt out. Transparency in decision-making, active partnership maintenance, equal partner participation, inclusiveness, and the performance of agreed obligations are additional important characteristics.

Focus of global health partnerships

Various partnerships have been formed at the global level to deal with specific health issues and challenges. These include partnerships for product development, the improvement of access to health products, global coordination and financing, and health systems strengthening.

Partnerships for product development

The goal of product development partnerships is to develop safe, effective vaccines, drugs and diagnostics for a range of diseases, and to deliver them as quickly and as cheaply as possible where they are needed. Partnerships that focus on product development

collaborate to varying degrees with pharmaceutical and biotech companies to reduce health inequities that affect the poor. Examples of this type of partnership include the Medicines for Malaria Venture (MMV), and the International AIDS Vaccine Initiative (IAVI). Partners working with the MMV are presented in Box 15.2.

Improvement of access to health products partnerships

Improvement of access to health products partnerships seek to create strong, health supply chains to improve upon the situation of systems plagued with stock outs, expired medicines, and unreliable delivery, by structuring and creating demand-driven operations geared towards delivering medicines and health commodities to the sick and dying. The GAVI and the Accelerating Access Initiative (AAI) are examples of this type of partnership. Partners working with GAVI are presented in Box 15.3.

Box 15.2 Medicines for Malaria Venture partnership.

GHP Description	Partners	Goal
Medicines for Malaria Venture (MMV) (established as a foundation in Switzerland in 1999); Currently a leading product-development partnership (PDP) in the field of antimalarial drug research and development	About 300 partners in over 50 countries from the public and private sector including governments (e.g., Ministries of Health in Zambia, Malawi, Uganda etc.), research and academic institutions (Boston, Cornell, and Yale University, etc.) and international organizations (WHO, GFTAM, Roll Back Malaria, etc.)	To reduce the burden of malaria in endemic countries by discovering, developing, and facilitating the delivery of new, effective, and affordable antimalarial drugs

---

Box 15.3 The Global Alliance for Vaccines and Immunization.

GHP Description	Partners	Goal
Global Alliance for Vaccines and Immunization (GAVI) (created in 2000 and is based in Geneva, Switzerland)	Gates Foundation, WHO (for scientific expertise), Unicef (for its procurement system), World Bank (for financial knowhow), the vaccine industry (for its market knowledge), developing country government (to play a lead role in proposal development for support and immunization program management and financing), and the pharmaceutical industry (to provide consistent, sustainable supply of quality vaccines and related technologies needed by developing countries)	To accelerate and create equal access to new and underused vaccines for children living in the world's poorest countries, so as to save lives and protect health

Global coordination and financing mechanisms partnerships

These partnerships generally conduct overarching coordination of initiatives or provide funding for health products procurement. They sometimes focus on research and development (R&D). The Stop TB Partnership, Roll Back Malaria Partnership, GAVI, GFTAM, and the 3 by 5 Initiative are examples of global coordination and financing mechanisms. Partners working with RBM and GFTAM are presented in Box 15.4).

Health systems strengthening partnerships

Health systems strengthening partnerships as their name implies, have health systems strengthening as their main objective. Improvement of access to health products partnerships also seek to strengthen health systems. Principal examples of this type of partnership include GAVI and the African Comprehensive HIV/AIDS Partnership (ACHAP) in Botswana supported by Merck, the Merck Foundation, and the Bill and Melinda Gates Foundation. Partners working with GAVI and ACHAP are presented in Box 15.5.

Box 15.4 The Roll Back Malaria Partnership and the Global Fund to Fight AIDS, TB and Malaria.

GHP Description	Partners	Goal
Rollback Malaria (RBM) (initiated in May 1998, by the Director-General of WHO as a new effort to roll back malaria)	More than 500 malaria endemic countries, their bilateral and multilateral development partners, the private sector, nongovernmental and community-based organizations, foundations, and research and academic institutions	To coordinate global action against malaria. The Malaria Advocacy Working Group (MAWG) coordinates RBMs advocacy to increase resource allocations for malaria prevention, treatment, and operational research
Global Fund to Fight AIDS, TB and Malaria (GFTAM) (created in 2002)	Governments, donors, civil society, the private sector, foundations, UN, representatives of communities living with and affected by the three diseases, etc.	To attract and disburse funds to prevent and treat AIDS, TB, and malaria globally. The GFTAM provides 25% of all International financing for AIDS

Box 15.5 The Global Alliance for Vaccines and Immunization and the African Comprehensive HIV/AIDS Partnership (ACHAP).

GHP Description	Partners	Goal
Global Alliance for Vaccines and Immunization (GAVI)	Gates Foundation, WHO, UNICEF, World Bank, governments of developing countries, pharmaceutical industry, research, and technical health institutions	To improve the ability of health systems to carry out immunization, raise rates of coverage in low- and middle-income countries, and promote uptake of underused vaccines
The African Comprehensive HIV/AIDS Partnership (ACHAP, created in 2000 and is based in Botswana)	Bill and Melinda Gates Foundation, Botswana Harvard Partnership, Botswana Ministry of Finance and Development Planning, Botswana Ministry of Health, Botswana Ministry of Labor and Home Affairs, Botswana Ministry of Youth, Sport and Culture, Botswana National AIDS Coordinating Agency, Central Medical Stores (CMS), Harvard School of Public Health, UNAIDS, University of Botswana, US President's Emergency Plan for AIDS Relief (PEPFAR), World Bank, World Health Organization (WHO)	To support and enhance Botswana's response to the HIV/AIDS epidemic through a comprehensive approach that includes HIV/AIDS prevention, treatment, care, support, and impact mitigation

Box 15.6 **The Global Fund to Fight AIDS, TB, and Malaria and the Global Forum for Health Research.**

GHP Description	Partners	Goal
Global Fund to Fight AIDS, TB and Malaria (GFTAM)	Governments, donors, civil society, the private sector, foundations, UN, and representatives of communities living with and affected by the three diseases	To advocate for HIV, TB, and malaria with a particular interest in scaling up programs for HIV antiretroviral therapy
Global Forum for Health Research (Created in 1998)	Governments policy makers, multilateral organizations, bilateral aid donors, international foundations, national and international NGOs, women's organizations, research-oriented bodies, and private sector companies	To correct the 10/90 disequilibrium and to focus research on issues that affect the majority of the world's population, particularly the poor, by providing research funds and through public-private sector collaboration Research initiatives include those on malaria, TB, domestic violence against women, and cardiovascular diseases

Public advocacy and research partnerships

These partnerships seek to draw global attention to critical global health issues and aim at strengthening health research capacity to enable local researchers and institutions develop the scientific knowledge and skills needed to address local health issues effectively. The RBM Partnership, GFTAM, and the Global Forum for Health Research are examples of this type of partnership. Partners working with GFTAM and Global Forum for Health Research are presented in Box 15.6).

Actors and funders of global health partnerships

Actors and funders of GHPs provide additional development assistance channels and resources for disease prevention, control, treatment, and care around the world. They range from bilateral and private NGOs, to academic and global multilateral organizations, each providing varied amounts of funds and support to global health efforts and initiatives (see Tables 15.1, 15.2, and 15.3).

Bilateral donors

Developed countries or bilateral donors provide funding to low- and middle-income countries to advance health and socio-economic development. These entities are usually involved in advocacy, knowledge generation, and financing. They also set priorities, influence agreements, and provide technical assistance. Examples of bilateral donors include Australia (AusAID), Denmark (DANIDA), France (AFD), Luxemburg (Lux-Development), Sweden (Sida), and Japan (JICA). In 2011, DANIDAs development assistance to low- and middle-income countries increased to 0.85% of its GNI (DKK 15.98 billion, or $2.68 billion) (Ministry of Foreign Affairs of Denmark, n.d.). Denmark is one of the five countries in the world whose total development assistance to developing countries exceeds the United Nations (UN) target of 0.7% of gross national income (GNI).

Multilateral organizations

Multilateral organizations are organizations formed between three or more countries to work on issues that relate to all the countries in the partnership. Multilateral organizations include UN agencies, financial institutions, and regional groupings.

United Nations agencies

Many UN agencies engage in advocacy, knowledge generation and dissemination, health financing, setting of global health standards, and other key functions. These agencies include the Joint United Nations Program on HIV/AIDS (UNAIDS), the United Nations High Commission for Refugees (UNHCR), United Nations Children's Fund (Unicef), the World Bank, and the World Health Organization (WHO).

Table 15.1 Major actors in global health partnerships.

Actor	Number of partnerships
1. World Health Organization(WHO)	43
2. United Nations Children's Fund(Unicef)	21
3. World Bank	18
4. Bill and Melinda Gates Foundation	16
5. US Centers for Disease Control and Prevention(CDC)	15
6. Glaxo Smith Kline (UK)	13
7. UNDP/WB/WHO Special Program for Research and Training in Tropical Diseases (TDR)	13
8. US Agency for International Development(USAID)	12
9. Merck & Co., Inc.	11
10. Sanofi-Pasteur (merger of Aventis-Pasteur and Sanofi)	9
11. UK Department for International Development(DFID)	9
12. Joint United Nations Program on HIV/AIDS (UNAIDS)	8
13. London School of Hygiene and Tropical Medicine	8
14. Pfizer Inc.	8
15. Médecins Sans Frontières (MSF)	7
16. Novartis	7
17. Bristol-Myers Squibb Company	6
18. Canadian International Development Agency (CIDA)	6
19. Carter Center	6
20. Program for Appropriate Technology in Health (PATH)	6

Source: The partnerships database by the Initiative on Public-Private Partnerships for Health. From: http://www.ide.go.jp/English/Publish/Download/Jrp/pdf/142_5.pdf (accessed October 30, 2016).

Unicef's advocacy activities and support for improved water and sanitation culminated in the passage of the Water for the World Act (HR 2901) in December 2014. Unicef works in over 190 countries and territories with governments, multilateral organizations, civil society organizations, and with the corporate sector to provide children and families with safe drinking water and improved sanitation facilities.

The WHO engages in a number of diverse GHPs. Its decision to participate in a GHP is determined by whether the partnership or collaborative arrangement (i) demonstrates a clear added value in terms of mobilizing partners, knowledge, and resources, (ii) has a clear goal that ties in with WHO priorities; (iii) supports national development objectives; (iv) ensures adequate participation of relevant stakeholders; and (v) clearly delineates partner roles. The WHO will serve as host organization for a GHP if its role in the partnership will be that of strategic and technical collaborator, member, and full participant in the steering body of the partnership, and if decisions of the partnership are consistent with its rules and policies. World Health Organization GHPs range from small, single-product collaborations with industries, to large entities hosted by UN agencies, and private not-for-profit organizations such as the Global Buruli Ulcer Initiative, Global Collaboration for Blood Safety, Global Collaboration for Development of Pesticides for Public Health, Global Outbreak Alert and Response Network, and the International Treatment Access Coalition. As host of the Global Buruli Ulcer Initiative, WHO convenes key actors involved in buruli ulcer on a routine basis to share information, coordinate disease control and research efforts, and to monitor progress. As a result, buruli ulcer has received global visibility and attracted resources to combat it.

Financial institutions

Financial institutions lend or grant money to countries to promote health and development. Such institutions include the African Development Bank (AfDB), Asian Development Bank, Inter-American Development

Table 15.2 Major Funders of Global Health Partnerships.

Funder	Contribution ($)
1. Bill and Melinda Gates Foundation	4 645 724 419
2. United Kingdom, government of	2 928 720 000
3. France, government of	2 664 751 427
4. US Agency for International Development(USAID)	1 539 500 000
5. Italy, government of	1 000 000 000
6. Norway, government of	808 221 757
7. United States, government of	566 420 000
8. European Commission	563 870 813
9. Canada, government of	324 220 000
10. UK Department for International Development(DFID)	299 421 096
11. Netherlands government of	265 835 059
12. Spain, government of	240 000 000
13. Japan, government of	200 000 000
14. Canadian International Development Agency (CIDA)	137 391 162
15. Bristol-Myers Squibb Company	115 000 000
16. Sweden, government of	107 040 000
17. Bill and Melinda Gates Foundation Challenge Grant	100 000 000
18. Swedish International Development Agency (SIDA)	73 026 600
19. Eli Lilly & Co.	70 000 000
20. Merck & Co. Inc.	50 000 000

Source: The partnerships database by the Initiative on Public-Private Partnerships for Health. From: http://www.ide.go.jp/English/Publish/Download/Jrp/pdf/142_5.pdf (accessed October 30, 2016).

Table 15.3 Distribution of GHPs by Disease.

Disease/condition	No. of GHP
Communicable diseases	2
Counterfeit and substandard drugs	2
Dengue	2
Diarrhea dehydration	1
Diseases of the poor	1
Guinea worm (dracunculiasis) disease	1
HIV/AIDS	20
Human African trypanosomiasis	4
Leprosy	2
Malaria	18
Reproductive health	5
Sexually transmitted infections	7
Tuberculosis(TB)	10
Vitamin A deficiency	1

Source: The partnerships database by the Initiative on Public-Private Partnerships for Health. From: http://www.ide.go.jp/English/Publish/Download/Jrp/pdf/142_5.pdf (accessed October 30, 2016).

Bank, and the World Bank. In support of global health, the World Bank funds several global health programs that focus on HIV/AIDS prevention, nutrition, and family planning. Through the New Partnership for Africa's Development Infrastructure Project Preparation Facility (NEPAD-IPPF), the AfDB provides grants to African countries through Regional Economic Communities (RECs), Power Pools (PPs), and other specialized regional institutions for a number of projects including cross-border infrastructure projects in energy, transboundary water, and transport (African Development Bank, 2015).

Regional grouping – European Union (EU)

European Union (EU) Member States focus their development assistance on agriculture, fisheries, science and technology, energy, industry, transportation, education, culture, broadcasting, social policy, consumer protection, the environment, finance, and foreign policy. The United Kingdom, Italy, France, and Germany are four examples of the 28 EU member countries. In response to the highly pathogenic Asian avian influenza (HPAI) crisis of 2009 caused by the A (H5N1) virus, the EU created a global partnership, with actors such as the UN, development organizations, and more than 120 nations to address the outbreak (European Union, 2016).

International nongovernmental organizations

International NGOs are private organizations that pursue activities in many countries to relieve suffering, promote the interests of the poor, and to protect the environment. These organizations are not part of the government and often work for social and public health benefit and not for profit. They include Save the Children, Doctors without Borders (Médecins Sans Frontières), Oxfam, CARE, Program for Appropriate Technology in Health (PATH), Foundations, the private sector, think tanks, and universities.

Save the Children

This organization seeks to provide children with a healthy start, the opportunity to learn, and protection from harm. It works in 120 countries including the United States. In 2013, GlaxoSmith Kline (GSK) and Save the Children formed a partnership that enabled them to pool their expertise, resources, and influence to save the lives of one million children globally. Together, they invested in the strengthening of healthcare infrastructure in low-income countries and helped fund training for over 5000 health workers in West and Central Africa, Haiti, and Yemen.

Doctors without Borders (Médecins Sans Frontières)

This international humanitarian aid organization helps people worldwide, especially those in countries where the health need is greatest, by delivering emergency medical aid to people affected by conflict, epidemics, disasters, or excluded from health care. It comprises 24 associations bound together as Médecins Sans Frontières (MSF) International and is based in Switzerland. This organization has programs in over 65 countries and is committed to medical ethics and human rights. During the 2014 Ebola outbreak in West Africa, MSF partnered with Medical Team International to expand health facilities and bed capacity for Ebola patients, improve health worker training on community health and education promotion, and to provide technical support and prepare

the stressed health ministries of Nigeria and Senegal to handle potential Ebola outbreaks.

CARE International

CARE International is one of the largest international relief and humanitarian organizations in the world. It has 880 poverty-fighting development and emergency projects in 95 countries. Headquartered in the United States, CARE focuses on addressing the underlying causes of poverty, empowering women and girls, responding to emergencies, fighting world hunger, improving health, educating communities, and advocating for change to address poverty. For over 60 years, CARE has partnered with the United States Agency for International Development (USAID) to implement programs in over 84 countries in various sectors including health, gender, climate change, and water (CARE, 2016).

Program for Appropriate Technology in Health

The Program for Appropriate Technology in Health is an international nonprofit organization that collaborates with diverse public- and private-sector partners to provide appropriate health technologies to populations in need. It focuses on emerging and epidemic diseases, health technologies for low-resource settings, maternal and child health, reproductive health, and vaccines and immunizations. This organization partners with governments, civil-society institutions, corporations, foundations, social entrepreneurs, individuals, as well as multilateral institutions to develop and introduce appropriate solutions to tackle health issues in developing countries.

Foundations

The Bill and Melinda Gates Foundation is the largest private foundation in the world. It gives high priority to global health programs with the aim of enhancing healthcare and reducing extreme poverty across the world. Its areas of emphasis include discovery and translational sciences, enteric and diarrheal diseases, family planning, HIV/AIDS, malaria, neglected infectious diseases, nutrition, pneumonia, and TB. The foundation's partners include GFTAM, Presidents Emergency Plan for AIDS Relief (PEPFAR), Malaria Control and Evaluation Partnership in Africa (MACEPA), GAVI Alliance, Meningitis Vaccine Project (MVP), and WHO. Since 2005, the foundation has supported MACEPA and PATH to work with the government of Zambia and other partners to set standards for comprehensive malaria control.

African Medical and Research Foundation (AMREF)

The African Medical and Research Foundation (AMREF) is an international African organization headquartered in Kenya, Nairobi. It focuses on research, capacity building, maternal and child health, fighting diseases, water and sanitation, clinical and diagnostic services research, and advocacy (African Medical Research Foundation, 2016). The foundation partners with the London School of Hygiene and Tropical Medicine, Harvard and Johns Hopkins Universities, and Medical Institutes on various projects. It receives substantial funding from donor countries such as Canada, Sweden, the United Kingdom, and the United States. Currently, AMREF works with over 100 poor and marginalized rural and urban slum communities, district health authorities, and Ministries of Health and Education in Ethiopia, Kenya, Rwanda, Somalia, South Africa, Sudan, Tanzania, and Uganda (African Medical Research Foundation, 2016).

The private sector

These are organizations that are part of the economy, but are run by private individuals or groups for profit. They include pharmaceutical companies such as Merck, Pfizer, and GlaxoSmithKline, tobacco companies such as Phillip Morris and Japan Tobacco, and food companies such as makers of infant formula.

Think tanks and universities

These often bring researchers together to work on global health issues. Some are involved in teaching, research, and the practice of global health, while others provide technical assistance on the design, monitoring, and evaluation of global health projects.

Successes of global health partnerships

Smallpox

Smallpox was officially eradicated from the world in 1980, following the implementation of the global Smallpox Eradication Program from 1966–1980. This feat was achieved through vaccination campaigns, surveillance, and prevention measures carried out by WHO in partnership with the United States Centers for Disease Control and Prevention (CDC), the erstwhile Union of Soviet Socialist Republics (USSR), and UN Member States (World Health Organization, 2010).

Poliomyelitis

In 1988, poliomyelitis (polio) was prevalent in 125 countries with an estimated 350 000 cases. Through the Global Polio Eradication Initiative established in 1988, wild polio cases as of December 9, 2015, stood at 66 in only two countries – Afghanistan (17) and Pakistan (49), thanks to the implementation of routine immunization, supplementary immunization campaigns, surveillance of possible outbreaks, and global partnerships (Centers for Disease Control and Prevention, 2015).

Guinea worm disease

In 1986, WHO declared guinea worm as one of the diseases to be eliminated globally. Since then, the Carter Center, together with Unicef, CDC, WHO, national governments in sub-Saharan Africa and Asia, the donor community, NGO's, foundations, and the private sector have joined forces to combat the disease. As of December 2015, the global incidence of guinea worm was 22 human cases in four countries (Chad: nine, Mali: five, South Sudan: five, and Ethiopia three), compared to an estimated 3.5 million cases in 21 countries in 1986 (Carter Center, 2016).

The concept of global health governance

Until the 1990s, international health and international health governance prevailed. This type of governance was relatively simple as it comprised few actors and clear lines of responsibility. With globalization, the disease landscape changed, and so did the number of actors. Globalization ushered in global health and its governing framework, global health governance (GHG). Unlike its predecessor, GHG involves a myriad of actors, uncoordinated activities, and most often, unclear responsibilities.

Global health governance is the use of formal and informal institutions, rules, and processes by states, intergovernmental organizations, and non-state actors, to deal with challenges to health that require cross-border collective action effectively. It is also how a global society "steers" itself to achieve common goals by establishing a set of rules, norms, principles and procedures to structure cooperation among global partners (Gostin, 2009).

Purpose of global health governance

Global health governance ensures accountability by developing systems of checks and balances that foster transparency and accountability to ensure equity and fairness in all aspects of health service delivery. It enhances synergy across partnerships, helps to coordinate and provide program leadership and direction, and introduces effective regulatory mechanisms to reduce waste, improve management, and minimize opportunities for corruption. Distinct from national governance, GHG has no overall government at the global level. Populations are organized into sovereign nation states, with no hierarchical political authority, and collaborations are among states and nonstate actors. There are no fixed mechanisms for mobilizing collective action such as tax collection. Global health governance focuses on public and private entities and partnerships and is only effective when there is agreement and compliance between the entities that govern and those that are governed.

Challenges of global health partnerships and governance

Projects targeted and funded by GHPs do not always align with recipient country priorities. The fear of losing a potential funding opportunity, causes recipient country governments to accept them without pushing back. At times recipient countries struggle to absorb GHP funding. This is often due to the fact that they do not receive adequate technical assistance from their partners on how to develop programs to utilize the funds provided. The nonadherence to country protocols by GHPs has the tendency to burden recipient countries with parallel duplicative processes and projects.

Poor communication between GHPs and recipient countries, lean GHP secretariats with inadequate financial and human resources to perform tasks required, and the lack of GHP in-country presence to facilitate the prompt receipt of answers to pressing questions are additional GHP challenges. The unclear delineation of roles and responsibilities causes in-country development partners to be confused about their roles and responsibilities, and the utilization of performance-based funding as mechanism to determine future funding, although a good approach, often creates uncertainty and anxiety about future funding.

Implementing GHP initiatives is sometimes a waste of time and effort as recipient countries are sometimes compelled to redraw their annual operational health plans in the middle of the fiscal year and try to synchronize them with the grant calendars of GHPs. An assessment of GHPs undertaken by the Bill and Melinda Gates Foundation and McKinsey & Company found that, GHPs stipulate certain practices, but generally do not handle shifts in policy and technology adequately. For example, when it comes to HIV/AIDS therapy, PEPFAR requires partner countries to use FDA-approved antiretroviral medicines and when it comes to malaria treatment, GFTAM promotes WHO policy on Artemisinin Combination Therapy (ACT). From the Gates, McKinsey and Company assessment, it came to light that GHPs also tend to use a common approach for all countries without taking cognizance of their diversity.

Global health governance challenges include the issue of sovereignty, which prevents national governments from fulfilling their obligations, the lack of clear mechanisms for holding state and non state actors accountable for their actions or inactions, weak or absent strategic direction, and the issue of how to mobilize, coordinate and focus the large and diverse set of global health actors around a clear mission, common objectives, effective approaches, sustained action, and the promotion of mutual accountability.

Further GHG challenges manifest in the form of the marginalization of specific stakeholders in decision making, mistaken assumptions about the efficiency of the public and private sectors, inadequate resources to carry out partnership activities and to pay for alliance costs, and the inadequate utilization of recipient country assets (Buse *et al.*, 2007).

Global action and strategies

To tackle GHP and GHG challenges, scholars and development partners have put forth a few recommendations. To address the challenges associated with nonalignment of health priorities, GHPs need to assess country needs and ensure that their initiatives mutually align. To foster greater transparency, all partners, especially those marginalized within the partnership, must be given the opportunity to participate in decision making. The capacity of recipient countries need to be built by GHPs, so they can develop good health plans and programs and thereby, be ready to receive and properly utilize funds provided. There needs to be effective coordination, shared governance strategy, and clearly defined lines of authority between partners. Grants provided for projects should include resources for their implementation, and secretariats tasked with providing administrative support for GHP implementation must be adequately staffed and funded so as to be able to effectively discharge their duties.

Strong in-country coordinating mechanisms and communication norms need to be established to aid coordination efforts. This is likely to improve communication between countries and their partners. To ensure that all parties know and understand their roles and responsibilities, a memorandum of understanding that sufficiently spells out roles and responsibilities needs to be crafted and signed by partners. Countries should be afforded some flexibility to adapt to new policies and technologies.

In considering the aforementioned strategies to improve upon GHP interactions between parties, it must be noted that GHPs are often implemented in countries with limited resources and infrastructure, therefore their successful implementation will very much depend on the collaboration of the global health community.

Discussion points

1 What is the purpose of GHPs and GHG?
2 What are some examples of GHPs? What is their focus?
3 What benefits if any are to be gained from GHPs? Explain your response.
4 Discuss two successes of GHPs.
5 What is the essence of GHG? Is it useful in the twenty-first century?
6 Discuss some of the challenges inherent in GHPS and GHG.
7 What is the difference between GHPs and GHG?
8 List and describe three characteristics essential for good partnerships.
9 What is WHO's role in GHPs and governance?
10 What are some of the actions that can be taken to address challenges associated with GHPs and GHG?

REFERENCES

African Medical Research Foundation. (2016) *Amref Health Africa's Strategic Priorities*, http://amref.org/what-we-do/amref-strategic-directions/#sthash.r1v2kb3n.dpuf (accessed October 29, 2016).
African Development Bank (2015) *African Development Bank Approves Ruzizi III Hydropower Plant Project, bringing Green Energy to Burundi, DRC and Rwanda*, http://www.afdb.org/en/news-and-events/article/afdb-approves-ruzizi-iii-hydropower-plant-project-bringing-green-energy-to-burundi-drc-and-rwanda-15275/ (accessed October 29, 2016).
Bill and Melinda Gates Foundation and McKinsey Company (2005) *Global Health Partnerships: Assessing Country Consequences*, http://www.who.int/healthsystems/gf16.pdf (accessed October 29, 2016).
Buse, K., and Harmer, A. M. (2007) Seven habits of highly effective global public–private health partnerships: Practice and potential. *Social Science and Medicine* **64**(2), 259-271.
CARE (2016) *CARE Partnering with USAID – Delivering Sustainable Impact*, http://www.care.org/our-impact/usaid-technical-project-briefs (accessed October 29, 2016).
Carter Center.(2016) *Guinea Worm Disease: Worldwide Case Totals*, http://www.cartercenter.org/health/guinea_worm/case-totals.html (accessed October 29, 2016).
Centers for Disease Control and Prevention. (2015) *Updates on CDC's Polio Eradication Efforts*, http://www.cdc.gov/polio/updates/ (accessed October 29, 2016).
Conway, M. D., Gupta, S., & Prakash, S. (2006) Building better partnerships for global health. *The McKinsey Quarterly* (December), 1–8.i
European Union. (2016) *Health*, https://eeas.europa.eu/diplomatic-network/health/2348/health_en (accessed October 29, 2016).
Ministry of Foreign Affairs of Denmark (n.d.) *Danish Development Cooperation – in the Top League*, http://um.dk/en/danida-en/activities/
World Health Organization (2010) *The Smallpox Eradication Programme – SEP (1966-1980)*, http://www.who.int/features/2010/smallpox/en/ (accessed October 29, 2016).

FURTHER READING

Gostin, L. M., E. (2009) Grand challenges in global health governance *British Medical Bulletin* **90**, 7–18.
Nishtar, S. (2004) Public – private 'partnerships' in health – a global call to action. *Health Research Policy and Systems* **2**(5), https://health-policy-systems.biomedcentral.com/articles/10.1186/1478-4505-2-5 (accessed October 30, 2016).
Shotwell, S. L., (2007) Product development and IP strategies for global health product development partnerships, in *Intellectual Property Management in Health and Agricultural Innovation: A Handbook of Best Practices* (eds. A. Krattiger, R. T. Mahoney, L. Nelsen, *et al.*). MIHR, Oxford and PIPRA: Davis, CA.

16

Evaluating global health projects

Learning objectives

By the end of this chapter, you will be able to:

✓ Define evaluation;

✓ Discuss the rationale for evaluating global health projects;

✓ List and explain the components of an evaluation framework for global health;

✓ Identify and explain at least two evaluation standards for global health;

✓ Distinguish between the two main types of evaluation;

✓ Discuss the functions of a logic model;

✓ Discuss the relevance of an evaluation plan;

✓ Identify and discuss at least two challenges associated with the evaluation of global health projects;

✓ Describe global action and strategies for the successful evaluation of global health projects.

Summary of key points

Although project cycles have an evaluation component, it is often ignored due to a myriad of factors including the lack of financial resources and skilled personnel, previous disappointing experience with evaluation outcomes, and a nonappreciation of the value of evaluation. While neglecting to conduct evaluation during or after a project's implementation was not much of an issue a few decades ago, these days it is a big issue, as funding agencies want to know the outcomes of the projects they funded so they can report back to their constituents. This change in circumstances has put evaluation on the project management landscape and has changed attitudes towards evaluation. Through evaluation, project staff and other stakeholders obtain information that can be used to improve upon project design, implementation, and decision making. This chapter provides an overview of project evaluation. It discusses

Global Health: Issues, Challenges, and Global Action Lecture Notes, First Edition. Elizabeth A. Armstrong-Mensah.
© 2017 John Wiley & Sons Ltd. Published 2017 by John Wiley & Sons Ltd.

key concepts and the rationale for evaluating global health projects, presents a framework for evaluating global health projects, and reviews the standards for project evaluation. It also describes the various types of evaluation, in addition to logic model and evaluation plan design. Some challenges associated with conducting evaluation in the real world are revealed together with global efforts to facilitate the effective evaluation of global health projects.

The concept of evaluation

Evaluation, according to Rossi *et al.* (2004) is the "use of social research procedures to systematically investigate the effectiveness of social intervention programs that are adapted to their political and organizational environments and designed to inform social action in ways that improve social conditions." For Michael Scriven, evaluation is "the investigation of the merit, worth, or significance of an object." In other words, evaluation is the assessment of the overall quality, value, or importance of a program, project, or intervention. To the World Health Organization (WHO), evaluation is the "systematic examination and assessment of features of an initiative and its effects, in order to produce information that can be used by those who have an interest in its improvement or effectiveness."

In very simple terms, evaluation according to Patton, is the systematic and objective assessment of a project at various stages of maturity (planning, implementation, or completion) utilizing social science research methods to identify needs, understand what it set out to do, and to determine the extent to which it achieved what it set out to do (Patton, 1987).

Although the definitions of evaluation presented above vary, a common thread that runs through them all is the fact that evaluation is not an afterthought, but a planned systematic activity implemented from the onset of a project to track processes and effectiveness, so as to accurately identify areas to be improved upon. The definitions also allude to the fact that conducting evaluation to measure project performance involves thinking ahead about intended outcomes and the indicators that will help define success. To be useful, evaluations need to be conducted on time and provide credible information.

Key evaluation concepts

Like various fields of study, evaluation also has a set of terminologies. Familiarizing with these terminologies provides a better understanding of the field. Some evaluation terms are presented and described in Box 16.1.

Box 16.1 Evaluation terminologies.

Term	Description
Activity	An event or action undertaken through the utilization of project inputs to produce specific outputs. *Example*: an activity for a global health educational project could be the development of a course syllabus.
Baseline Assessment	The existing situation before project implementation against which change or progress can be compared. Baseline data should be collected in a manner that allows the same type of data to be collected after project implementation, so results can be compared and judgments made about the extent of change that occurred, or the lack thereof. *Example:* If the goal of a global health educational project is to ensure that students who take the Introduction to Global Health class at Armstrong University improve their global health knowledge, the baseline assessment among other things should include information on the level of student knowledge of the subject prior to taking the class.
Effect	The intended or unintended change that occurs as a result of the implementation of a project.

Effectiveness	The extent to which a project's objectives are achieved or expected to be achieved.
Efficiency	The extent to which a project is delivered in a timely and cost-effective manner.
Goal	A broad general description of what a project seeks to achieve.
	Example: the goal of a global health educational project may be to increase student enrollment for the Introduction to Global Health class.
Impact	The net long-term outcome that can be attributed to a project. It answers the question "what would have happened to the target group if the project had not been implemented?" Impact may be intended, unintended, positive, negative, primary, or secondary.
Indicator	A qualitative or quantitative variable that provides a means to measure progress towards a project goal or objectives. It answers the question "How will we know whether what we planned has actually occurred?" Indicators tell us whether a project is meeting its goals or objectives and whether improvements are necessary.
	There are different types of indicators. Input indicators which measure inputs used for project implementation; process and output indicators which measure whether planned activities took place; outcome indicators which measure whether desired short-term and medium-term outcomes have been achieved and; impact indicators which measure whether desired long-term outcomes have been achieved.
	A good indicator should be SMART: it should be *Specific* – unambiguous and clear, *Measurable* – able to be measured and the cost for measurement appropriate, *Achievable* – required data can be actually collected, *Relevant* – has relevance for project manager and stakeholders, and *Time bound* – when an objective should be achieved. Indicators can be derived from a logic model or from project objectives.
	Example: An objective of a global health educational project may be: By the fall of 2016, increase the number of students taking the Introduction to Global Health class from 50 to 100. The indicator for this objective may be number of students enrolled in the Introduction to Global Health class in the fall of 2016.
Input	Resources invested for the implementation of project activities.
	Example: Inputs needed to conduct a global health class may include faculty, reading materials, and audiovisual equipment.
Monitoring	The systematic and continuous collection of project data. Monitoring involves tracking, documenting, and summarizing project progress and performance against expected results. Monitoring efforts may track program inputs, activities, and outputs.
Objective	An objective is a detailed description of an outcome, or what is to be achieved for a target group by a project. A good objective must be SMART (it should be *Specific* – what is to be done and for whom, *Measurable* – how much change is expected, *Attainable* – possible to achieve within the specified timeframe, *Relevant* – related to the desired project goal and *Time bound* – when objectives will be accomplished).
	Example: By August 2016, increase the number of students taking the Introduction to Global Health class from 50 to 100.
Outcome	A desired change as a result of project implementation. An outcome may be positive, negative, neutral, intended, or unintended.
	Example: An example of an outcome may be the proportion of under five children with diarrhea who receive oral rehydration therapy.
Output	The direct product of an activity. When done properly, outputs should lead to outcomes.
	Example: services, dosage, and products associated with a project.
Stakeholders	People or entities who care about or are affected by a project, such as beneficiaries; people involved with the operations including funding agencies, partners, project staff and managers, and the users of the evaluation. When it comes to stakeholders, the primary questions are "Who cares?" and "What do they care about?"

Rationale for evaluating global health projects

To address the health issues confronting the global community, a number of projects have been and are currently being implemented all over the world. While some of these projects focus on child and maternal health, others focus on the provision of potable water and improved sanitation facilities. The primary purposes of these efforts often range from improving upon the health status of populations, to preventing, controlling, and treating diseases and adverse health conditions.

The implementation of global health projects by themselves do not provide any information about whether they achieved their intended goals, objectives, or desired outcomes. The systematic and continuous collection, analysis, and interpretation of data through monitoring and evaluation, bridges the gap by providing information at specific points in time about a project's performance, outcome, and or impact.

Given the cultural, economic, environmental, and infrastructural differences between countries, global health projects that work well in certain countries do not always lend themselves to replication in others. Thus, project managers and other relevant stakeholders have to adapt them to meet the realities of countries, so scarce resources can be prudently used and desired goals achieved. Conducting formative evaluation enables needs to be properly identified so projects are steered in the right direction and design gaps eliminated.

Through the regular and systematic monitoring and evaluation of global health project processes, unforeseen problems associated with project implementation are exposed at an early stage, thus allowing for timely remedial action to be taken so as to improve the chances of achieving desired outcomes prior to project completion. The evaluation of global health project implementation, enables project staff to assess project efficiency and effectiveness, prioritize the allocation of resources, and to gather accurate information about the strengths and weaknesses of a project.

Evaluating the outcomes of global health projects enables project staff to demonstrate project progress, success, or the lack thereof so funding agencies and other relevant stakeholders can make informed decisions about whether to continue with their implementation, increase funding, or terminate them. Evaluation findings have implications for project management, policy formulation, and advocacy.

The assessment of global health projects hold project staff accountable to their target populations and to funding agencies, as they have to provide evidence to show how time and other resources allocated were used in project implementation. Through impact evaluation of global health projects, the overall long-term effects of a project are assessed and cause-and-effect relationships established. Where it can be proven that a project indeed led to desired changes in a target population, lessons learned and best practices can be disseminated and used as the basis for the replication of similar future projects (MEERA, n.d.).

Program evaluation framework

The utilization of a set of well-thought-out and clearly defined steps is essential for assessing global health projects. The United States Centers for Disease Prevention and Control (CDC) has a framework for evaluating public health programs. This framework can also be used to assess global health projects (see Figure 16.1). The framework comprises six steps: (i) engage stakeholders, (ii) describe the program, (iii) focus

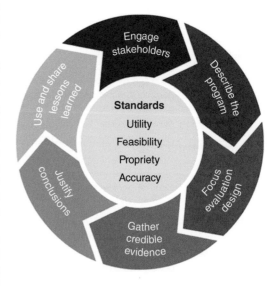

Figure 16.1 Program evaluation framework.
Source: Centers for Disease Control and Prevention (1999).

the evaluation design; (iv) gather credible evidence, (v) justify conclusions, and (vi) ensure use and share lessons learned. Although the components of the framework are presented linearly, they in reality do not always occur in that manner (Centers for Disease Control and Prevention, 1999).

Step 1: Engage stakeholders

The first step of the evaluation framework is stakeholder engagement. Stakeholders are people or groups of people involved in project operations (such as program staff, funding agencies, and management), those served or affected by the project beneficiaries, and the intended users of evaluation findings. Thus, it is crucial to involve them from the onset in the evaluation effort and to determine the extent of their participation before, during, and after an evaluation. As there are different types of stakeholders with different interests, it is important to work with them to prioritize what should be evaluated. Taking cognizance of stakeholder concerns and involving them in the evaluation process has the tendency to improve evaluation planning, build trust, ensure buy-in, establish consensus and ownership of evaluation results, and provide unique opportunities for the dissemination and utilization of findings. Stakeholder participation in evaluation can help with the identification or development of questions to be answered by an evaluation, determine what will be considered credible information, and help with the interpretation of the data collected.

Step 2: Describe the program

After stakeholders have been identified and engaged, the next step is to describe the project. This is often done through the design of a logic model to show relationships between project elements and expected change. A description of the project should include information on the need for the project expressed in its goals, objectives, and desired outcomes (short, intermediate, or long term), the nature and scale of the issue to be addressed, the population affected, activities or actions to be undertaken, partners to bring about the desired change, and confounders that may influence project success or failure. The description of the project should also include information on the resources that will be used to implement activities, the stage or level of project maturity (planning, implementation, and effects), as this will have implications for the type of evaluation to be conducted, and a description of the context and setting of the project including history, geography, politics, social, and economic conditions.

Step 3: Focus the evaluation design

After describing the project to be evaluated, the next step is to put together a written evaluation plan to anchor the evaluation. Focusing the evaluation involves planning in advance where an evaluation is headed and isolating what needs to be done to get there. Specifically, it involves ensuring that stakeholders are aware of and understand the goals, strategy, and purpose of the project. It also involves identifying users and establishing uses of the evaluation, developing relevant, appropriate, and useful evaluation questions, selecting appropriate methods that will help to gather evidence to answer each evaluation question, and agreeing on who will do what *a priori*.

Specifying the purpose of an evaluation justifies why it should be conducted and therefore guards against it being steered in several different directions. The rationale for conducting an evaluation ranges from obtaining information about the appropriateness of a programs design, especially if it is new, to finding out how a project is operating. Knowledge of who will use evaluation results beforehand ensures that evaluation questions are prioritized and tailored to meet the needs of the user. Indicating how evaluation findings will be used prior to conducting an evaluation assures that results will be disseminated and applied.

Evaluation efforts must be driven by a question or set of questions that stakeholders want answers to about a project. Evaluation questions define the boundaries of an evaluation by indicating which aspect of a project will be evaluated. Stakeholders must be involved in the identification, development, and prioritization of evaluation questions. The type of evaluation questions to be answered are influenced by a number of factors including the type of evaluation to be conducted and the level of project maturity and have implications for the method(s) that will be used to collect data. The methods used will determine the extent of stakeholder involvement and the type of data to be collected will determine the sources of information, data collection instruments to be used, and the data-management systems needed.

Social science research methods are often used to collect evaluation data. The selection of methods of data collection should be based on the extent to which they provide needed information to answer stakeholder questions. Qualitative or quantitative methods of data collection may be used, however, given their limitations, it is advisable to use both methods when conducting an evaluation. Methods initially selected for data collection may be changed if unforeseen circumstances arise. Prior to conducting an evaluation, there must be agreement among all parties involved about their roles and responsibilities. This will prevent potential conflicts.

Step 4: Gathering credible evidence

Indicators help to determine the type of information to be collected to answer evaluation questions. If the evaluation question is input oriented, input indicators should drive the data collection process. Where the question is process related, process indicators that show the extent to which planned activities took place among others should steer the data collection process, and where the question focuses on output, output indicators that provide information on the output of an activity should guide data collection. Outcome indicators should steer data collection on the extent to which the objectives of a project or its "results" have been achieved, and impact indicators should drive data collection on the long-term effects and impact of a project.

Data to answer evaluation questions should be collected in a manner that is conceived as credible, relevant, and believable by the primary users of findings. User standards for what constitutes credibility should be considered. Thus, if a survey or key informant interview is viewed as a credible method of obtaining information by evaluation users, they should be considered. The sources relied on for information, such as people or documents, the data collection process, the expertise of data collectors, and data management should also be appropriate and credible. Regarding the quality and amount of information to be collected, a criteria and threshold should be established from the onset. Logistically, cultural issues and preferences around the way questions are asked and how data are collected should be considered within the context and setting of the project. The privacy and confidentiality of data sources must be protected.

Step 5: Justifying conclusions

Justifications for the conclusion of an evaluation must be derived from the evaluation conducted and compared to predetermined values and standards defined by stakeholders as what constitutes success. Evaluation conclusions may be arrived at by isolating important findings to identify patterns (analysis), or by combining sources (synthesis) of information to reach an understanding of the project. To understand an evaluation's conclusion, information collected must be interpreted so it makes sense. Stakeholder

involvement can help with this effort. Justifying an evaluation's conclusion also involves making judgments about the worth, merit, or significance of a project. Judgments and recommendations are made after findings are interpreted and compared with preselected standards of success.

Step 6: Ensuring use and sharing lessons learned

After an evaluation has been conducted, conscious and appropriate steps must be taken to ensure that findings are used by users and other stakeholders and that best practices and lessons learned are disseminated in a timely manner. Decisions about how evaluation findings will be used should be discussed from the onset, when an evaluation is being planned and designed. To ensure potential use, draft findings should be shared with a majority of relevant stakeholders and feedback invited. Recommendations provided should be advisory and not instructive. Evaluation results may be communicated through a variety of means and not just through formal reports. Methods employed should be determined by users or stakeholders. To avoid surprises and rejection of reports, the layout should be discussed beforehand with users and stakeholders, and findings should be objectively communicated.

Program evaluation standards

To conduct evaluations that are accurate, free from bias, and balanced, evaluators must observe and be guided by certain standards. First is the standard of utility, which focuses on ensuring that information obtained from an evaluation is useful to users and other stakeholders, enough to answer evaluation questions, is easy to understand, properly interpreted, and is delivered in a timely manner. The second standard is feasibility, which ensures that an evaluation will be realistic, prudent, diplomatic, and frugal. Third is the standard of propriety, which underscores the need for evaluation to be legally and ethically conducted with regard for those involved in, or affected by the evaluation, and fourth is the standard of accuracy, which seeks to ensure that an evaluation will reveal and convey adequate information about the worth or merit of the project being evaluated. (Centers for Disease Control and Prevention, 1999).

Types of evaluation

There are two main types of evaluation: formative and summative evaluation. Formative evaluation is undertaken during the development and implementation phase of a project. It helps to improve project design and implementation. Formative evaluation includes needs assessments and process or implementation evaluation and is often conducted by internal evaluators. Summative evaluation on the other hand, is conducted at the end of a project. It helps to determine the effectiveness of a project and to make judgments on the extent to which a project is achieving its set goals and objectives. Summative evaluation is often conducted by external evaluators for the benefit of external decision makers. Summative evaluation includes outcome and impact evaluations. Figure 16.2 provides an overview of the types of evaluation and when they occur in the life of a project.

Needs assessment

Needs assessments are generally conducted to identify and close existing gaps between a current situation and a desired end state of affairs. Needs assessments enable evaluators to assess whether there is a need for a new project or whether those already in progress should continue. Needs assessments involve a few steps: First, relevant stakeholders are identified and involved in the assessment-planning process. This enhances buy-in and ensures the potential utilization of results. Second, a needs assessment plan is developed, which includes a list of relevant assessment questions to be asked and information on how data will be collected, analyzed, reported, disseminated, and used. Third, the potential target group for the assessment is defined, taking their assets or resources into consideration. Fourth, data are collected from credible sources and analyzed. Fifth, judgment is made to determine if there are gaps between the current and desired end state and solutions identified with stakeholders. Sixth, needs assessment results are disseminated and action items implemented.

Process evaluation

Process evaluation focuses on project implementation and operation. It helps to determine if project activities are being implemented as indicated in the project design or logic model, and whether a project

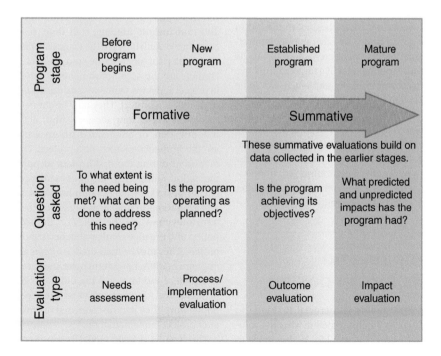

Figure 16.2 Types of evaluation.
Sources: Norland (2004); Pancer and Westhues (1989); Rossi *et al.* (2004).

is operating as planned. Process evaluation allows for the assessment of project inputs, activities, outputs, and reach of services to target populations, and consequently, exposes challenges in the life of a project before its completion, so corrective action can be taken. Process evaluation reveals the strengths and weaknesses in project design, promotes project accountability, and helps with the identification of best practices for future project implementation.

Outcome evaluation

Outcome evaluation assesses the effects of a project on a target population in the short to medium term. It measures changes in knowledge, attitudes, skills, behavior, and policy, and the extent to which project objectives have been achieved. To conduct effective outcome evaluation, baseline data must be collected and used as the basis for comparison.

Impact evaluation

Impact evaluation assesses net change in wellbeing, both intended and unintended, which can be directly attributed to the implementation of a project. It provides strong and reliable evidence on performance and the extent to which a program achieved its desired outcomes. At the global level, impact evaluation exposes what works and what does not in the bid to improve upon global health status or population welfare. To measure impact, a counterfactual has to be established; what would the lot of a target group have been if the project had not been implemented? To be able to attribute the achievement of desired changes unequivocally to a particular project, an intervention and comparison group have to be created, so potential influences on outcomes beside that of the project can be eliminated. Impact evaluation is conducted a year or more after a project has been completed, to measure long-term effects. It is sometimes conducted after the implementation of an intervention.

Logic model and evaluation plan design

Developing a logic model is a crucial first step to project evaluation as it helps to define what to evaluate at what stage of a project's life. It also helps to identify or develop appropriate indicators to be measured. It is pertinent to note that creating a logic model does not necessarily mean that a project will be monitored and evaluated. Developing an evaluation plan to which the project team is committed, can ensure that a project is monitored and evaluated.

Logic model

A logic model is graphic depiction of what a project should look like. It summarizes key project elements and shows the logical relationship between the resources that are invested to implement a project and the activities to be undertaken to achieve outputs and desired outcomes. A logic model serves as a planning, management, and communication tool. As a planning tool, a logic model bridges the gap between the issue to be addressed by a project and desired change. As a management tool, it helps to clarify, track, and monitor project operations, processes, and functions. As a communication tool, a logic model describes a project to all involved. A logic model should be created prior to project implementation and should be a one-page document. It should contain information on assumptions and potential external factors that may affect a project's implementation.

Components of a logic model

A logic model comprises inputs, activities, outputs, and outcomes. Inputs are the investments or resources that go into the implementation of a project and may include funding, staff time, research, and equipment. Activities are the actual events or actions undertaken to achieve desired project outcomes. Outputs are the accomplishments or direct products of project activities. Outcomes are the desired changes or results of a project. They may be short-term, intermediate-term, or long-term, positive, negative, neutral, intended, or unintended. Short-term outcomes are the immediate effects of a project. They may be measured during the first 3 years of project implementation. Short-term outcomes manifest in the form of changes in knowledge, attitudes, skills, motivation, and aspirations that occur as a result of a project. Midterm outcomes are the behavior, decision-making, policy, and practice changes that occur as a result of a project. They may be measured 3–5 years after project implementation. Long-term outcomes are the effects of a project and impact is the ultimate consequence or difference a project makes in the life of a target population. They may be measured five years or more after project implementation.

The logic of a logic model is represented by the direction and flow of arrows. The arrows explain the theory of change from the left to the right of the model and are informed by research, evidence, or practice. Assumptions and external factors influence

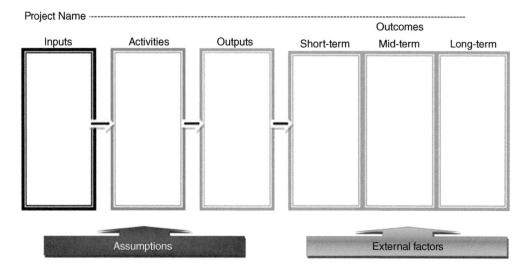

Figure 16.3 Sample logic model template.

the implementation of a project. Assumptions are the beliefs we have about the project, its context, and the way we think the project will work. External factors are the environment in which the program exists. Figure 16.3 is a sample logic model template.

Evaluation plan

A monitoring and evaluation (M&E) plan is a written document that describes how a project will be monitored and evaluated. It guides what is to be monitored and evaluated along the path of a logic model and includes key evaluation questions to be answered, the type of data to be collected to answer evaluation questions, how and when information will be collected, and who will be responsible for their collection. An evaluation plan also describes how information collected will be analyzed, interpreted, and disseminated.

An evaluation plan clarifies the steps needed for evaluation, sets the stage for project evaluation, builds project M&E ownership and helps to determine project evaluation costs. An evaluation plan should be developed from the onset and should as much as possible be based on a project's logic model. It must be rigid and yet flexible to accommodate change and reality, and should not be ignored during project implementation.

The basic components of an evaluation plan include:

- Purpose of the evaluation. (Why is the evaluation being conducted?)
- Intended users of the evaluation. (Who will use the evaluation findings? Who is the audience of the evaluation findings?)
- Intended uses of the evaluation. (How will findings be used?)
- Evaluation questions. (What do stakeholders want to know about a project? What questions do they want to address?)
- Logic model. (What are the projects components and desired outcomes?)
- Indicators. (What specific indicators or measures will help answer the evaluation question?)
- Data collection plan. (What data sources and methods will be used to collect data? Who will be responsible for collecting what data and how frequently?)
- Data analysis plan. (How will collected data be analyzed and interpreted?)
- Communication plan. (How will findings be communicated and disseminated?)

Real-world evaluation challenges

There are many challenges when it comes to conducting evaluations of global health projects. Some of these challenges range from the weak evaluation capacity and outright nonappreciation of the relevance of evaluation, to the issue of political demands.

Weak evaluation capacity

Many project personnel do not have the knowledge or skills to conduct project evaluations as such, after a project is completed, there is no available information on how the project fared or whether it affected the population it targeted. The lack of evaluation skills also negatively affects accountability, as project managers are unable to adequately account for and show what they used the funding they received to accomplish.

Lack of baseline data

In many instances, evaluators are hired to evaluate global health projects long after implementation has began. As the evaluation effort is an afterthought, there is often no baseline data or comparison group to enable judgments to be made about a project's impact or effectiveness.

Time constraints

Where consultants who have limited time are hired to conduct an evaluation, there could be issues with the quality, credibility, and timeliness of reporting. For evaluation findings to be useful, they must be conducted within the stipulated time frame and results disseminated on time. Added to the time constraint challenge is the utilization of inexperienced personnel to collect and analyze data. This may extend the data collection period unduly and compromise the integrity of the data collected, as analyzed data may be fraught with substantial errors.

Limited financial resources

Budgetary constraints often dictate whether an evaluation will be conducted or not. In situations where project funds are limited, evaluation is often eliminated in favor of other project activities. In other situations where there is a budget for evaluation, it is often inadequate and therefore tends to cause evaluations to be oversimplified, hence potentially reducing the reliability of results obtained.

Cultural insensitivity

Lack of cultural competence causes some evaluators, especially expatriates, to conduct evaluations from an ethnocentric perspective. This is often reflected in how they involve local stakeholders in the evaluation process, select data collection methods, and interpret findings (Centers for Disease Control and Prevention, 2014).

Political demands

In some instances, evaluators are unduly pressured by certain stakeholders to only concentrate on the evaluation questions they want answered, to definitely use certain methods they prefer to gather data, and to define success according to their standards regardless of how it impacts other stakeholder needs or interests. On occasion, evaluators are asked by high ranking stakeholders to doctor negative evaluation findings, or face the risk of having their evaluation findings not accepted or used.

Global action and strategies

Currently, many organizations see the utility of M&E and are using a variety of mechanisms, such as needs assessments, workshops, and on-the-job training to enhance the monitoring and evaluation capacity of their staff. At the global level, WHO works in close collaboration with partners, such as the Joint United Nations Program on HIV/AIDS (UNAIDS), World Bank, the United Nations Children Fund (Unicef), the Centers for Disease Control and Prevention (CDC), and the United States Agency for International Development (USAID) to strengthen and improve upon health sector M&E systems and capacity of countries. To address the baseline data situation where baseline data are unavailable, some evaluators have caused baseline conditions to be reconstructed retrospectively by engaging community members through participatory methods so as to obtain information through recall or have utilized relevant documentary (secondary) data sources. On very few occasions where budgets, skill, and time have permitted, feasible comparison groups have been formed to enable sound judgements to be made about evaluations.

To address the issue of time constraints, external consultants are now being served with well thought out terms of reference, which clearly delineate how much time is needed to conduct various components of an evaluation assignment and when reports should be submitted. Regarding data collection and time constraints, great effort is going into the hiring of highly qualified and trained data collectors, statisticians, and analysts.

To handle budgetary constraints for evaluation, some project staff and stakeholders have found it imperative to reduce the amount of data to be collected and to focus primarily on those necessary to answer evaluation questions. Rather than collect primary data, they have depended on secondary data where they are available. Where the sample size is considered too large and therefore requires more resources, it has been cut down. This step does reduce costs, but cutting the sample size too much has the tendency to affect the statistical significance of results.

To address the culture and evaluation issue, some evaluation specialists have in recent times developed and disseminated guidelines for making evaluations more culturally sensitive. Such guidelines include Ellen Taylor-Powell's "Ways to make your projects more culturally sensitive". Among other things, Taylor-Powell's guidelines call on evaluators to take time to explore any cultural issues that might affect their evaluation, and to engage members of all cultural groups in the evaluation design and implementation process. To handle stakeholder pressures and demands to ensure that stakeholder conflicting interests are amicably sorted out and prioritized, and to ensure that evaluation ethics are upheld, some evaluators are conducting stakeholder analyses.

Discussion points

1 What is evaluation and what are its functions?
2 How different is formative evaluation from summative evaluation?
3 Provide a brief description of the following terms:
   a Needs assessment
   b Evaluation plan
   c Logic model
   d Monitoring
   e Stakeholder
4 What are the components of a logic model? Describe each component.
5 What is an evaluation plan and why is it relevant?
6 List and describe four components of an evaluation plan?
7 What framework can be used to evaluate global health projects?
8 What are some of the challenges involved in evaluating global health projects?
9 What actions can be taken to address challenges associated with the evaluation of global health?
10 Describe process, outcome, and impact evaluation? At what point in a project's life are they conducted?

REFERENCES

Centers for Disease Control and Prevention (1999) Framework for program evaluation in public health. *Morbidity and Mortality Weekly Report* **48**(RR11), 1–40.

Centers for Disease Control and Prevention (2014) *Practical Strategies for Culturally Competent Evaluation*, US Department of Health and Human Services, Atlanta, GA.

MEERA (n.d.) *Evaluation: What Is It and Why Do It?* (n.d.) http://meera.snre.umich.edu/evaluation-what-it-and-why-do-it (accessed October 29, 2016).

Norland, E. (2004) From education theory to conservation practice. Paper presented at the Annual Meeting of the International Association for Fish and Wildlife Agencies, Atlantic City, NJ.

Pancer, S. M. and Westhues, A. (1989) A developmental stage approach to program planning and evaluation. *Evaluation Review* **13**, 56–77.

Patton, M. Q. (1987) *Qualitative Research Evaluation Methods*, Sage, Thousand Oaks.

Rossi, P. H., Lipsey, M. W., and Freeman, H. E. (2004) *Evaluation: A Systematic Approach*, Sage, Thousand Oaks, CA.

FURTHER READING

European Commission (2004) *Program Cycle Management Guidelines*, http://ec.europa.eu/europeaid/sites/devco/files/methodology-aid-delivery-methods-project-cycle-management-200403_en_2.pdf (accessed October 30, 2016).

Johnson, B. and Christensen, L. (2008) *Educational Research: Quantitative, Qualitative, and Mixed Approaches*, Sage, Thousand Oaks, CA.

Joint Committee on Standards for Educational Evaluation (1994) *Program Evaluation Standards: How to Assess Evaluations of Educational Programs* (2nd edn.). Sage, Thousand Oaks, CA.

Wynn, B. O. (2005) *Challenges in Program Evaluation of Health Interventions in Developing Countries*, RAND Corporation, Santa Monica, CA, http://www.rand.org/pubs/monographs/MG402.html (accessed October 30, 2016).

Index

Note: Page numbers in *italic* refer to figures, those in **bold** to tables.

Global Health: Issues, Challenges, and Global Action Lecture Notes, First Edition. Elizabeth A. Armstrong-Mensah.
© 2017 John Wiley & Sons Ltd. Published 2017 by John Wiley & Sons Ltd.

Printed and bound by CPI Group (UK) Ltd, Croydon, CR0 4YY

06/12/2023

08203128-0001